AF411561

ANGER, HOSTILITY, AND THE HEART

Edited by

Aron Wolfe Siegman
University of Maryland Baltimore County

Timothy W. Smith
University of Utah

LAWRENCE ERLBAUM ASSOCIATES, PUBLISHERS
1994   Hillsdale, New Jersey   Hove and London

Copyright © 1994 by Lawrence Erlbaum Associates, Inc.
All rights reserved. No part of the book may be reproduced in any form, by photostat, microform, retrieval system, or any other means, without the prior written permission of the publisher.

Lawrence Erlbaum Associates, Inc., Publishers
365 Broadway
Hillsdale, New Jersey 07642

Library of Congress Cataloging-in-Publication Data

Anger, hostility, and the heart / edited by Aron Wolfe Siegman, Timothy W. Smith.
        p.   cm.
    Includes bibliographical references and index.
    ISBN 0-8058-1194-X (alk. paper)
    1. Coronary heart disease—Psychosomatic aspects.   2. Anger.
3. Hostility (Psychology).   4. Type A behavior.   I. Siegman, Aron Wolfe.   II. Smith, Timothy W.
    [DNLM: 1. Anger.   2. Coronary Disease—etiology.   3. Coronary Disease—psychology.   4. Hostility.   5. Psychophysiology.   WG 300 A587   1994]
    RC685.C6A59   1994
    616.1′208—dc20
    DNLM/DLC
    for Library of Congress   92-48546
                                                                                              CIP

Books published by Lawrence Erlbaum Associates are printed on acid-free paper, and their bindings are chosen for strength and durability.

Printed in the United States of America
10 9 8 7 6 5 4 3 2 1

CONTENTS

INTRODUCTION

Aron Wolfe Siegman
University of Maryland Baltimore County

Timothy W. Smith
University of Utah

It is only 7 years since Margaret Chesney and Ray Rosenman (1985) presented us with their book, *Anger and Hostility in Cardiovascular and Behavioral Disorders*, and one can reasonably ask: Is there a need for yet another book on the same topic? Our justification for presenting this edited book is that Chesney and Rosenman offered theirs just about the time that Dembroski and associates (Dembroski & MacDougall, 1985; Dembroski, MacDougall, Williams, Haney, & Blumenthal, 1985) proposed the hypothesis that hostility was the "toxic" component of the then extremely popular Type A behavior pattern construct, although at the time the evidence regarding its validity was still quite scant. Since then, research not only on the role of hostility but also on that of anger in the etiology and course of coronary heart disease (CHD) has mushroomed. Moreover, there has been considerable progress in our knowledge of the neurohormonal correlates of anger and hostility that are likely to play a role in the pathogenesis of CHD. This is not to imply that the evidence in support of a positive relationship between anger and hostility, and CHD is unanimously positive, or that all the steps that are involved in the translation of anger and hostility into the CHD disease process have been clearly established. Far from it. We do believe, however, that this is the appropriate time in the history of coronary-prone behavior research to take stock: to identify the basic questions that need further elucidation and to provide direction for where we go from here. Even in the absence of definitive answers, it is becoming increasingly clear what the basic questions are, and we have promising leads for the solution of many of these questions.

Although there is a surprising consensus among our contributors about the nature of the critical issues and about the directions for future research, they each bring to bear a somewhat different perspective. Hopefully, this book makes a modest contribution by providing the reader with a variety of perspectives on what we know and what we still need to know, and by becoming a useful source for promising research hypotheses.

The first chapter in this book, by Siegman, attempts to place the current concern with the role of anger and hostility in CHD in a historical context. It is clear that, in some form or another, the hypothesis that there is a relationship between anger and hostility, especially the former, and CHD has been around since ancient times, and yet, until very recently, the biomedical community viewed attempts to link psychosocial variables to CHD with suspicion: as interesting bits of folk wisdom having no serious scientific merit. Perhaps the current, more receptive attitude on the part of many, if not all, in the biomedical community to the possible role of behavioral factors in CHD can be attributed to the fact that we have at least begun to identify the mechanisms through which anger and hostility may become translated into atherosclerosis and CHD. Most importantly, technological advances have made it possible to test these processes in the laboratory, both with humans and with animal models. Moreover, this is all happening at an ever accelerating pace.

The latter part of chapter 1 traces the development from a concern with global Type A to a focus on hostility and, more recently, on anger, as potential behavioral risk factors in coronary artery disease (CAD) and CHD. Although it is now generally accepted that we need to distinguish between anger (essentially an affective construct) and hostility (primarily an attitudinal construct), the early literature failed to recognize this distinction. In fact, it is still not clear whether they should be viewed as relatively independent risk factors or whether hostility lowers the threshold for anger and thus affects CHD.

In chapter 2, Tim Smith outlines the major conceptual issues that run through the literature on anger, hostility, and health, and identifies areas where reformulation of models and refined research strategies are needed. Among others, he discusses the distinctions among anger, hostility, and aggression, the problems of assessment, and the fact that only some forms of anger and hostility may be toxic, as far as CHD is concerned. Most of these issues are taken up in greater detail by other contributors in subsequent chapters. Thus, Barefoot and Lipkus (chapter 3) present a comprehensive review of the various instruments—both objective, paper-and-pencil questionnaires and interview-based procedures—that have been used to assess anger and hostility, their psychometric problems, and recent efforts—including those now taking place at Duke University—to introduce greater objectivity in the interview-based assessment procedures.

The basic question is: Is there, in fact, a demonstrable empirical relationship between anger–hostility and CHD? Chapter 4, by Helmers, Posluzny, and Krantz, reveals why the answer to this question is less easy to come by than would be expected on first glance. Complicating factors include: (a) defining and measuring CHD, (b) determining what are the proper endpoints (myocardial infarction [MI], sudden cardiac death, or angiographic evidence of CAD), and above all, (c) the need to address a host of methodological issues. In case control studies, it is typically impossible to tell whether hostility is a cause, or perhaps a consequence, of the disease. Angiographic studies have been criticized on the grounds that the patients referred for such examinations typically suffer from severe CHD symptoms or are otherwise seriously at risk for an MI, and that one cannot readily generalize from findings obtained with such patients to more healthy individuals. Pickering (1986) pointed out that even some of the established risk factors for CHD, such as high blood pressure (BP) levels, frequently are not associated with severity of CAD in angiographic studies. Such findings moved Pickering to question the use of angiographic patients for the study of CHD risk factors and instead to recommend the use of patients referred for thallium testing, on the assumption that they tend to be less severely ill. However, our own experience suggests that, although the proportion of patients with no serious CHD history is clearly lower among patients referred for angiographic studies than among patients referred for thallium stress tests, the latter group, too, contains a significant proportion of patients with histories of severe MIs or of coronary bypass surgery. At least one thallium stress test study (Kahn et al., 1982) found that covarying previous MIs can seriously affect the results. However, this problem can be solved by eliminating the patients with such histories from the analysis.

When the assessment of anger and hostility is based on interview behavior rather than on questionnaire responses, the best available studies (including two prospective studies) suggest that anger–hostility is indeed a significant risk factor for CHD. Thus, although the evidence is highly suggestive, better studies are needed. Perhaps, we are ready for yet another major prospective study—we certainly know much more than we did until recently about the methodological pitfalls to be avoided.

One of the oldest theories about how behavioral variables become translated into CHD involves repeated and/or exaggerated episodes of cardiovascular reactivity, with *reactivity* defined as a person's systolic blood pressure, diastolic blood pressure, or heart rate during a task minus baseline scores. Chapter 5, by Kent Houston, reviews the empirical findings on the relationship between various trait measures of anger and hostility and cardiovascular reactivity (CVR). Houston finds that the results vary as a function of both the task and the methods used to assess the anger and hostility. The expected positive relationship between the Cook–Medley Ho-scale and CVR was obtained in studies in which the participants were involved in *interpersonally* stressful tasks, but was not found when the task was of an impersonal nature or was nonstressful. This is not particularly surprising, because the Ho-scale seems to tap an interpersonal dimension: cynicism and mistrust. Results of studies that used the Structured Interview (SI) to assess anger and hostility are inconsistent, despite the fact that this measure has been quite successful in predicting CHD endpoints. Houston suggests that the subjective nature of scoring anger and hostility from the SI may account for the inconsistent finding. Yet another possibility is that early studies did not distinguish between the experience of anger and hostility versus their expression. Recent evidence indicates that only the latter (the Hostile-style subscore of PoHo) is related to disease endpoints. Some exceptions notwithstanding, the majority of the studies reviewed by Houston are consistent with the position that only indices that measure the tendency to express anger, not those of neurotic anger, are associated with heightened reactivity. Moreover, it should be noted that experimental animal and human studies provide strong support for the hypothesized positive relationship between the expression of anger and heightened reactivity (chapters 7 and 9), even though studies using paper-and-pencil measures of the disposition to express one's anger do not always show a positive relationship with hyperreactivity. Finally, the author points out that the majority of studies in this area have been conducted with young White males. Clearly, we need more studies on the roles of gender and race in the relationships among anger, hostility, and cardiovascular reactivity.

At the beginning of chapter 6, Williams states:

> As documented in the other chapters of this book, the 1980s witnessed a stunning and accelerating rate of progress in research aimed at elucidating the role of hostility and anger in the etiology and course of coronary heart disease and other serious illnesses. To sustain this momentum it will be necessary to begin the process of integrating the research on hostility and disease with the growing corpus of basic research concerned with the neurochemistry of behavior (i.e., hostility/anger) and with the molecular biology underlying pathogenesis of the diseases associated with hostility and anger.

Williams responds to this challenge by showing how the biobehavioral correlates of hostility (i.e., high cholesterol production and enhanced catecholamine reactivity) affect the molecular biology of macrophage activation so as to accelerate the atherogenic process. He then proceeds with the exciting suggestion that the complete array of biobehavioral characteristics found in hostile persons is the result of a single neurochemical factor: diminished brain serotonin function. This is the same conclusion reached by Kaplan, Botchin, and Manuck (chapter 7) on the basis of different types of evidence. The convergence is exceedingly encouraging. The only difference is that Williams addresses the role of serotonin in hostility, and Kaplan et al. discuss the role of serotonin in actual aggressive behavior. Further research will have to ascertain whether hostile attitudes per se are sufficient or whether these changes are driven by the actual *expression* of anger. The authors of both chapters provide very interesting suggestions for the testing of their hypotheses.

Attempts to establish with a reasonable degree of certainty the relationship between anger and hostility, on the one hand, and the intervening physiological mechanisms and the resulting disease processes, on the other, is hampered by many factors, not the least of which is that some of these relationships can be assessed only with invasive procedures that cannot be ethically applied to asymptomatic individuals. An obvious alternative strategy is the use of animal models. Kaplan, Manuck, and their associates have been pioneers in the use of such models (i.e., using macaque monkeys) for evaluating behavioral influences on atherosclerosis. These monkeys are particularly suitable for testing the hypothesis that the overt expression of anger (i.e., aggressive behavior) is a risk factor for CHD, because their aggressive behavior is very similar to that of humans. In a series of experiments, Kaplan et al. found that dominant social status and heart rate responsivity potentiate atherosclerosis in cynomolgus monkeys. The authors point out that such monkeys also exhibit a tendency for intense aggression. Aggression can contribute to the development of atherosclerotic lesions with accompanying activation of the sympathetic nervous system and subsequent increases in heart rate, blood pressure, and circulating catecholamines. Additionally, a review of the literature leads the authors to speculate that serotonergic drive is involved in the modulation of aggression, and that animals with low serotonergic drive are likely to exhibit extreme levels of aggressive behavior, which places them at risk for atherosclerosis and CHD.

Chapter 8 provides a theoretical approach to the relationship between personality and disease. Although we now have numerous empirical studies investigating the relationship between discrete personality variables and disease outcomes, seldom are they accompanied by a conceptual analysis of the linkage between the two. Contrada provides such an analysis. Although the focus is on the anger–hostility–CHD relationship, he provides a general framework for conceptualizing personality–disease relationships. The key feature of his approach is an integration of personality theory and stress theory. According to Contrada, the stress response is essential for understanding how psychological processes get translated into disease processes. However, individual differences in personality structure and in personality processes impact stress appraisal and the nature of the coping response. Moreover, the transactional perspective spelled out by Smith in chapter 2 is employed by Contrada to construct a more complete understanding of the personality–disease relationship.

In chapter 9, Siegman discusses the complex, multidimensional nature of anger and hostility and, like others, suggests that not all of their dimensions are necessarily associated with CHD. Early contradictory findings in regard to the cholesterol–CHD relationship led researchers to conclude that not all of cholesterol's components are toxic and drove them to search for which cholesterol components might be the toxic ones. It is suggested that a similar search is necessary with respect to anger and hostility. Some components of anger and hostility (or some ways of coping with anger and hostility) may be toxic, whereas others may not, and some may even be protective. Siegman reviews the evidence regarding the effects of experiencing anger, expressing anger, and repressing anger on CHD, and concludes that, of these three ways of coping with anger, the expression of anger is related most clearly and consistently to CHD and its risk factors. Similarly, of these three ways of coping with anger, the expression of anger is the most clearly related to the physiological processes that are involved in the pathogenesis of CHD. However, the expression of anger, too, needs to be further refined: purely cognitive verbal expressions versus full-blown affective expressions.[1] In discussing the harmful effects of expressing anger on the cardiovascular system, the reference is to the full-blown, affective expression of anger with all of its nonverbal and paraverbal manifestations, and not to the mere verbal communication of angry feelings. Such purely verbal discussions may, in fact, have positive consequences, in that they could provide insight into the causes of such affective explosions and suggest means for their cognitive control. Finally, although the repression of anger also has negative health consequences, they are mostly in terms of immune-related diseases and do not prominently involve the cardiovascular system.

Recently, a number of investigators have suggested that hostile individuals may be at risk for CAD and CHD, because such individuals engage in a lifestyle that puts them at risk for coronary disease. They may smoke or drink more, or may have other habits that make them coronary-prone (e.g.,

---

[1]The construct of expressed aggression as conceptualized by Siegman (chapter 9) and by Stoney and Engebretson (chapter 11) is similar to the concept of provoked aggression (Olweus, 1986), or anger-produced aggression (Rule & Nesdale, 1976), or impulsive aggression (Berkowitz, 1974), all of which need to be distinguished from instrumental aggression. Another way of articulating this distinction is in terms of "hot" versus "cold" aggression. The failure to consider this distinction is probably responsible for the confusion and the contradictory findings that characterize the frustration–aggression and catharsis literatures. If we make the not unreasonable assumption that the frustration–aggression hypothesis as well as the catharsis hypothesis address the problem of impulsive, or provoked, or hot aggression, and not instrumental aggression, then many of the studies that purport to test these hypotheses are simply irrelevant because they use an instrumental aggression paradigm. It is suggested that in relation to CHD, too, the significant risk factor is hot, provoked aggression, not cold instrumental aggression. In this context, it is of interest to note that Olweus (1986) reported that only provoked aggression shows a direct relationship with testosterone production, which has been identified (Williams, 1989) as one of the hormones that mediates the anger–CHD relationship. There may very well be considerable data in the social psychological aggression literature, that could be of help in clarifying the anger–hostility–CHD relationship.

Scherwitz & Rugulies, 1992; Siegman, Anderson, Herbst, Boyle, & Wilkinson, 1992). Ilene Siegler (chapter 10) provides a systematic review of the literature on the relationship between hostility and the major demographic and lifestyle variables that have been implicated in CHD. The overriding impression is that the evidence in regard to this health behavior model (i.e., that lifestyle variables mediate the hostility–CHD relationship) is contradictory, as it is in regard to many other hypotheses reviewed in these chapters.

Siegler alludes to the fact that the varying ways in which anger and hostility are defined and assessed by different investigators may be at the root of some of the discrepancies. Siegman and associates (1992) showed that the experience of anger versus the expression of anger relate differentially to a variety of lifestyle risk factors, and Stoney and Engebretson (chapter 11) show how males tend to score higher than females on some aspects of anger and hostility but not on others. Additionally, Siegler demonstrates how the anger and hostility–health behavior relationship is also a function of how the latter is defined—which also tends to vary from study to study. The review provides useful information about which relationships are worth pursuing further and which are not, and it identifies the methodological issues that need to be addressed if the results are to have any validity.

Chapter 11, by Stoney and Engebretson, explores the role of anger and hostility as potential mediators of gender differences in relation to CHD. As pointed out earlier, cardiovascular and physiological reactivity has been posited as the mechanism by which behavioral tendencies become translated into coronary disease processes. If the threshold for anger arousal and hostility is lower in males than in females—and there is some prima facie evidence that it is—we may have one explanation for the fact that men experience twice the age-adjusted mortality and morbidity rates from CHD as women. Before reviewing the literature relevant to this hypothesis, the authors propose a model for conceptualizing the various components of the anger–hostility domain. Throughout this introduction, we have posited a distinction between the experience of anger and the expression of anger and hostility. Stoney and Engebretson accept this fundamental distinction, with the former referring to the emotional experience of anger and hostility, and the latter to the behavioral manifestations of anger and hostility. However, they have added a third dimension: attitudinal hostility, which refers to the cognitive experience of anger and hostility. They recognize that these distinctions are somewhat artificial because, in life, they interact with one another in different ways. Additionally, they suggest that within the expression of anger and hostility category we need to distinguish between communicative expression and aggressive expression. The latter refers to the verbal or physical expression of anger and hostility, with the intent of inflicting harm, whereas the former refers to the nonthreatening expression of anger and hostility.

On the basis of, admittedly, a limited number of studies, the authors reach the following conclusions. First, males and females experience a similar level of experiential anger; second, males have a higher level of attitudinal hostility relative to females; and third, females express their anger in a communicative fashion to a greater degree than males, but are less likely to express their anger in an aggressive fashion, relative to males. Given the apparent gender differences in relation to the expression of anger–hostility and hostile attitudes, and given the evidence of significant relationships (a) between the expression of anger–hostility and CHD endpoints; and (b) between hostile attitudes and cardiovascular reactivity, as well as other CHD risk factors, it is not at all unreasonable to suggest that gender differences in anger–hostility may account for the gender differences in CHD. Clearly, this is an important area for further research.

Whereas the chapters reviewed thus far are concerned with the possible role of anger and hostility in the pathogenesis of CHD, chapter 12, by Deffenbacher, is concerned with intervention, presenting a detailed manual for anger reduction techniques. Research on the role of anger and hostility in CHD has proceeded without much attention to the extensive research literature on aggression conducted by social psychologists. Similarly, scant attention has been paid by behavioral medicine scientists to the available clinical literature on anger. True, clinicians were preoccupied with the contributions of anxiety and depression to a variety of psychiatric disorders, at the expense of considering the dysfunctional consequences of anger and their role in psychopathology. In his chapter, Deffenbacher provides criteria for the diagnosis of dysfunctional anger, its assessment, and its treatment. He also reviews the research literature, a good deal of which was conducted in his laboratory, which shows that cognitive interventions, relaxation techniques, or their combination produce robust and long-lasting beneficial effects. Social and communication skills training also appears to be an appropriate intervention, at least for interpersonally prompted anger.

Lest we get carried away by utopian and/or social engineering impulses, we close this introduction by quoting Deffenbacher's concluding paragraph:

> The goal of intervention should be *anger management*, not anger elimination. It is idealistic to believe that anger will or can ever be eliminated. Frustration, pain, injustice, and disagreement will continue. People become ill, jobs are lost, relationships end, others are inconsiderate and obnoxious. Even when anger regarding these events is well managed, a realistic residue of mild anger (e.g., frustration, disappointment, annoyance, irritation) remains, and difficult choices remain to be made and implemented. Acceptance and tolerance of these events are among the developmental and existential tasks of life. However, employing anger management strategies such as those described in this chapter can help patients lower their anger and move more freely and more healthfully through life, a life that still may be realistically painful and frustrating at times.

REFERENCES

Berkowitz, L. (1974). Some determinants of impulsive aggression: Role of mediated associations with reinforcements for aggression. *Psychology Review, 81,* 165–176.

Chesney, M. A., & Rosenman, R. H. (Eds.). (1985). *Anger and hostility in cardiovascular and behavioral disorders.* Washington, DC: Hemisphere.

Dembroski, T. M., & MacDougall, J. M. (1985). Beyond global Type A: Relationships of paralinguistic attributes, hostility, and anger-in to coronary heart disease. In T. Field, P. McCabe, & N. Schneiderman (Eds.), *Stress and coping* (pp. 223–241). Hillsdale, NJ: Lawrence Erlbaum Associates.

Dembroski, T. M., MacDougall, J. M., Williams, R. B., Haney, T. L., & Blumenthal, J. A. (1985). Components of Type A, hostility, and Anger-In: Relationship to angiographic findings. *Psychosomatic Medicine, 47,* 219–233.

Kahn, J. P., Kornfeld, D. S., Blood, D. K., Lynn, R. B., Heller, S. S., & Frank, K. A. (1982). Type A behavior and the thallium stress test. *Psychosomatic Medicine, 44,* 431–436.

Olweus, D. (1986). Aggression and hormones: Behavioral relationship with testosterone and adrenaline. In D. Olweus, J. Block, & M. Radke-Yarrow (Eds.), *Development of antisocial and prosocial behavior* (pp. 51–72). New York: Academic Press.

Pickering, T. C. (1986). Should studies of patients undergoing coronary angiography be used to evaluate the role of behavioral risk factors for coronary heart disease. *Journal of Behavioral Medicine, 8,* 203–213.

Rule, B. G., & Nesdale, A. R. (1976). Emotional arousal and aggressive behavior. *Psychological Bulletin, 83,* 851–863.

Scherwitz, L., & Rugulies, R. (1992). Life style and hostility. In H. S. Friedman (Ed.), *Hostility coping and health* (pp. 77–98). Washington, DC: American Psychological Association.

Siegman, A. W., Anderson, R. A., Herbst, J., Boyle, S., & Wilkinson, J. (1992). Dimensions of anger-hostility and cardiovascular reactivity in provoked and angered men. *Journal of Behavioral Medicine, 15,* 257–272.

Williams, R. B. (1989). Biological mechanisms mediating the relationship between behavior and coronary heart disease. In A. W. Siegman & T. M. Dembroski (Eds.), *In search of coronary-prone behavior: Beyond Type A.* Hillsdale, NJ: Lawrence Erlbaum Associates.

1

FROM TYPE A TO HOSTILITY TO ANGER: REFLECTIONS ON THE HISTORY OF CORONARY-PRONE BEHAVIOR

Aron Wolfe Siegman
University of Maryland Baltimore County

Research on the contribution of psychological factors to coronary heart disease (CHD) has changed from a preoccupation with the role of the Type A behavior pattern (TABP) to that of hostility, and more recently to that of anger. This chapter will trace the origin and rationale for these shifts, and will place these developments within the broader framework of behavioral medicine. Although terms like *behavioral medicine, psychosomatic medicine*, and *holistic medicine* each have their own unique connotations, they share the assumption that the mind influences the body,[1] that expectations and cognitions, emotions, and personality traits play a significant role in the development, maintenance, and treatment of physical diseases. This point of view represents a major paradigm shift from that which dominated the thinking of the biomedical community until very recently. Nevertheless, this brief and admittedly selective review intends to demonstrate that this new psychosomatic, holistic perspective has its roots in antiquity, and existed throughout history, alongside other paradigms and models. Conflicting models existed side by side, and the tension that was generated by such conflicting models frequently led to the emergence of new models. At times, progress was slow and incremental, at other times it occurred in quantum leaps, and sometimes it was preceded by serious regressions. Progress in this regard, like progress in science in general, is probably best represented by an ellipse rather than by

---

[1]For a contemporary psychological perspective on the mind–body relationship, see Miller (1990).

a straight line. Perhaps there is validity to Hegelian dialectics, at least insofar as scientific progress is concerned.

BODY AND MIND IN ANTIQUITY

The concept that strong negative emotions and the aggravations that are encountered in the course of everyday life (stress, in contemporary parlance)
can adversely affect one's health, indeed one's very survival, was well understood as far back as Biblical times. When Jacob's sons wanted to take their
youngest sibling, Benjamin, with them to Egypt, Jacob refused to let Benjamin go because if anything were to happen to Benjamin on the way, he, Jacob,
would die from grief[2] (Genesis 42:38). A dictum of Talmudic origin maintains
that a hurried walking style is damaging to one's eyesight[3]—shades of Type
A. The rabbis of the Talmud were aware not only of the damaging health
consequences of strong negative emotions and stress but also of the benefits
of positive emotions and experiences.[4] They were also aware of beneficial
consequences of strong social support. A Talmudic dictum maintains that visit-
ing and spending time with the sick relieves them of one sixtieth of their
illness (Tractate Nedarim 39b). In discussing the ability of a certain medication to reverse an eye disease common in animals, the Talmud suggests that
its effectiveness is contingent on the animal being treated in a tranquil, pastoral
environment and on it being in the company of other animals (Tractate Be-
horot 39a). In general, the rabbis of the Talmud had a profound appreciation
of the importance of social support. This is reflected in the Talmudic laws
that make it incumbent on the members of the community to entertain a
newly married bride and groom and to comfort the bereaved.

To the best of my knowledge, there is no reference in the Talmud specifically linking anger to heart disease, but there are numerous references regarding the devastating effects of anger on a person's physical and spiritual
well-being. The rabbis base their warnings about the undesirable consequences of anger on a verse in Ecclesiasties (11:10): "Remove anger from
your heart and evil from your body . . ." that the rabbis interpret in terms
of a cause–effect relationship. *If* you will remove anger from your heart, *then*
your body will be spared evil (illness, pain). A similar thought is expressed
by the Psalmist when he exclaims (6:7): "My eye is dimmed by anger,"
although in Biblical Hebrew the same word that connotes anger also con-

---

[2]Like so many Biblical verses, this one too lends itself to an alternative interpretation, namely,
that he, Jacob, would go to his grave grieving.

[3]Diseases of the eye are common in the Middle East today. The frequent Talmudic references to such diseases suggest that this was also the case in antiquity.

[4]There are references in the Talmud (Gittin 42b) to the effects of positive and negative mood
states on weight gain and loss.

notes mental torment and anguish. Moreover, the Psalmist's earlier plea (6:2): "God heal me," can be, and has been, interpreted to refer to that which ails the Psalmist's spirit. The very fact that Biblical Hebrew allows, nay, demands such dual interpretations bears witness to the thoroughly holistic world view of biblical man. Even a cursory reading of this particular psalm as well as other psalms reveals how the author moves freely from the physical to the mental-spiritual and vice versa. The aforementioned verse (Psalms 6:7) is undoubtedly the source of the later Rabbinic dictum that anger is damaging to one's eyesight (Midrash Aggadah, Toledot 27a). When Rabbi Zeira, a Talmudic scholar who lived about 300 C.E., was asked by his students to what he attributed his longevity, he replied: "I have never lost my temper in dealing with the members of my family" (Tractate Taanit 20a). Similarly, Rabbi Joshua ben Hananya, a first and second century (C.E.) scholar, maintained that hostility and hatred of one's fellow man were among the factors that shorten one's lifespan (Tractate Avot 2:15).

I have dwelt on these ancient Biblical and Rabbinic texts primarily because of my first-hand acquaintance with this literature, and not because the holistic approach to health and illness that is reflected in these texts was unique to ancient Israel. Quite to the contrary, it was the dominant view of the ancient world in general. For example, suggestion and other behavioral interventions were widely practiced in the temples of ancient Greece that were dedicated to Aesculapius, the god of healing (see Ullman & Krasner, 1969, pp. 109–110). Until recently, it was assumed that the patients who visited these temples suffered from mental illness. However, given the fact that the stadium in the temple in Epidaurus had a 12,000 seating capacity—and there were numerous such shrines throughout ancient Greece—it is more reasonable to assume that these shrines ministered to the physically ill as well. True, with the ascendancy of a more empirical scientific approach in ancient Greece, increasingly less attention was being paid to the role of psychological factors in physical diseases. But even so, there were those who lamented the loss of the holistic approach. As noted in Charmides by Plato, Socrates stated, "Let no one persuade you to cure his headache until he has first given you his soul to be cured, for this is the great error of our day in the treatment of the human body, that physicians separate the soul from the body." Clearly, then, the holistic approach to explaining and treating disease is not a modern discovery.

With the rise of modern scientific medicine during the Renaissance, however, the holistic paradigm—which readily acknowledges the role of emotional factors in health and illness—was replaced by another paradigm. According to this new paradigm, only physical factors initiate physical disease processes, which in turn are to be treated by physical means such as surgery and drugs. The spectacular success of modern scientific medicine, especially in controlling infectious diseases, reinforced this point of view. Even during the new scientific era, however, there were those who, for a variety of reasons, acknowledged the role of psychological factors in physical disease. Thus, in 1628, William Harvey, the father of cardiovascular physiology, wrote: "A mental disturbance provoking pain, excessive joy, hope or anxiety extends to the heart, where it affects its temper, and rate, impairing general nutrition and vigor" (1628/1928, p. 106). Dr. J. Archer, the noted 17th-century physician, wrote: "The observations I have made in the practice of physicks these several years have confirmed me in this opinion, that the origin or cause of most men and women's sickness, disease and death, is first some great discontent which brings a habit of sadness of mind" (Archer, 1673). Heberden (1772), who was one of the first to clearly describe the symptoms of angina pectoris, implicated strong emotions, especially anger, in CHD. Similar views were held by Fothergill (1781) and Wardrop (1851), and Trousseau (1882) went as far as to propose that outbursts of anger could precipitate sudden death in CHD patients. John Hunter, the 18th-century pioneer in cardiovascular surgery and pathology, who suffered from emotion-related bouts of angina, used to say: "My life is in the hands of any rascal who chooses to put me in passion" (cited in DeBakey & Gotto, 1977). In fact, he died from a heart attack soon after a heated exchange at a faculty meeting at the Royal College of Physicians in Glascow, Scotland. It is of interest to note that these early writers emphasized the role of anger in the pathogenesis of CHD, while in more recent times anger has taken a back seat to such constructs as the TABP and hostility.

TWENTIETH-CENTURY PRECURSORS OF BEHAVIORAL MEDICINE

The clinical work of Sigmund Freud and his followers, especially that of Alexander, French, and associates (Alexander, 1950; Alexander, French, & Pollack, 1968), and the physiological research of Cannon (1932), contributed to the re-emergence of the holistic paradigm. Based on their clinical experience, psychoanalysts like French and Alexander claimed that psychological conflicts can trigger or at least contribute to disease processes. In this psychoanalytic version of psychosomatic medicine, specific conflicts were linked to specific diseases. Thus, conflicts about expressing anger were linked to heart disease, conflicts about dependency needs to ulcers, and repressed depression to dermatological disorders (Alexander et al., 1968). These various somatic manifestations were said to represent symbolic expressions of underlying repressed psychological conflicts. Unfortunately, empirical tests of these psychoanalytically inspired hypotheses were inconsistent at best.

The psychoanalytic explanations of psychosomatic disorders (or psychophysiological disorders, as they are now referred to) were lacking a physiologically credible rationale of how psychological events become translated into physical disease processes. This was provided by Cannon's (1932) research on the fight–flight response. His investigations showed that the fight–flight phenomenon involves a number of adaptive physiological responses, such as increased blood pressure, the release of epinephrine, and corticosteroids. Although adaptive in the short term, in that these physiological changes prepare the body to engage in the intense motor activity that is required for the fight–flight response, their chronic activation can cause tissue damage and disease. Furthermore, the threats faced by modern man, such as loss of job, divorce, and chronic disease, are not resolved by intense physical activity, increasing the potential tissue damage of the fight–flight response. Of course, we now know that fight and flight are the behavioral (action) manifestations of anger and fear. The emotions, then, play a key role in the transformation of psychological events into disease processes. Of the three major negative emotions, namely, fear, depression, and anger, it is the latter that is most uniquely associated with dangerously high blood pressure elevations (Siegman, 1992). Anger, then, is a logical candidate for being a behavioral risk factor for coronary heart disease—but this gets us ahead of our story.

THE TYPE A BEHAVIOR PATTERN AND CORONARY HEART DISEASE

The search for "psychological" risk factors in coronary heart disease (CHD) was driven primarily by the fact that the traditional risk factors, such as habitual cigarette smoking, high blood pressure, hyperlipidemia, obesity, parental history of CHD, account for less than 50% of CHD cases (Jenkins, 1978; Keys, 1970; Rosenman, 1983). During the 1950s, two cardiologists, Friedman and Rosenman, identified a complex of behaviors that they considered to be risk factors for CHD. These behaviors include extreme ambition and competitiveness, impatience, aggressive and hostile behavior, and a sense of time pressure. These behaviors were labeled as the Type A coronary-prone behavior pattern (TABP). By way of summary, the Type A individual was described by Friedman and Rosenman as "a person who is aggressively involved in a chronic, incessant struggle to achieve more and more in less and less time, and, if required to do so, against the opposing efforts of other things or other persons" (Friedman & Rosenman, 1974; Rosenman & Friedman, 1974). Most often, the Type B behavior pattern is defined negatively, that is, the absence of Type A characteristics. Occasionally, investigators (e.g., Siegman & Dembroski, 1989) suggested a somewhat more positive definition of the Type B behavior pattern, for example, when they refer to this behavior pattern in terms of a "relaxed" lifestyle, but, so far, there is no precise conceptualization and definition of the Type B behavior pattern similar to that of the Type A behavior pattern. It is important to point out that from the very beginning, anger, hostility, and aggressive behavior were considered to be part of the TABP, although by no means its only or even its most prominent constituents. The idea that Type A like behaviors may be related to CHD did not originate with Friedman and Rosenman. The contribution of these investigators consists of their efforts to operationalize and measure the Type A behavior pattern, so that its hypothesized role in CHD could be investigated in a scientifically convincing manner.

Rosenman and Friedman developed a structured interview (SI) designed to assess the TABP. (Over the years, Rosenman and Friedman took somewhat divergent approaches to the administration and scoring of the SI, but more about this later.) Having developed the SI, the two investigators were now ready to launch a major prospective epidemiological study—the Western Collaborative Group Study (WCGS)—to test the hypothesized TABP–CHD link. The study included 3,154 men, ages 39–59, who were administered the SI and who were followed for 8.5 years. The results of this study disclosed that, relative to the Type Bs, the Type As were slightly more than twice as likely to show clinical manifestations of CHD (Rosenman, et al., 1975). This increased risk for CHD in Type A men remained significant after multivariate statistical adjustment for the traditional risk factors. Moreover, the amount of risk associated with the TABP was about the same as that conferred by the traditional risk factors.

Other research revealed that the TABP was related to the severity of coronary artery disease (CAD) documented by autopsy in the WCGS (Friedman, Rosenman, Straus, Wurm, & Kositchek, 1968), and through cardiac catheterization by independent investigative groups (Blumenthal, Williams, Kong, Schanberg, & Thompson, 1978; Frank, Heller, Kornfeld, Sporn, & Weiss, 1978; Zyzanski, Jenkins, Ryan, Flessas, & Everist, 1976).

By the late 1970s, the evidence in support of the hypothesized TABP–CHD link was sufficiently persuasive to convince an NIH sponsored review panel that the TABP was associated with increased risk for CHD "over and above that imposed by age, systolic blood pressure, serum cholesterol, and smoking and [that increased risk due to TABP] appears to be of the same order of magnitude as the relative risk associated with any of these factors" (Review Panel on Coronary-Prone Behavior and Coronary Heart Disease, 1981, p. 1199).

Early results of the Recurrent Coronary Prevention Project (Friedman et al., 1986) also provided support for the hypothesized Type A–CHD relationship. In this project, MI survivors were randomly assigned to a behavioral intervention procedure designed to modify Type A behavior or to one of two control groups. Initial results showed that the behavioral intervention produced marked reduction in Type A behavior and that recurrence of MI in the treatment group was only about 13%, compared to 21% and 28% in the two control groups. These findings provided a strong boost to the hypothesized Type A–CHD relationship.

THE EMERGENCE OF NEGATIVE FINDINGS

It is somewhat ironic that just about the time when general textbooks in abnormal and social psychology began to cite the link between the TABP and CHD as evidence of a causal relationship between psychosocial variables and disease, and just as the biomedical community appeared ready for the first time to accept a psychosocial variable as an independent risk factor for CHD (Cooper, Detre, & Weiss, 1981), evidence began to appear that challenged the validity of the presumed relationship between the TABP and CHD. Perhaps the most damaging evidence in this regard was the results of the Multiple Risk Factor Intervention Trial (MRFIT) study (Shekelle et al., 1985). Like the WCGS, this study was a large-scale prospective investigation, but it failed to replicate the relationship between SI-derived Type A designation and CHD (in a subset of 3,110 participants), despite great efforts on the part of the investigators to make the assessment of the TABP comparable to the WCGS. Although the MRFIT study differed from the WCGS in that its subjects were selected on the basis of being at risk for CHD, it should be noted that in the WCGS the TABP predicted CHD at all levels of risk (Rosenman et al., 1964). Moreover, MRFIT was not alone in casting doubt on the presumed relationship between SI-derived Type A and CHD. Thus, a number of studies (Arrowood, Uhrich, Gomillion, Popio, & Raft, 1982; Dembroski, MacDougall, Williams, Haney, & Blumenthal, 1985; Dimsdale, Hackett, & Hutter, 1979; Krantz, Sanmarco, Selvester, & Matthews, 1979; Scherwitz et al., 1983; Siegman, Feldstein, Tommaso, Ringel, & Lating, 1987) failed to replicate earlier findings of a relationship between SI-derived Type A designation and severity of coronary occlusion. Also, a recent study (Ragland & Brand, 1988) of subsequent mortality among 257 patients who survived a clinically confirmed primary event during the first phase of the WCGS unexpectedly showed that Type A patients died at a lower rate than their Type B counterparts. It should be noted, however, that, along with the many recent negative findings, one also finds an occasional positive finding. Thus, in a recent study (Williams et al., 1988) SI-derived Type A scores were found to be positively related to CAD among younger patients in a large angiographic sample, although the relationship was not particularly strong. As a result of these negative findings, some investigators (e.g., Dembroski & Czajkowski, 1989; Siegman & Dembroski, 1989, pp. ix–x) called for a major change in direction in coronary-prone behavior research. They urged that from here on the focus in coronary-prone behavior research should be on variables other than global Type A.

Thus, in their book, *In Search of Coronary-Prone Behavior: Beyond Type A*, Siegman and Dembroski (1989) stated that:

> Notwithstanding the evidence against global Type A as a risk factor for CHD, research should continue to examine whether some of the components of the multidimensional TABP are related to clinical manifestations of CHD, and that such research should be guided by the distinction between the construct of TABP and the concept of coronary-prone behavior. This distinction recognizes that many of the attributes contained in the conceptual definition of the global TABP may not be related to CHD and as such are simply benign correlates of the pattern. In fact, some elements of TABP may even be protective and only a few, even perhaps one, may be "toxic" in its effects. In addition, the concept of coronary-prone behavior raises the possibility that behavioral attributes not included in the traditional definition of TABP may qualify as coronary-prone tendencies. (p. ix)

Others, like Williams and associates (Williams et al., 1991), although acknowledging that global Type A accounts at best for only a small percentage of CHD variance, continue to investigate the contribution of global Type A to CHD, but mostly in interaction with other variables.

EXPLANATIONS FOR THE NEGATIVE FINDINGS REGARDING GLOBAL TYPE A

Two types of explanations have been offered to account for the increasingly negative findings regarding the global Type A–CHD relationship. One set of explanations focuses on methodological problems of the SI, the other on the Type A construct.

The questions that make up the SI deal with hard driving, competitive, time urgent, impatient, and hostile behaviors (i.e., behaviors that constitute the conceptual definition of the TABP construct). Over the years, there have been some changes in the content of the questions, but they are minor, and it is not likely that they affect a person's ultimate classification. However, the changes that have taken place over the years in the administration of the SI present a more serious problem. Originally, in the WCGS, the interviewer's demeanor was correct and professional, but not especially challenging and confrontational (Scherwitz, 1989). However, in his 1978 article, Rosenman emphasized the importance of interviewer challenge, although the article is not very specific on how to implement this challenge, besides indicating that occasionally the interviewer should interrupt the interviewee and challenge the interviewee's responses with statements such as "Why?" and "Why not?" More specific guidelines were provided in a subsequent article by Chesney, Eagleston, and Rosenman (1980). According to this article, the questions in the SI are to be asked in a crisp, abrupt, and staccato style, and the challenging remarks, which are designed to evoke competitiveness and self-justification, are to be presented in a rapid-fire manner. The rationale for conducting the interview in such a highly confrontational manner is that it is designed to elicit a behavioral sample of the interviewee's response to challenge (Chesney et al., 1980). The evidence suggests that in MRFIT some interviewers were considerably more challenging and confrontational than others (Scherwitz, 1989). This is not a minor issue, because the evidence indicates that such variations in interviewer demeanor affect the interviewee's Type A designation (Siegman, Feldstein, Simpson, Barkley, & Kobren, 1984). Furthermore, the evidence suggests that a less confrontational and challenging interview, such as was conducted in the WCGS, is more effective in predicting CHD than an interview that is conducted in a relentlessly challenging and confrontational manner (Scherwitz, 1989; Siegman, Feldstein, Tommaso, Ringel, & Lating, 1987). In other words, it is suggested that the inconsistent findings may reflect inconsistencies in the administration of the SI. Another issue concerns the scoring of the SI. From the beginning, Rosenman (1978) was very clear that the scoring of the SI is to be based not so much on the content of the interviewee's responses as on the interviewee's expressive vocal behavior, or vocal stylistics, during the SI. The scoring criteria include short response latencies, loud speech, explosive speech, rapid accelerated speech, and frequent interruptions of the interviewer. It is not quite clear, however, precisely how much weight is to be given to evidence of hostility. If SI scorers are now giving more weight to vocal style and less weight to hostility references than they used to in the WCGS, and there is reason to believe that this is what has been happening at least among scorers trained in the Rosenman tradition, then we may have yet another explanation for the increasingly negative findings. Moreover, it is not at all clear that there is consistency in this regard across scorers.

Another set of explanations for the negative, contradictory findings regarding the global Type A–CHD relationship, rests on a critique of the Type A construct. It is argued that the multidimensional nature of the Type A construct makes failure to demonstrate a significant relationship between the TABP and CHD almost inevitable. Recall that the TABP encompasses such diverse behaviors as ambition, hostility, and a hurried lifestyle. Exaggerated behavior in any one of these categories could earn one a Type A designation. However, it has never been demonstrated that they all are equally coronary-prone. Different combinations of these behaviors could earn one a Type A designation, although only some of these may be coronary-prone, others may not, and yet others may even be protective.

THE DECONSTRUCTION OF THE
TYPE A CONSTRUCT

Theodore M. Dembroski must be given considerable credit for moving the field away from global Type A and focusing its attention on hostility as the toxic component in the TABP construct. He insisted that further progress in identifying coronary-prone behavior depends on decomposing the Type A construct into its constituent components (Dembroski & MacDougall, 1983, 1985). Based on previous research by Matthews, Glass, Rosenman, and Bortner (1977), and findings by Williams and associates, discussed shortly, Dembroski felt that the potential for hostility is the most likely candidate as the "toxic" component of Type A. The study by Matthews et al. (1977) was based on 62 new cases of CHD and 124 matched controls of the WCGS. Comparisons were made in relation to over 40 SI-derived Type A relevant variables. Significant discriminators between cases and controls were potential for hostility, anger directed outward, experience of anger more than once a week, irritation at waiting in lines, vigorous answers, and explosive responses. In the absence of a multivariate analysis, it is impossible to say which of the aforementioned are independent risk factors and which owe their relationship with CHD to the fact that they are confounded with other CHD risk factors. The findings obtained by the Duke University group, led by Redford Williams, Jr., that MMPI-derived Hostility (Ho) Scale scores correlate significantly with severity of coronary artery disease (CAD) (Williams et al., 1980, 1985), contributed to Dembroski's position that the potential for hostility is likely to be the toxic component of the Type A complex. Dembroski proceeded to develop a component scoring system for the SI, which includes a potential for hostility (PoHo) component, and the following three hostility subcomponents: hostile content, intensity of hostility, and hostile style. The other components are: explosive voice, short latencies, rapid accelerated speech, loud speech, competition for control, and Anger-In (Dembroski & MacDougall, 1983, 1985). In several cross-sectional angiographic studies, Dembroski and associates (Dembroski et al., 1985; MacDougall, Dembroski, Dimsdale, & Hackett, 1985) found significant associations between SI-derived clinical ratings of the potential for hostility and extent of coronary artery disease, although global Type A scores were not significantly related to disease status. The most recent and, perhaps, the most convincing evidence for the conclusion that hostility is the toxic component in the Type A complex comes from a reanalysis of the MRFIT findings, which showed that clinical ratings of the potential for hostility derived from the SI were significantly associated with incidence of CHD, although global Type A scores (also derived from the SI) showed no such significant relationship (Dembroski, MacDougall, Costa, & Grandits, 1989; Shekelle et al., 1985). A reanalysis of data from the WCGS, in which the authors compared 250 initially healthy CHD cases and 500 matched controls, also found that clinical ratings of the potential for hostility were the only SI-derived component that predicted CHD in multivariate analyses (Hecker, Chesney, Black, & Frautschi, 1988). These interview-derived ratings of hostility were also found to predict all cause mortality in a 22-year follow-up of WCGS subjects.

Of course, the many prospective and cross-sectional studies that found significant relationships between Cook–Medley (1954) Hostility (Ho) scale scores and CHD endpoints contributed significantly to the shift in focus from global Type A to hostility (for a review of this literature, see Helmers, Posluszny, & Krantz, this volume).

The key question is whether the Type A behavior pattern contributes to one's risk for CHD over and above the unique risk conferred by hostility. This has been recognized by Rosenman (1985, p. 109):

> Although TAB has been found (Rosenman et al., 1964) and confirmed (Rosenman & Chesney, 1982) to be a risk factor for CHD, there is considerable evidence that it may be the anger/hostility dimension of TAB that confers coronary-proneness (Matthews et al., 1977; Spielberger et al., to be published; Jenkins, 1966). This emotional characteristic also was found to relate significantly to the incidence of CHD in the Framingham Study (Haynes et al., 1980), but only spuriously apart from TAB because the Framingham Type A Scale was directed primarily at the impatience and accelerated pace of activities of TAB and a separate scale was used to assess the anger/hostility dimension. The same problem appears to arise with the studies that used scales derived from the MMPI (Cook & Medley, 1954; Hathaway & McKinley, 1967) to measure hostility and found predictive correlations with the incidence of CHD (Shekelle et al., 1983; Barefoot et al., 1983) as well as with the severity of coronary atherosclerosis (Williams et al., 1980; Blumenthal et al., 1978). The finding of a relationship of "hostility to the severity of coronary atherosclerosis in the studies of Shekelle and Barefoot led them to infer that this behavior was independent of TAB. Unfortunately, these authors had failed in their studies to administer the SI to assess either the TAB of their subjects or its hostility–anger dimensions, thus leading to a somewhat spurious conclusion that such behaviors are independent of TAB, when they may in fact be dominant Type A behaviors that relate TAB to CHD (Matthews et al., 1977; Spielberger et al., in press)."

However, contrary to Rosenman's claim, correlational studies, and reanalyses of the two major prospective studies, the WCGS and MRFIT, found significant relationships between SI-derived clinical ratings of the potential for hostility and CAD and CHD endpoints in the absence of significant relationships between global Type A and disease endpoints. In this context, it should be noted that a recent study (Williams et al., 1988) did find a significant positive relationship between global Type A and severity of CAD, but only in younger, not in older patients. Perhaps failure to consider the moderating role of age accounts for some of the aforementioned negative findings regarding global Type A and CHD. However, even the positive relationship between Type A and CAD reported by Williams et al. (1988) was not particularly strong, and may have been mediated by hostility.

A brief comment is in order on the significant relationships that were obtained by the Friedman group in their Recurrent Coronary Prevention Project between VCI-derived Type A scores and CHD endpoints. Although both the Rosenman group and the Friedman group use the structured interview for the assessment of the TABP, over time, differences developed between these two groups of investigators both in relation to the administration and the scoring of the interview. The Friedman group videotaped the interview so they could use both auditory and visual cues for determining Type A scores. Consequently, they refer to their interview as the Videotaped Clinical Interview (VCI). At one time a major difference between the two involved the interviewer's demeanor during the interview, with the interviewer behaving in a much more provocative and challenging manner in the SI than in the VCI administration. However, this excessive level of challenge on the part of the interviewer during the administration of the SI has abated during recent years, so the two have become much more similar in that respect as well (Scherwitz, 1989). At the present time, the major difference between the SI and the VCI is in the cues that are used to determine a respondent's Type A score. As pointed out earlier, in the SI, which is audiotaped, the interviewees are assigned a global Type A score primarily on the basis of vigorous vocal stylistics (e.g., brief response latencies, loud and rapid accelerated speech, frequent interruptions, etc.). Auditors are specifically instructed to ignore content (Rosenman, 1978). By way of contrast, in the VCI, which is both audio- and videotaped, a respondent's Type A score is based on content as well as on vocal style, but also on motor behavior, posture, and facial expressions (i.e., on both verbal and nonverbal cues). In the VCI, respondents are assigned a Time–Urgency and a Hostility score, which are then combined into a global Type A score. A recent comparison (Siegman, Dembroski, Anderson, Perlstein, & Lating, 1990) of the SI and VCI derived global Type A scores in a group of 41 male undergraduates failed to obtain a significant relationship between the two. This is not especially surprising because, in the VCI, scorers are instructed to consider content, whereas, in the SI, they are instructed to ignore it. Furthermore, VCI scorers rely on visual cues, which are not available to SI scorers. On the other hand, the VCI-derived Hostility scores and the SI-derived Potential for Hostility scores did correlate significantly with each other [$(r) = .55, p < .0001$]. Consequently, it may very well be that hostility mediates the significant relationship VCI-derived Type A scores and the recurrence of MIs reported by the Friedman group.

Of course, none of the aforementioned is to be taken to mean that hostility is the sole coronary-prone behavior. In a recent thallium stress test study, Siegman, Lating, Johnston, and Boyle (see Siegman, this volume) found a significant positive relationship between the patients' SI-derived Verbal Competition scores and their severity of perfusion defects scores. Now, the frequency of interrupting one's conversational partner, which is the major constituent of the Verbal Competition category, is an expressive correlate of dominance and assertiveness (Siegman, 1987, p. 368). Perhaps this personality trait, which is conceptually related to the original definition of the Type A construct, is yet another independent risk factor for CHD. This conclusion is supported by the results of a recent study by Houston, Chesney, Black, Cates, and Hecker (1992). Clearly, this is an issue that needs to be pursued further.

THE DECONSTRUCTION OF THE HOSTILITY CONSTRUCT

Although the weight of the evidence indeed indicates that hostility is a risk factor for CHD (Dembroski & Czajkowski, 1989; Dembroski & Williams, 1989; Matthews, 1988; Siegman, this volume), there also were some negative findings (e.g., McCranie, Watkins, Brandame, & Sisson, 1986). It must be recognized, however, that hostility too is a multidimensional construct, and that only some of its dimensions may be coronary prone (Siegman, Dembroski, & Ringel, 1987). The multidimensional nature of hostility is supported by the results of several factor analytic studies of the Buss–Durkee Hostility Inventory (BDHI) conducted in our laboratory and elsewhere (Bendig, 1962; Buss & Durkee, 1957; Edmunds & Kendrick, 1980; Sarason, 1961; Siegman, Dembroski, & Ringel, 1987). The BDHI consists of several rationally constructed subscales: Physical Aggression (Item example: When I really lose my temper, I am capable of slapping someone), Verbal Aggression (When I get mad, I say nasty things), Indirect Aggression (When I am mad, I sometimes slam things), Irritability (I am irritated a great deal more than people are aware of), Negativism (When someone is bossy, I do the opposite of what he asks), Suspicion and Resentment. Factor analyses of the BDHI items, or of the BDHI subscales, have consistently identified two factors. The first is defined by items or subscales that measure the frequency with which the individual experiences feelings of hostility, including feelings of mistrust and suspicion. The first factor, then, is a measure of the experience of hostility. This factor has substantial positive correlations with indices of trait anxiety or neuroticism (Siegman, Dembroski, & Ringel, 1987) and, therefore, can be viewed as a measure of *neurotic* hostility. The second factor is defined by items and subscales that measure the *expression* of anger–hostility that occurs in response to provocation. These findings prompted Siegman et al. (1987) to ascertain whether these two components of hostility have the same or different relationships with CAD. The results of a study (Siegman et al., 1987) with angiographic patients showed that only the expression of anger–hostility, not its mere experience, is positively related to the severity of CAD. Other investigations showed that the same differential relationship obtains in relation to physiological and hormonal factors that have been implicated in the pathogenesis of CHD, such as cardiovascular reactivity, platelet formation, and testosterone levels in response to challenge and stress (Siegman, this volume). In each case, only the expression of anger–hostility, not its mere experience, is positively related to the above mediating risk factors. Clearly then, hostility too is a multidimensional construct, and only the expression of hostility seems to be toxic as far as CAD and CHD are concerned.

These findings raise problems about some of the other instruments that have been used to assess hostility, such as Dembroski's SI-derived clinical hostility ratings, the VCI-derived clinical hostility ratings, and the Cook–Medley (1954) Hostility (Ho) scale, all of which measure both the expression of anger-hostility and the experience of hostility, but in different degrees. Thus, in a recent study (Siegman et al., 1991), Dembroski's SI-derived potential for hostility (PoHo) ratings correlated .45 ($p < .01$) with the expression of anger-hostility and only .29 (n.s.) with the experience of hostility. On the other hand, the VCI-derived hostility ratings correlated only .28 (n.s.) with the expression of anger–hostility, but .37 ($p < .05$) with the experience of hostility. Finally, the Ho scale correlated .42 ($p < .01$) with the expression of anger–hostility and .70 ($p < .0001$) with the experience of hostility.

Given these findings, one is tempted to call for the development of "purer" measures of hostility, measures that do not confound the experience with the expression of hostility. However, such a call must be tempered by the fact that there is no convincing evidence that relatively pure measures of the expression of hostility—such as the relevant BDHI scales—are better predictors of CHD than measures that confound the expression with the experience of hostility—such as the Ho-scale—but more about this later in this chapter.

There is also the issue of validity. Not every measure that has hostility in its title is necessarily a valid measure of that construct. Let us consider the Ho scale. Is it really a measure of hostility? Even a quick perusal of Ho scale items suggests that this scale is probably most accurately described as a measure of mistrust and cynicism—a conclusion that was confirmed by more formal factor analytic studies of this scale (Costa, Zonderman, McCrae, & Williams, 1986; Greenglass & Julkunen, 1989). Based on their findings, Costa et al. (1986) concluded that the term "hostility" is somewhat misleading as a description and that a better label might be "cynical mistrust." Although clearly a measure of cynicism, the Ho scale apparently also taps other characteristics. Relying on the face validity of the Ho scale items, Barefoot, Dodge, Peterson, Dahlstrom, and Williams (1989) attempted an a priori, rational classification of these items. Six subsets were identified: Cynicism, Hostile

Attribution, Hostile Affect, Aggressive Responding, Social Avoidance, and Other. Three of these subsets, namely, Cynicism, Hostile Affect, and Aggressive Responding, predicted mortality (from all causes) in a prospective study of law school students. Moreover, the sum of these three subsets were appreciably better able to predict mortality than any of its components or than the total Ho scale. Recall, however, that in this study the authors tried to predict mortality from all causes, not just from CHD. If there are different behavioral risk factors for different diseases (e.g., hostility for CHD and cynical mistrust for cancer), then we can understand why the sum of the three subsets was a better predictor of mortality from all causes than any one subset of items.

Thus far, we know very little about differential relationships between various behavioral risk factors and different CHD endpoints, such as sudden cardiac death, atherosclerosis, angina, and so on. Consider, however, the possibility that expressed anger–hostility is primarily associated with sudden cardiac death, the experience of anger–hostility with atherosclerosis, and cynical mistrust with yet another CHD endpoint. If such were indeed the case, then the strength of the Ho scale in predicting CHD may be precisely in the fact that it measures these various coronary-prone behaviors.[5] Alternatively, these various components may interact with each other, perhaps in a mutually reinforcing manner, to produce CHD. The clarification of these questions may be a long way off. In the interim, however, we need to be concerned with the more easily resolved problem: the validity of our independent measures. For example, if cynical mistrust is, indeed, an independent risk factor for CHD, there may be better (i.e., more valid) ways of assessing this dimension than by means of the Ho scale—an issue that is now being addressed in our laboratory. (For a more detailed discussion of these and other assessment issues, see Barefoot, this volume.)

THE RETURN OF ANGER

Of the three major negative emotions, fear–anxiety, sadness–depression, and anger, psychologists have paid the least attention to anger. Even though clinicians surely must be aware of the important role that anger plays in their patients' lives, there has been relatively little explication of its development and of its precise role in different psychopathologies. Although *DSM III* discusses the role of anxiety in various psychopathological syndromes in some detail, there is very little to be found about the role of anger.

However, the search for behavioral risk factors in cardiovascular diseases

---

[5]Of course, this is not an endorsement of confounded scales. Separate unconfounded scales of the various contributing factors to CHD should be equally good or better predictors.

has generated a new interest in anger and its somatic consequences. As far back as 1939, Franz Alexander suggested that the repression of anger is associated with chronic elevations in blood pressure and ultimately with essential hypertension (EH). Because empirical support for this hypothesis has been inconsistent (for a review of this literature, see Diamond, 1982; Julius, Schneider, & Egan, 1985; Manuck, Morrison, Bellack, & Polefrone, 1985), the early interest in anger as a cause of CHD began to wane. Several decades later, anger—but this time not in its repressed form—reemerged as part of the TABP. Rosenman and Friedman's original conceptualization of the TABP (Rosenman, 1978; Rosenman et al., 1964) clearly included anger as part of the TABP construct. However, with the success of the Cook–Medley Ho scale and Dembroski's SI-derived clinical ratings of the potential for hostility in predicting CHD, the interest of coronary-prone behavior researchers shifted to hostility, with anger becoming submerged or totally ignored. However, even a cursory examination of the criteria on which the SI-derived clinical judgments of hostility are based readily reveals that these judgments involve both anger and hostile attitudes. One attempt to identify the psychological attributes reflected in SI-derived Potential-for Hostility ratings yielded the following attributes: anger experience, anger expression, hostile attitudes. Indeed, in recent publications, Dembroski and associates (1989) refer to their SI-derived index as a measure of "anger–hostility." The same is true of the Buss–Durkee Factor II scales. Originally, they were referred to as *hostility* scales (Siegman et al., 1987). Here, too, however, even a cursory examination of the items in these scales reveals that many are concerned with anger (e.g., When I get mad, I say nasty things; When I really lose my temper, I am capable of slapping someone), which led me to relabel them as (the expression of) *anger* or *anger–hostility* scales (see Siegman, this volume).

Psychologists distinguish between anger, hostility, and aggression, with the first referring to affect, the second to attitudes, and the last to destructive behavior. However, these distinctions have been ignored in the earlier coronary-prone behavior literature. Given the physiological and neurohormonal manifestations of anger, it should come as no surprise that anger may play a significant role in the development of CHD. It has long been known that anger is associated with heightened levels of cardiovascular arousal, which has been identified as the mechanism that translates behavior into coronary heart disease processes (Kaplan, Botchin, & Manuck, this volume; Williams, 1989). Anger is also associated with increased rates of testosterone production and platelet formation, which are also involved in the pathogenesis of CHD (Williams, 1989). However, we need to distinguish between different forms of anger. There is a substantial body of evidence that suggests that only the expression of anger, not its mere experience, is associated with heightened levels of CVR (Siegman, this volume). Neither is the repression of anger related to CV hyperreactivity, at least not in terms of BP reactivity, or to CHD, although it has other negative health consequences (Siegman, this volume). Just as we need to distinguish between different dimensions of hostility, we also need to distinguish between different modes of coping with anger and their coronary consequences.

What emerges from the previous discussion is that, to begin with, we need to clear the ground conceptually. We need to distinguish between anger, hostility, and aggressive behavior, and between all of these and cynical mistrust, and we need to determine how these constructs relate to each other. Next, we need to develop valid and reliable measures of these constructs. If it is the case that all of these constructs are related to CHD—a not unlikely possibility given the available data—we will want to know whether they are, indeed, independent relationships. Are the relationships between hostility, cynical mistrust, and CHD due to the fact that cynical individuals are prone to become angry and to express it vigorously, or are they independent relationships? In a similar vein: We now know that high Ho scale scorers (i.e., cynical, mistrusting individuals) tend to have a coronary-prone lifestyle, involving excessive alcohol consumption, overeating, and so forth (see Siegler, this volume). It is important, therefore, to establish whether or not the contribution of cynical mistrust to CHD is independent of these lifestyle variables. We also need to know more about the relationship between anger, hostility, and these lifestyle variables. In a study with male undergraduates that was recently completed in our laboratory, we found a positive association between the experience of anger–hostility and smoking, the consumption of caffeine, and sleep deprivation. No such associations obtained between the expression of anger and these coronary-prone lifestyle variables. This would suggest that the expression of anger is a risk factor for CHD, independent of these lifestyle variables. A related issue involves the role of social support. It is not unreasonable to assume that angry, hostile, or mistrusting individuals are not likely to enjoy the positive, buffering experiences that are provided by good social support systems. However, more empirical research is needed on how social support is affected by these CHD risk factors.

Of course, explanations involving anger, hostility, cynicism, and lifestyle variables need not be mutually exclusive—in fact, they probably are mutually reinforcing. Finally, we need to know much more about the mediating mechanisms and pathophysiologies that are involved in these various relationships.

ACKNOWLEDGMENT

The preparation of this chapter and some of the research reported herein were supported by a grant from the National Heart, Lung, and Blood Institute (HL-036027).

REFERENCES

Alexander, F. G. (1930). Emotional factors in essential hypertension. Presentation of a tentative hypothesis. *Psychosomatic Medicine, 1,* 175–179.

Alexander, F. G. (1950). *Psychosomatic medicine.* New York: Norton.

Alexander, F. G., French, T. M., & Pollack, G. H. (1968). *Psychosomatic specificity: Experimental study and results.* Chicago: The University of Chicago Press.

Archer, J. (1673). *Every man his own doctor.* London.

Arrowood, M., Uhrich, K., Gomillion, C., Popio, K., & Raft, D. (1982). New markers of coronary-prone behavior in a rural population. *Psychosomatic Medicine, 119,* 44–119.

Barefoot, J. C., Dodge, K. A., Peterson, B. L., Dahlstrom, W. G., & Williams, R. B., Jr. (1989). The Cook–Medley Hostility scale: Item content and ability to predict survival. *Psychosomatic Medicine, 51,* 46–57.

Bendig, A. W. (1962). Factor analytic scales of covert and overt hostility. *Journal of Consulting Psychology, 26,* 200.

Blumenthal, J. A., Williams, R. S., Kong, Y., Shanberg, S. M., & Thompson, L. W. (1978). Type A behavior pattern and coronary atherosclerosis. *Circulation, 258,* 634–639.

Buss, A. H., & Durkee, A. (1957). An inventory for assessing different kinds of hostility. *Journal of Consulting Psychology, 21,* 343–349.

Cannon, W. B. (1932). *The wisdom of the body.* New York: Norton.

Chesney, M. A., Eagleston, J. R., & Rosenman, R. H. (1980). The Type A structured interview: A behavioral assessment in the rough. *Journal of Behavioral Assessment, 2,* 255–272.

Cook, W., & Medley, D. (1954). Proposed hostility for Pharisaic-virtue skills of the MMPI. *Journal of Applied Psychology, 38,* 414–418.

Cooper, T., Detre, T., & Weiss, S. M. (1981). Coronary-prone behavior and coronary heart disease: A critical review. *Circulation, 63,* 1199–1215.

Costa, P. T., Jr., Zonderman, A. B., McCrae, R. R., & Williams, R. B., Jr. (1986). Cynicism and paranoid alienation in the Cook and Medley Ho scale. *Psychosomatic Medicine, 48,* 283–285.

DeBakey, M., & Gotto, A. (1977). *The living heart.* New York: Charter Books.

Dembroski, T. M., & Czajkowski, S. M. (1989). Historical and current developments in coronary-prone behavior. In A. W. Siegman & T. M. Dembroski (Eds.), *In search of coronary-prone behavior: Beyond Type A* (pp. 21–39). Hillsdale, NJ: Lawrence Erlbaum Associates.

Dembroski, T. M., & MacDougall, J. M. (1983). Behavioral and psycho-physiological perspectives on coronary-prone behavior. In T. M. Dembroski, T. H. Schmidt, & G. Blumchen (Eds.), *Biobehavioral bases of coronary heart disease* (pp. 106–129). New York: Karger.

Dembroski, T. M., & MacDougall, J. M. (1985). Beyond global Type A: Relationships of paralinguistic attributes, hostility, and anger-in coronary heart disease. In T. Field, P. McCabe, & N. Schneiderman (Eds.), *Stress and coping.* Hillsdale, NJ: Lawrence Erlbaum Associates.

Dembroski, T. M., MacDougall, T. M., Costa, P. T., & Grandits, G. A. (1989). Components of hostility as predictors of sudden death and myocardial infarction in the Multiple Risk Factor Intervention Trial. *Psychosomatic Medicine, 51,* 514–522.

Dembroski, T. M., MacDougall, J. M., Williams, R. B., Haney, T. L., & Blumenthal, J. A. (1985). Components of Type A, hostility, and anger-in: Relationship to angiographic findings. *Psychosomatic Medicine, 47,* 219–233.

Dembroski, T. M., & Williams, R. B. (1989). In N. Schneiderman, P. Kaufman, & S. M. Weiss (Eds.), *Handbook of research methods in cardiovascular behavioral medicine.* New York: Plenum.

Diamond, E. L. (1982). The role of anger and hostility in essential hypertension and coronary heart disease. *Psychological Bulletin, 92,* 410–433.

Dimsdale, J. F., Hackett, T. P., & Hutter, A. M. (1979). Type A behavior and angiographic findings. *Journal of Psychosomatic Research, 23,* 273–276.

Edmunds, G., & Kendrick, D. C. (1980). *The measurement of human aggressiveness.* West Sussex, England: Ellis Horwood.

Fothergill, J. (1781). *Complete collection of the medical and philosophical works.* London.

Frank, K. A., Heller, S. S., Kornfeld,, D. S., Sporn, A. A., & Weiss, M. B. (1978). Type A behavior pattern and coronary angiographic findings. *Journal of the American Medical Association, 240,* 761–763.

Friedman, M., & Rosenman, R. H. (1974). *Type A behavior and your heart.* New York: Knopf.

Friedman, M., Rosenman, R. H., Straus, R., Wurm, M., & Kositchek, R. (1968). The relationship of behavior pattern to the state of the coronary vasculature. A study of 51 autopsy subjects. *American Journal of Medicine, 244,* 525–538.

Friedman, M., Thoresen, C. E., Gill, J. J., Ulmer, D., Powell, L., Price, V., Brown, B., Thompson, L., Rabin, D. D., Breall, W. S., Gourg, E., Levy, R. A., & Dixon, T. (1986). Alteration of Type A behavior and its effect on cardiac recurrences in post myocardial infarction patients: Summary results of the Recurrent Coronary Prevention Project. *American Heart Journal, 112,* 653–665.

Greenglass, E. R., & Julkunen, J. (1989). Construct validity and sex differences in Cook–Medley hostility. *Personality and Individual Differences, 10,* 209–218.

Harvey, W. (1928). *Exercitatio anetomica de motu cordis et sanguinis* [An anatomical exercise concerning the movement of heart and blood]. London: Baillieve, Tindall, & Cox. (Facsimile of original 1628 edition)

Heberden, W. (1772). Some account of a disorder of the breast. *Medical Transactions Royal College of Physicians, 2,* 59.

Hecker, H. L., Chesney, M. A., Black, G. W., & Frautschi, N. (1988). Coronary-prone behaviors in the Western Collaborative Group Study. *Psychosomatic Medicine, 50,* 153–164.

Houston, B. K., Chesney, M. A., Black, G. W., Cates, D. S., & Hecker, M. H. L. (1992). Behavioral clusters and coronary heart disease risk. *Psychosomatic Medicine, 54,* 447–466.

Jenkins, C. D. (1979). *Jenkins Activity Survey.* New York: Psychological Corporation.

Julius, S., Schneider, R., & Egan, B. (1985). Suppressed anger in hypertension: Facts and problems. In M. A. Chesney & R. H. Rosenman (Eds.), *Anger and hostility in cardiovascular and behavioral disorders* (pp. 127–137). Washington, DC: Hemisphere.

Keys, A. (1970). Coronary heart disease in seven countries: XIII multiple variables. *Circulation, 41,* 138–144.

Krantz, D. S., Sanmarco, M. I., Selvester, R. H., & Matthews, K. A. (1979). Psychological correlates of progression of atherosclerosis in men. *Psychosomatic Medicine, 41,* 467–476.

MacDougall, J. M., Dembroski, T. M., Dimsdale, J. E., & Hackett, T. P. (1985). Components of Type A, hostility, and anger-in: Further relationships to angiographic findings. *Health Psychology, 4,* 137–152.

Manuck, S. B., Morrison, R. L., Bellack, A. S., & Polefrone, J. M. (1985). Behavioral factors in hypertension: Cardiovascular responsivity, anger, and social competence. In M. A. Chesney & R. H. Rosenman (Eds.), *Anger and hostility in cardiovascular and behavioral disorders* (pp. 149–172). Washington, DC: Hemisphere.

Matthews, K. A. (1988). Coronary heart disease and Type A behavior: Update on and alternative to the Booth-Kewley and Friedman (1987) quantitative review. *Psychological Bulletin, 104,* 373–380.

Matthews, K. A., Glass, D. C., Rosenman, R. H., & Bortner, R. W. (1977). Competitive drive, pattern A, and coronary heart disease: A further analysis of some data from the Western Collaborative Group Study. *Journal of Chronic Diseases, 30,* 489–498.

McCranie, E. W., Watkins, L., Brandsma, J., & Sisson, B. (1986). Hostility, coronary heart disease (CHD) incidence, and total mortality: Lack of association in a 25-year follow-up study of 478 physicians. *Journal of Behavioral Medicine, 9,* 119–125.

Miller, N. E. (1990). How the brain affects the health of the body. In K. D. Craig & S. M. Weiss (Eds.), *Health enhancement, disease prevention, and early intervention.* New York: Springer.

Ragland, D. R., & Brand, R. J. (1988). Type A behavior and mortality from coronary heart disease. *New England Journal of Medicine, 318,* 65–69.

Review Panel on Coronary-Prone Behavior and Coronary Heart Disease (1981). Coronary-prone behavior and coronary heart disease: A critical review. *Circulation, 63,* 1199–1215.

Rosenman, R. H. (1978). The interview method of assessment of the coronary-prone behavior pattern. In T. M. Dembroski, S. Weiss, J. Schillar, S. G. Haynes, & M. Feinlieb (Eds.), *Coronary prone behavior.* New York: Springer-Verlag.

Rosenman, R. H. (1983). Current status of risk factors and Type A behavior pattern in the pathogenesis of ischemic heart disease. In T. M. Dembroski, S. M. Weiss, J. L. Shields, S. G. Haynes, & M. Feinlieb (Eds.), *Coronary prone behavior.* New York: Springer-Verlag.

Rosenman, R. H. (1985). Health consequences of anger and implications for treatment. In M. A. Chesney & R. H. Rosenman (Eds.), *Anger and hostility in cardiovascular and behavioral disorders* (pp. 103–125). Washington, DC: Hemisphere.

Rosenman, R. H., Brand, R. J., Jenkins, C. D., Friedman, M., Strauss, R., & Wurm, M. (1975). Coronary heart disease in the Western Collaborative Group Study: Final follow-up experience of 8½ years. *Journal of the American Medical Association, 223,* 872–877.

Rosenman, R. H., & Friedman, M. (1974). Neurogenic factors in pathogenesis of coronary heart disease. *Medical Clinics of North America, 58,* 269–279.

Rosenman, R. H., Friedman, M., Straus, R., Wurm, M., Kositchek, R., Hahn, W., & Wethessen, N. T. (1964). A predictive study of coronary heart disease: The Western Collaborative Group Study. *Journal of the American Medical Association, 189,* 15–22.

Sarason, I. (1961). Intercorrelations among measures of hostility. *Journal of Clinical Psychology, 17,* 192–195.

Scherwitz, L. (1989). Type A behavior assessment in the Structured Interview: Review, critique, and recommendations. In A. W. Siegman & T. M. Dembroski (Eds.), *In search of coronary-prone behavior: Beyond Type A* (pp. 117–148). Hillsdale, NJ: Lawrence Erlbaum Associates.

Scherwitz, L., McKelvain, R., Laman, C., Patterson, J., Dutton, L., Yusim, S., Lester, J., Kraft, I., Rochelle, D., & Leachman, R. (1983). Type A behavior, self-involvement, and coronary atherosclerosis. *Psychosomatic Medicine, 45,* 47–57.

Shekelle, R. B., Hulley, S., Neaton, J., Billings, J., Borhani, N., Gerace, T., Jacobs, D., Lasser, N., Mittlemark, M., & Stamler, J. (1985). MRFIT Research Group: The MRFIT behavior pattern study. II. Type A behavior pattern and incidence of coronary heart disease. *American Journal of Epidemiology, 122,* 559–570.

Siegman, A. W. (1987). The telltale voice: Nonverbal messages of verbal communications. In A. W. Siegman & S. Feldstein (Eds.), *Nonverbal behavior and communication* (2nd ed.). Hillsdale, NJ: Lawrence Erlbaum Associates.

Siegman, A. W. (1992, July). *The role of expressive vocal behavior in negative emotions: Implications for stress management.* Paper presented at XXV International Congress of Psychology, Brussels.

Siegman, A. W., & Dembroski, T. M. (Eds.) (1989). *In search of coronary-prone behavior: Beyond Type A.* Hillsdale, NJ: Lawrence Erlbaum Associates.

Siegman, A. W., Dembroski, T. M., Anderson, R. W., Perlstein, S., & Lating, J. (1990, April). *A comparison of videotaped and audiotaped scoring procedures of Type A and its components.* Paper presented at the annual meeting of the Society of Behavioral Medicine, Chicago, IL.

Siegman, A. W., Dembroski, T. M., & Ringel, N. (1987). Components of hostility and the severity of coronary artery disease. *Psychosomatic Medicine, 49,* 127–135.

Siegman, A. W., Feldstein, S., Simpson, S. M., Barkley, S., & Kobren, R. (1984, April). *Content and stress in the interview method for the assessment of Type A behavior.* Paper presented at the annual meetings of the Eastern Psychological Association, Baltimore, MD.

Siegman, A. W., Feldstein, S., Tommaso, C., Ringel, N., & Lating, J. (1987). Expressive vocal behavior and the severity of coronary artery disease. *Psychosomatic Medicine, 49*, 545–561.

Siegman, A. W., Perlstein, S. M., Anderson, R. W., Boyle, S., & Lating, J. (1991). A comparison of SI and VCI derived Type A and hostility measures. Manuscript submitted for publication.

Spielberger, C. D., Johnson, E. H., Russell, S. F., Crane, R. J., Jacobs, G. A., & Worden, T. J. (1985). The experience and expression of anger: Construction and validation of an anger expression scale. In M. Chesney & R. Rosenman (Eds.), *Anger and hostility in cardiovascular and behavioral disorders* (pp. 5–30). New York: McGraw-Hill.

Trousseau, A. (1982). *Clinical medicine.* Philadelphia.

Ullman, L. P., & Krasner, L. (1969). *A psychological approach to abnormal behavior.* Englewood Cliffs, NJ: Prentice-Hall.

Wardrop, J. (1851). *Diseases of the heart.* London.

Williams, R. B., Jr., (1989). Biological mechanisms mediating the relationship between behavior and coronary heart disease. In A. W. Siegman & T. M. Dembroski (Eds.), *In search of coronary-prone behavior: Beyond Type A* (pp. 195–205). Hillsdale, NJ: Lawrence Erlbaum Associates.

Williams, R. B., Jr., Barefoot, J. C., Haney, T. L., Harrell, F. E., Blumenthal, J. A., Pryor, D. B., & Peterson, B. (1988). Type A behavior and angiographically documented coronary atherosclerosis in a sample of 2,289 patients. *Psychosomatic Medicine, 50*, 139–152.

Williams, R. B., Jr., Barefoot, J. C., & Shekelle, R. B. (1985). The health consequences of hostility. In M. A. Chesney & R. H. Rosenman (Eds.), *Anger and hostility in cardiovascular and behavioral disorders* (pp. 173–185). New York: McGraw-Hill.

Williams, R. B., Jr., Haney, T. L., Lee, K. L., Kong, Y., Blumenthal, J., & Whalen, R. (1980). Type A behavior, hostility, and coronary atherosclerosis. *Psychosomatic Medicine, 42*, 539–549.

Williams, R. B., Jr., Suarez, E. C., Kuhn, C. M., Zimmerman, E. A., & Schanberg, S. M. (1991). Biobehavioral basis of coronary-prone behavior in middle-aged men: Part I. Evidence for chronic SNS activation in Type As. *Psychosomatic Medicine, 53*, 517–527.

Zyzanski, S. J., Jenkins, C. D., Ryan, T. J., Flessas, A., & Everist, M. (1976). Psychological correlates of coronary angiographic findings. *Archives of Internal Medicine, 136*, 1234–1237.

2

CONCEPTS AND METHODS IN THE STUDY OF ANGER, HOSTILITY, AND HEALTH

Timothy W. Smith
University of Utah

During the 1980s, many studies examined the association of chronic anger and hostility with cardiovascular morbidity and mortality (Helmers & Krantz, this volume; Smith, 1992). In fact, more empirical support for this psychosomatic hypothesis accrued during this period than had appeared in its entire previous history, despite the fact that the health consequences of anger and hostility have been discussed for centuries (Siegman, this volume). This empirical support came from cross-sectional studies of coronary artery disease (CAD; e.g., Dembroski, MacDougall, Williams, Haney, & Blumenthal, 1985) and prospective studies of initially healthy persons (e.g., Barefoot, Dahlstrom, & Williams, 1983; Hecker, Chesney, Black, & Frautschi, 1988). There is also converging evidence from animal studies implicating aggressive behavior and angerlike states in the development of CAD (Kaplan, Botchin, & Manuck, this volume; Manuck, Kaplan, Muldoon, Adams, & Clarkson, 1991) and the occurrence of acute manifestations of coronary heart disease (CHD), such as myocardial ischemia (Verrier, Hagestad, & Lown, 1987). The possible clinical relevance of these findings was suggested in the Recurrent Coronary Prevention Project (RCPP), in which group therapy for coronary-prone behavior significantly reduced recurrent cardiac events (Friedman et al., 1986). Although this intervention focused on the globally defined Type A pattern, chronic anger and hostility was a central issue in the treatment program (Thoresen & Powell, 1992).

Despite these supportive findings, there are inconsistencies in this literature (Helmers & Krantz, this volume; Smith, 1992). Several cross-sectional (e.g., Helmer, Ragland, & Syme, 1991) and prospective studies (e.g., Hearn,

Murray, & Luepker, 1989; McCranie, Watkins, Brandsma, & Sisson, 1986) failed to find an association between hostility and disease. Although methodological problems might account for these negative results (Siegler et al., 1990; Williams, 1987), the inconsistencies weaken the conclusions that can be drawn about this literature. Such inconsistencies also provide fuel for skeptics, many of whom dismiss the notion that personality traits and other psychological factors influence physical health (e.g., Angell, 1985).

Failures to replicate the association between chronic anger or hostility and disease are likely to have one of two effects on future work in this area. Conflicting results can provide the basis for refinement and heuristic reformulation of the research questions and methods, as explanations for differing results are articulated and tested. Ultimately, such a process leads to cumulative progress. However, in a critique of the course of behavioral science, Meehl (1978) noted that research topics are often characterized by cycles of waxing and waning activity. After a period of initial interest, inconclusive studies typically lead to the slow abandonment of an area, without resolution or reformulation of the original questions. After a period of inactivity, interest may be rekindled, but with a great chance of fading from view again rather than generating a more lasting, definitive scientific contribution. A skeptic might view the history of this research area traced by Siegman (this volume) as consistent with Meehl's critique. Inconsistencies in the current decade of research on anger, hostility, and health could be seen as portending its abandonment under the weight of lingering doubt and inconclusive findings, much like the failure to generate compelling empirical support led to the demise of psychoanalytically based models (e.g., Dunbar, 1943; Menninger & Menninger, 1936) earlier in this century (Holroyd & Coyne, 1987). Thus, the field is approaching a crossroads between substantive evolution and declining interest (Smith, 1992).

There is reason for optimism, however. As this volume clearly documents, the research is far more extensive and methodologically sophisticated than in previous periods of interest in the topic. Further, the research tools for studying all aspects of the problem continue to improve, and studies to date have not even taken full advantage of those methods currently available.

This chapter outlines the conceptual issues and questions running through the recent literature on anger, hostility, and health. As such, it serves as a guide or framework for much of what appears in later chapters. It also identifies areas where reformulation of models and refined research strategies are needed, although all of the following individual chapters provide such information as well.

CONCEPTUAL DEFINITIONS

One potential use of an empirically documented association between chronic anger or hostility and health is improved prediction of cardiovascular disease (CVD). If we were simply interested in more accurate estimates of CVD risk, it would not matter what dimension(s) our questionnaires or interviews actually measured. In other words, predictive utility does not require construct validity. However, research in this area is primarily intended to evaluate theories and models of psychosocial influences on health. As such, delineation of the hypothetical constructs assessed by research instruments used in this area is essential.

As discussed in the subsequent section on assessment and in the following chapter by Barefoot and Lipkus, construct validity is a central and active focus of measurement research on hostility. However, an often overlooked step in this process is the articulation of clear conceptual definitions. Cook and Campbell (1979) suggested that inadequate preoperational definition of constructs is a basic threat to the validity of research findings. Imprecise conceptual definitions are likely to result in similarly imprecise measurement procedures, thereby clouding the implications of subsequent research. Researchers in this area have rediscovered the difficulties in defining the central constructs of anger, hostility, and aggression encountered decades before by personality and social psychologists.

Anger, Hostility, and Aggression

Previous distinctions among emotion, cognition, and behavior (Buss, 1961; Spielberger et al., 1985) are very useful in this regard. From this perspective, anger refers to an unpleasant emotion ranging in intensity from irritation or annoyance to fury or rage. Angry affect, the subjective or experiential component of this emotion, is typically accompanied by physiological arousal, characteristic facial expression, and activation of action tendencies or impulses toward aggression. Anger is also characterized by a relational theme or script, consisting of the perception of being subjected to illegitimate or unfair interference or harm (Lazarus, 1991). The clearly cognitive nature of this theme or script and the behavioral nature of action tendencies underscore the difficulty in deriving completely distinct conceptual definitions of anger, hostility, and aggression. Like all emotions, anger can be seen as a time-limited state, or an enduring disposition or trait consisting of a general tendency to experience frequent and pronounced episodes of the emotional state of anger.

Most current approaches to the description and classification of emotions identify several other negative emotions that are similar to anger, as opposed to fear, sadness, or guilt, for example (Lazarus, 1991; Plutchik, 1980; Shaver, Schwartz, Kirson, & O'Connor, 1987). Contempt, or reproachful disdain, is a distinct emotion, but one which is clearly related to anger. Similarly, resentment refers to a feeling of indignation or ill will as a result of perceived mistreatment. Envy, jealousy, and disgust are more closely related to anger than to other negative emotions, although perhaps less so than contempt and resentment.

Also, the cognitive variable of hostility is multifaceted and difficult to define. It has been defined previously as the tendency to wish to inflict harm on others or the tendency to feel anger toward others (Chaplin, 1982), although these definitions clearly blur the distinctions among emotion, cognition, and behavior. In part, hostility entails a negative attitude toward others, consisting of enmity, denigration, and ill will. Cynicism is a closely related belief that other people are motivated by selfishness rather than by concern for others or by similar higher motives. Mistrust is an associated expectancy that people are unlikely to fulfill obligations and are frequent sources of mistreatment, provocation and harm, despite the fact that they might appear to be friendly and cooperative. Thus, as an enduring, general trait, hostility connotes a devaluation of the worth and motives of others, an expectation that others are likely sources of wrong doing, a relational view of being in opposition toward others, and a desire to inflict harm or see others harmed.

Aggression refers to overt behavior, typically defined as attacking, destructive, or hurtful actions. There have been many attempts to classify subtypes of aggressive behavior (Averill, 1982; Bandura, 1973; Megargee, 1985), usually in terms of its motivation or controlling stimuli. For example, aggression might reflect an impulsive response following frustration and the arousal of anger, or an attempt to influence others and obtain desired outcomes. Perhaps more important are the many varieties of aggressive actions. Harm can be inflicted verbally or physically. Physical aggression can be direct and active (e.g., assault) or indirect (e.g., gossip, making intrusive noises) and passive (e.g., failing to keep an appointment). Similarly, verbal aggression can consist of hateful insult, opposition, argumentativeness, rudeness, or sarcasm. These forms of aggression vary not only in the mode of their expression and their severity, but also in their frequency of occurrence. Although physical aggression is often contemplated, it is far less common than verbal aggression and carries far more severe social consequences (Averill, 1982).

Experience Versus Expression

As is clear elsewhere in this volume, an increasingly important conceptual distinction is that between the experience and expression of anger. These constructs typically refer to traits or dispositions. Taking into consideration the definitions previously mentioned, the experience of anger refers not only to subjective processes—primarily angry affect—but also related emotions (e.g., contempt, resentment) and the cognitive processes connoted by hostility. In contrast, the expression of anger refers to aggressive behavior subsequent to the arousal of anger. It is important to note that both terms imply the occurrence of anger. Thus, people at the extremes of both of these dimensions are prone to frequent and strong anger, but they might differ in their overt responses when they are angry.

Related constructs, such as anger coping styles, or the Anger-in versus Anger-out distinction, are similar to the experience versus expression of anger. These constructs typically refer to the extent to which people display anger outwardly, and the outward behaviors included in these schemes typically represent one or more types of aggression. It is important to further delineate, however, the nature of unexpressed anger. Failure to express anger through overt aggression could reflect automatic or voluntary inhibition of aggressive urges (i.e., repression or suppression), or it could reflect the enactment of alternative overt social responses, such as assertiveness. Earlier, psychodynamic approaches to unexpressed anger conveyed a hydraulic model of increasing internal pressure and energy-consuming inhibition. This model was the impetus for studies of the affective and psychophysiological effects of expression versus withholding of aggression (Hokanson, 1973). Unexpressed anger may or may not be associated with angry brooding—the internal rehearsal of the provoking events and aggressive fantasies.

Similarly, as noted previously, the expression of anger might reflect an uninhibited response to provoking or frustrating events, or it might reflect an effortful attempt to influence or control the individuals involved in such incidents. In short, if the distinction between the experience versus expression of anger is important to further progress in the area, then these constructs will require additional clarification.

This overview makes obvious the overlapping features of anger, hostility, and aggression. Given that personality traits are generally seen as having emotional, cognitive, and behavioral correlates and features, this overlap is not surprising. However, it is also true that individual elements within broadly defined traits might be differentially related to health or related through distinct mechanisms (Briggs, 1989; Carver, 1989). As a result, clear, conceptual distinctions among closely related processes are essential prerequisites for building models and testing their predictions.

ASSESSMENT OF ANGER AND HOSTILITY

As noted previously, conceptual models linking anger, hostility, and health cannot be tested without valid measures of the psychosocial variables. In the absence of established construct validity, neither positive nor negative results can be interpreted with confidence as relevant to the potential health consequences of anger and hostility. Positive results might reflect the adverse effects of anger and hostility or some other characteristic(s) tapped by the purported measures of these traits. Null results might reflect the absence of adverse effects or the fact that anger and hostility were not adequately assessed. Thus, clear evidence of construct validity is essential for definitive conclusions. Further, validity requires reliability. Given that studies in this area are concerned with chronic anger and hostility, reliability or stability of the assessment devices over time is relevant. Internal consistency of questionnaires and interrater agreement for interview-based methods are important psychometric considerations, as well.

Many of the assessment devices used in this area are lacking in some of these respects (see Barefoot & Lipkus, this volume; Smith, 1992). For example, the Cook and Medley (1954) Ho scale has an ill-defined internal structure (Contrada & Jussim, in press) with a heterogeneous pool of items. Further, although fairly stable during adulthood (Shekelle, Gale, Ostfeld, & Paul, 1983), scores initially assessed during late adolescence and early adulthood are much less stable over the course of subsequent decades (Siegler et al., 1990). Thus, the predictive utility of the scale may be reduced by its poor internal consistency and its temporal instability when younger subjects are followed over long periods of time, as is the case in many prospective studies.

The Uses of Construct Validation

The process of construct validation entails placing constructs and related measures in a theoretically derived framework. This framework or nomological net consists of hypothesized relationships among multiple constructs and multiple measures (Cronbach & Meehl, 1955). From the previous conceptual definitions, it is clear that a variety of emotional, cognitive, physiological, and behavioral processes would be part of the nomological net surrounding anger, hostility, and aggression. To be complete, however, tests of the construct validity of measures must include evidence that scales not only are closely related to other indices of the same construct (i.e., convergent validity) but also are clearly less closely related to other constructs (i.e., divergent or discriminant validity).

In addition to providing much needed information to be used in interpreting findings involving these assessment devices, studies of construct validity can extend knowledge of the nature and correlates of chronic anger and hostility. This information, in turn, can be quite useful in elaboration of the psychological underpinnings of these traits and in analyses of the mechanisms linking personality and disease. For example, studies of the behavioral and cardiovascular responses of hostile and nonhostile persons to various social situations (for reviews, see Houston, this volume; Smith & Christensen, 1992a) can suggest specific social motives or concerns underlying hostility (e.g., mistrust, dominance, etc.), as well as interpersonal and psychophysiological processes that might increase hostile persons' vulnerability to disease. Until recently, evidence of the construct validity of the Ho scale was sparse at best (Megargee, 1985). Although studies of the cognitive, affective, behavioral,

interpersonal, and psychophysiological correlates of this scale have done much
to clarify the nature of the construct it taps (see Smith, 1992; Smith & Christensen, 1992a, for reviews), other assessment devices are in need of further
evaluation.

Advantages and Disadvantages of Measures in Current Use

The selection of assessment devices for research in this area presents something of a dilemma. Some of the scales used in prospective studies have clear
psychometric limitations. These scales were often pressed into service because of their presence in databases collected years ago for other purposes.
Such samples provide opportunities for follow-up periods sufficiently long as
to permit sensitive tests of association with morbidity and mortality, without
the otherwise necessary wait of many years. Despite the limitations of these
measures, important evidence of their relevance to subsequent health is available as a result. More psychometrically sound measures of anger and hostility are available, but few of them have been included in large-scale prospective
studies. Thus, their relevance to health is unknown. The psychological
research on the Type A pattern accumulated a large body of findings with
the Jenkins Activity Survey (Jenkins, Zyzanski, & Rosenman, 1971), an assessment device that later proved to be unrelated to cardiovascular disease
in prospective studies (Matthews, 1988). As a result, much is known about
an individual difference variable that is apparently not useful in understanding the development of CVD. To avoid a repetition of this history, studies
of anger and hostility must proceed along two lines—continued psychometric evaluations of measures currently in use in epidemiological research, and
use of more sound scales and ratings in cross-sectional and prospective studies
of documented morbidity and mortality.

ROBUSTNESS OF THE ASSOCIATION

The inconsistent association between hostility and subsequent health is a trou-
bling feature of this literature. Although positive results predominate, additional studies are clearly needed to evaluate the robustness of this effect. Refinement of conceptual and operational definitions of the predictor variables as
discussed previously is likely to improve the yield of such efforts. However,
other considerations are important to maximize the resulting information.

Cautions in Cross-Sectional Research

Cross-sectional studies, despite the obvious difficulty of distinguishing psychosocial antecedents and consequences of disease, are still potentially useful in this area. However, likely selection confounds require special caution

in their design and interpretation (Matthews, 1988). For example, cases of sudden coronary death are obviously excluded in these analyses, limiting the generalizability of the findings and possibly weakening the results through the early death of some angry and hostile persons.

For some types of studies, such as those relying on the results of clinical diagnostic procedures (e.g., coronary angiograms, thallium stress testing), severely ill subjects will be overrepresented in the sample, given the fact that such diagnostic tests are reserved for probable CHD cases. The resulting restriction in range of disease severity is likely to weaken statistical tests of association. Finally, disease-free persons in these samples are not likely to be representative of the larger healthy population, as they have somehow been referred for costly and invasive tests despite their freedom from CVD. In samples of patients undergoing coronary angiography, individuals found to have little or no CAD are often characterized by high scores on measures of anxiety and other chronic dysphoric emotions. Presumably, symptoms of acute emotional distress were somehow interpreted as possible symptoms of CVD, resulting in the diagnostic evaluation (for a review, see Smith & Williams, 1992; Stone & Costa, 1990). To the extent that such individuals also experience anger and related emotions, this selection process could create an artifactual inverse association between the experience of anger and disease (Siegman, Dembroski, & Ringel, 1987).

Moderating Variables and Confounding Factors

In both cross-sectional and prospective studies, the inconsistent results might reflect the existence of one or more moderating variables. For example, the strength of the association between anger or hostility and health might vary as a function of the age of the study sample. Some evidence exists to support this assertion (Dembroski et al., 1989; Siegman, Dembroski, & Ringel, 1987). Chronic anger and hostility might be more or less unhealthy depending on characteristics of the individual's work environment. Jobs presenting repeated opportunities for interpersonal conflict, as compared to those involving more solitary working conditions, could potentiate the adverse effects of anger and hostility. Given strong influences of sociodemographic factors such as sex, race, and economic status on the experience and expression of anger and hostility, these variables might also influence the magnitude of association between personality factors and disease. Thus, some of the inconsistencies in the epidemiological literature might be explained through the systematic evaluation of moderating effects in future work.

Future tests of the association between anger or hostility and health must also consider the appropriate treatment of correlated risk factors. For example, as discussed later and elsewhere by Siegler (this volume), hostility is significantly associated with age, male sex, nonwhite race, lower socioeconomic status and education levels, smoking, less exercise, and elevated cholesterol (for reviews, see Siegler, this volume; Smith, 1992), all of which are established CHD risk factors. The common practice in studies of the association between hostility and health is to control these risk factors statistically in multivariate analyses so as to test the independent effects of hostility. This is a generally accepted approach to potential confounding factors or nuisance variables in correlational studies. However, this approach also might underestimate the effects of anger and hostility on health. For example, as discussed later, unhealthy behaviors might explain or mediate the association between hostility and health. In that light, simple statistical control of confounding factors such as smoking and inactivity eliminates a substantive effect of hostility on health. This approach also fails to take advantage of the opportunity to test a mediational conceptual model. Matthews (1989) suggested that psychosocial factors, such as anger and hostility, might mediate the association between demographic factors and health status. Here again, simple statistical control of correlated risk factors does not permit complete exploration of the possible causal pathways. This is not to suggest that the typical statistical procedures are inappropriate. Rather, it suggests that analyses in cross-sectional and prospective studies should be guided by conceptual models of the association between hostility and health, instead of focusing solely on the issue of simple increments in predictive utility beyond the effects of traditional risk factors (Smith, 1992).

MODELS OF MECHANISM

Evidence of a statistical association between the constructs of anger and hostility and subsequent health raises the question of mechanism. What is the link between these psychological characteristics and CVD? Several models have been proposed (for reviews, see Smith, 1992; Suls & Rittenhouse, 1990), and all deserve additional attention in future research. Several examples of these models are detailed in subsequent chapters, so the present review is brief. The models are not mutually exclusive, and some are explicitly integrative.

Reactivity, Social Relations, and Transactions

The *psychophysiological reactivity model* is perhaps the predominant view of the mechanism linking anger or hostility and CVD. As described by Williams and his colleagues (1985), hostile persons are likely to display two psychological responses that are accompanied by increased physiological arousal. These individuals are prone to experience anger and to engage in vigilant observation of their social environments as they scan for signs of impending mistreatment. Anger and vigilance are accompanied by sympathetically mediated increases in a variety of physiological parameters (e.g., blood pressure, circulating catecholamines). Heightened psychophysiological reactivity to social stressors is hypothesized to initiate and hasten the development of CAD and precipitate the appearance of symptoms of CHD (e.g., myocardial infarction, angina, etc.) among individuals with CAD. As reviewed by Houston (this volume) and elsewhere (Smith, 1992), the available evidence is relatively consistent with the basic hypothesis that hostile persons respond to potential stressors with larger increases in blood pressure and other indices of arousal, as compared to their more agreeable counterparts. However, there are inconsistencies in this portion of the literature as well, and the further link between reactivity and disease is not firmly established (for reviews, see Manuck, Kaplan, Muldoon, Adams, & Clarkson, 1991; Smith & Christensen, 1992b).

The *psychosocial vulnerability model* suggests that chronic anger and hostility are associated with a variety of unhealthy characteristics, such as low social support and high levels of interpersonal conflict at home and work (Smith & Frohm, 1985; Smith, Pope, Sanders, Allred, & O'Keeffe, 1988). This negative psychosocial profile, in turn, would confer an increased risk of disease (Krantz, Contrada, Hill, & Friedler, 1988; Syme, 1987). Of course, some psychophysiological process such as the sympathetically mediated responses described previously would still link this more stressful and less supportive environment and subsequent disease.

The *transactional model* (Smith & Pope, 1990) represents an integration and extension of the psychosocial and psychophysiological reactivity approaches. The reactivity model focuses on *responses* associated with anger and hostility, and the psychosocial vulnerability model focuses on the *correlates* of these traits. In addition to these features, the transactional model describes the social *consequences* or effects of anger and hostility. Briefly, this model views anger and hostility as stress-engendering processes. It is not coincidental that chronically angry and hostile persons experience more interpersonal conflict and less social support. Rather, the transactional model maintains that chronically angry and hostile persons create those features of their social environments, through their thoughts and actions. By mistrusting others, by expecting mistreatment, and by attributing hostile intent to others, hostile persons are prone to antagonistic and aggressive actions. Such behaviors are likely to increase interpersonal conflict and undermine social support. Once created, this divisive and unsupportive environment is likely to maintain anger, hostility, and aggression. Thus, the transactional model is founded on the notion that personal characteristics and the social environment are reciprocally determined (Bandura, 1977). Further, pathogenic physiological responses arise from two classes of situations. Hostile persons display heightened reactivity to the social stressors common to all persons, but also display these responses to the additional stressors they have created.

Biological Vulnerability

The somatopsychic or *constitutional vulnerability model* (Krantz & Durel, 1983) proposed a quite different mechanism linking personality traits and disease. Briefly, this perspective posits basic biological individual differences as causing the psychological and behavioral manifestations of anger, hostility, and aggression. This underlying biological factor, such as a hyperresponsive sympathetic nervous system, also confers vulnerability to CVD. Except for this underlying biological process, personality and disease are not seen as causally related. Rather, they are seen as coeffects of a single biologically based individual difference. In this volume, chapters by Williams and Kaplan, Botchin, and Manuck present detailed examples of this general perspective.

It is important to note that the constitutional vulnerability model and the preceding models are also not mutually exclusive. For example, even if they are biologically based, anger, hostility, and aggressive behavior are likely to have an adverse impact on the social environment. As a result, biologically vulnerable persons are likely to be exposed to what is especially for them an unhealthy environment. In contrast, biologically resilient persons would be at even less risk, because of the stress-reducing effect of their agreeable social style on the interpersonal climate. This type of integration is quite consistent with the general biopsychosocial perspective (Engel, 1977).

Health Behavior

A final model is based on the health behavior correlates of hostility. Leiker and Hailey (1988) proposed that hostile persons may be vulnerable to CVD by virtue of their poor health habits. As reviewed by Siegler (this volume) and elsewhere (Smith, 1992), there is some evidence that hostility is associated with smoking, inactivity, alcohol consumption, and other unhealthy behaviors. Hostile persons might also be less adherent to prescribed medical regimens, thereby increasing their medical risk (Lee et al., 1992). As noted previously, this mechanism is not necessarily inconsistent with other models.

In each case, preliminary evidence suggests that these models are plausible. All require additional research, however. Ultimately, complete path-analytic tests of personality, mediating mechanism, and health outcome associations are possible (Krantz & Hedges, 1987). However, such comprehensive research presents enormous challenges, and partial tests of components of the models are likely to be useful, given their preliminary status.

CONCEPTS AND METHODS
FROM PERSONALITY PSYCHOLOGY

From the preceding discussion, several challenges emerge as central in the future of research in this area. Conceptual definitions of the central constructs must be clarified and in some cases extended. Current assessment methods must be evaluated and new ones tested. The basic association between chronic anger and hostility must be examined in additional large prospective and cross-sectional studies. Finally, models of the mechanism(s) linking these personality characteristics and health must be refined and tested.

In each of these endeavors, concepts and methods from current personality research are likely to be useful. Three current areas within personality psychology seem particularly relevant: trait taxonomies, cognitive–social models of personality process, and biological approaches to personality.

Trait Taxonomies

In recent years, a consensus has emerged among personality researchers as to an adequate taxonomy of personality traits (Digman, 1990; John, 1990). The so-called "big five" approach includes extraversion, agreeableness, conscientiousness, neuroticism, and openness to experience. As several authors have argued (Costa & McCrae, 1987; Smith & Williams, 1992), this taxonomy is likely to make a significant contribution to personality and health research. For example, the trait of agreeableness versus antagonism corresponds closely to the conceptual description of hostility and its affective and behavioral correlates. Agreeable persons are seen as good-natured, soft-hearted, courteous, sympathetic, trusting, forgiving, warm, and compassionate. In contrast, antagonistic persons are described as irritable, distrustful, rude, selfish, uncooperative, suspicious, vengeful, cynical and stubborn (Costa, McCrae, & Dembroski, 1989).

Neuroticism is also a relevant trait, because the tendency to experience anger (i.e., trait anger) is one facet of this broader disposition to experience a variety of negative affects and thoughts, such as anxiety, sadness, insecurity, and self-doubt. However, many of the facets or components of neuroticism are conceptually distinct from anger, hostility, and aggression as they are typically defined. Further, the available research suggests that neuroticism is associated with somatic complaints, but not actual physical illness (Stone & Costa, 1990). This underscores the necessity to evaluate the individual components of broad, multifaceted personality traits (Briggs, 1989; Carver, 1989).

The traits within five-factor taxonomy can also be fruitfully employed in pairs as well as single dimensions. For example, traditional views of hostility as coronary-prone behavior might be more accurately described as consisting of high levels of antagonism and neuroticism, rather than antagonism alone. The combination of these characteristics includes people described as harsh, ill-tempered, demanding, angry, quarrelsome, intolerant, and irritable (Hofstee, de Raad, & Goldberg, 1992). Similarly, high levels of antagonism and extraversion characterize people described as domineering, combative, abrupt, and controlling. In contrast, people with high levels of antagonism combined with introversion (i.e., low levels of extraversion) are described as skeptical, aloof, unfriendly, and cynical. Thus, the use of multiple traits within the five-factor model can provide more precise conceptual and empirical descriptions.

This use of the five-factor model also evokes older approaches to the subclassification of hostility. Interpersonal approaches to personality have been based on a circumplex model consisting of two dimensions—hostility versus friendliness and dominance versus submission (Leary, 1957; Wiggins & Broughton, 1985). Hostility can be accompanied by dominant or submissive behavior, with a distinct pattern of correlates, antecedents, and consequences. The poles of the five-factor model trait of agreeableness versus antagonism corresponds roughly to friendly submissiveness and hostile dominance, respectively (McCrae & Costa, 1989). This interpersonal distinction augments the five-factor approach by suggesting likely patterns of interpersonal interactions, with possible psychosomatic consequences. For example, recurring attempts to exert social dominance and control are likely to elicit heightened cardiovascular reactivity (Smith, Allred, Morrison, & Carlson, 1989; Smith, Baldwin, & Christensen, 1990), especially among hostile persons (Smith & Brown, 1991). Angry, effortful attempts to influence and control others, rather than angry reactions alone might be a central social psychophysiological process linking hostility and health. This hypothesis has an obvious parallel in the Boman–Gray model of interactive effects of social dominance and social stress on atherogenesis in monkeys (Kaplan, Botchin, & Manuck, this volume; Manuck, Kaplan, Muldoon, Adams, & Clarkson, 1991).

In addition to providing conceptual refinements in describing and understanding anger, hostility, and health, the five-factor taxonomy and interpersonal approaches provide important assessment technologies. Developed and refined over many years, these instruments include several reliable and valid self-report and rating scales (for a review, see Digman, 1990; John, 1990). These scales would be useful in clarifying the constructs assessed by currently used measures of chronic anger and hostility (cf. Costa, McCrae, & Dembroski, 1989), as well as in future cross-sectional and prospective studies of health outcomes.

Cognitive–Social Models of Personality Process

The taxonometric approaches described previously are most useful in the assessment and description of traits. They are less directly relevant for explicating the processes by which different types of individuals (e.g., hostile vs. friendly) select, perceive, interpret, and respond to their social environments. Cantor (1990) contrasted the "having" versus "doing" aspects of trait versus process approaches to personality. The taxonometric approaches provide important detail and organization in the description of individual differences, or characteristics, that people have. Other aspects of recent theory and research in personality psychology are available for use in attempts to understand the psychological mechanisms or processes involved in the expression of these individual differences as people select, interpret, and respond to social situations. These process-oriented approaches are useful in psychological models of the effects of anger and hostility on health. For example, Contrada (this volume) describes how recent theory and research on the cognitive–mediational approaches to stress and adjustment can be used as an integrative framework to describe the effects of personality and emotion on health.

An earlier example of this approach is the work of Dodge and his colleagues on aggressive behavior in children (e.g., Dodge & Coie, 1987). Aggressive children are more likely to attribute hostile intent to others' actions and select aggressive behaviors as responses to the perceived provocation. This analysis has clear relevance in attempts to understand differing physiological and behavioral responses of hostile and nonhostile persons to various social situations. Preliminary studies have supported the basic hypothesis that hostility is associated with a distinct style of processing social information and interpreting the actions of others (Allred & Smith, 1991; Pope, Smith, & Rhodewalt, 1990; Smith, Sanders, & Alexander, 1990).

The general cognitive–social perspective (Cantor, 1990; Cantor & Kihlstrom, 1987; Dweck & Leggett, 1988) describes personality traits as consisting of individual differences in social appraisal processes, internal representations (i.e., schemas) of the self and other people, representations of recurring types of relationships or interactions (i.e., scripts), personal goals or tasks, and self-evaluation processes. Cognitive descriptions of chronic anger and hostility, using these types of constructs, have been offered by theorists in several different contexts (Beck & Freeman, 1990; Lazarus, 1991).

The cognitive–social perspective explicitly recognizes the reciprocal association between personality and the social environment. Clearly, personality influences the subjective experience of the social environment through the cognitive processes described previously. However, personality characteristics are likely to shape objective aspects of the social environment through their impact on the selection of social situations, the unintentional evocation of social reactions to interpersonal behavior, and behavioral tactics employed in conscious attempts to influence or manipulate others (Buss, 1987). Thus, the cognitive–social perspective is likely to make a significant contribution to the extension and evaluation of the psychophysiological reactivity, psychosocial vulnerability, and transactional models described previously. The explication of these cognitive–social processes might also help to refine therapeutic intervention techniques, by providing a detailed description of maladaptive processes and likely points of change.

Biological Perspectives

In recent years, personality psychologists have renewed their attention to biological underpinnings of personality (Buss, 1990). Three general issues have been central in this work, all of which are potentially relevant to future research on anger, hostility, and health. First, psychophysiological analyses of basic mechanisms presumed to underlie personality traits have become increasingly refined and sophisticated. As such, the literature on the psychophysiological tests of models originally proposed by Eysenck (1967), Gray (1973), and others provides several guides to efforts to test the recently proposed psychobiological models of hostility (Kaplan, Botchin, & Manuck, this volume; Williams, this volume). This body of theory and research might also suggest additional psychobiological traits as possible diatheses.

Second, recent advances in behavioral genetics research can provide increasingly sophisticated tests of the basic hypothesis that the angry, hostile, and aggressive traits are, in part, genetically transmitted. Recent modeling methods in behavioral genetics research can also evaluate the assumption that these psychological traits covary with genetically influenced biological processes, such as hypothesized brain mechanisms involving serotonin (Plomin, Chipuer, & Loehlin, 1990). In addition, these modeling procedures provide a unique opportunity to disentangle genetic and environmental bases of anger and hostility (Reiss, Plomin, & Hetherington, 1991).

Finally, evolutionary perspectives on personality offer a unique context for understanding the possible origins and nature of anger and hostility (Buss, 1984). This school of thought also offers another point of integration for the human and animal research reviewed in this volume. As with the tools of the taxonometric/descriptive and cognitive–social process perspectives in current personality psychology, biological approaches can inform our efforts to understand the psychosomatic process.

CLOSING COMMENT:
A VIEW FROM THE CROSSROADS

The central issues emerging from this overview define needed areas of conceptual refinement and redoubled research efforts. Clarification of key constructs and models, evaluation and enhancement of assessment procedures, additional tests of the basic association with CVD, and further exploration of underlying mechanisms represent the major foci of needed progress. Should the results of such work support the basic psychosomatic hypothesis, ongoing research on development, prevention, and therapeutic modification of anger and hostility would become even more important topics than they already are. Although the agenda is clear, the skepticism fueled by inconsistencies in this literature could contribute to a decline in interest and activity.

As noted previously, 40 years ago the psychoanalytic model of the influence of anger and hostility on health faced a similar crossroads. At that time, interest in those models waned, as the medical research on CVD made rapid advances in other directions and psychological science pursued other topics.

There is reason to predict that this history will not be repeated. Current personality theory and research methods provide a much more scientifically sound foundation than was available previously. Developments in basic biological research on CVD and stress physiology have helped to articulate plausible connections between psychological factors and illness, and have supplied invaluable methodological tools. Advances in the design and analysis of cross-sectional, clinical, and prospective epidemiological studies now permit much more definitive tests of the basic association. Compelling animal models permit experimental manipulation of central variables in these models, as a complement to human observational studies. Finally, sophisticated procedures have been developed to evaluate the clinical efficacy of related interventions. Thus, the 1990s presents the opportunity to generate conclusive tests of one of the oldest hypotheses linking psychological processes and physical health.

REFERENCES

Allred, K. D., & Smith, T. W. (1991). Social cognition in cynical hostility. *Cognitive Therapy and Research, 15*, 399–412.

Angell, M. (1985). Disease as a reflection of the psyche. *New England Journal of Medicine, 312*, 1570–1572.

Averill, J. R. (1982). *Anger and aggression: An essay on emotion.* New York: Springer-Verlag.

Bandura, A. (1973). *Aggression: A social learning analysis.* Englewood Cliffs, NJ: Prentice-Hall.

Bandura, A. (1977). *Social learning theory.* Englewood Cliffs, NJ: Prentice-Hall.

Barefoot, J. C., Dahlstrom, W. G., & Williams, R. B., Jr. (1983). Hostility, CHD incidence, and total mortality: A 25-year follow-up study of 255 physicians. *Psychosomatic Medicine, 45*, 59–63.

Beck, A. T., & Freeman, A. (1990). *Cognitive therapy of personality disorders.* New York: Guilford Press.

Briggs, S. R. (1989). The optimal level of measurement for personality constructs. In D. M. Buss & N. Cantor (Eds.), *Personality research for the 1990s* (pp. 246–260). New York: Springer-Verlag.

Buss, A. H. (1961). *The psychology of aggression.* New York: Wiley.

Buss, D. M. (1984). Evolutionary biology and personality psychology: Toward a conception of human nature and individual differences. *American Psychologist, 39,* 1135–1147.

Buss, D. M. (1987). Selection, evocation, and manipulation. *Journal of Personality and Social Psychology, 53,* 1214–1221.

Buss, D. M. (1990). Toward a biologically informed psychology of personality. *Journal of Personality, 58,* 1–16.

Cantor, N. (1990). From thought to behavior: "Having" and "doing" in the study of personality and cognition. *American Psychologist, 45,* 735–750.

Cantor, N., & Kihlstrom, J. F. (1987). *Personality and social intelligence.* Englewood Cliffs, NJ: Prentice-Hall.

Carver, C. S. (1989). How should multifaceted personality constructs be tested? Issues illustrated by self-monitoring, attributional style, and hardiness. *Journal of Personality and Social Psychology, 56,* 577–585.

Chaplin, J. P. (1982). *Dictionary of psychology* (rev. ed.). New York: Dell.

Contrada, R., & Jussim, L. (1992). What does the Cook-Medley hostility scale measure? *Journal of Applied Social Psychology, 22,* 615–627.

Cook, T. D., & Campbell, D. T. (1979). *Quasi-experimentation: Design and analysis issues for field studies.* Chicago: Rand McNally.

Cook, W. W., & Medley, D. M. (1954). Proposed Hostility and Pharisaic-Virtue scales for the MMPI. *Journal of Applied Psychology. 38,* 414–418.

Costa, P. T., Jr., McCrae, R. R., & Dembroski, T. M. (1989). Agreeableness versus antagonism: Explication of a potential risk factor for CHD. In A. W. Siegman & T. M. Dembroski (Eds.), *In search of coronary-prone behavior* (pp. 41–64). Hillsdale, NJ: Lawrence Erlbaum Associates.

Costa, P. T., Jr., & McCrae, R. R. (1987). Personality assessment in psychosomatic medicine. In T. M. Wise (Ed.), *Advances in psychosomatic medicine* (pp. 71–82). Basel, Switzerland: Karger.

Cronbach, L. J., & Meehl, P. E. (1955). Construct validity in psychological tests. *Psychological Bulletin, 52,* 281–302.

Dembroski, T. M., MacDougall, J. M., Costa, P. T., Jr., & Grandits, G. A. (1989). Components of hostility as predictors of sudden death and myocardial infarction in the Multiple Risk Factor Intervention Trial. *Psychosomatic Medicine, 51,* 514–522.

Dembroski, T. M., MacDougall, J. M., Williams, R. B., Jr., Haney, T. L., & Blumenthal, J. A. (1985). Components of Type A, hostility, and anger-in: Relationship to angiographic findings. *Psychosomatic Medicine, 47,* 219–233.

Digman, J. M. (1990). Personality structure: Emergence of the five-factor model. *Annual Review of Psychology, 41,* 417–440.

Dodge, K. A., & Coie, J. D. (1987). Social information processing factors in reactive and proactive aggression in children's peer groups. *Journal of Personality and Social Psychology, 53,* 1146–1158.

Dunbar, H. F. (1943). *Psychosomatic diagnosis.* New York: Hoeber.

Dweck, C. S., & Leggett, E. L. (1988). A social–cognitive approach to motivation and personality. *Psychological Review, 95,* 256–273.

Engel, G. L. (1977). The need for a new medical model: A challenge for biomedicine. *Science, 196,* 129–136.

Eysenck, H. J. (1967). *The biological basis of personality.* Springfield, IL: Charles C. Thomas.

Friedman, M., Thoresen, C. E., Gill, J. J., Ulmer, D., Powell, L. H., Price, V. A., Brown, B., Thompson, L., Rabin, D. D., Breall, W. S., Bourg, E., Levy, R., & Dixon, T. (1986). Alteration of Type A behavior and its effects on cardiac recurrences in post myocardial infarction patients: Summary results of the Recurrent Coronary Prevention Project. *American Heart Journal, 112,* 653–665.

Gray, J. A. (1973). Causal theories of personality and how to test them. In J. R. Royce (Ed.), *Multivariate analysis and psychological theory* (pp. 409–463). New York: The Academic Press.

Hearn, M. D., Murray, D. M., & Luepker, R. V. (1989). Hostility, coronary heart disease, and total mortality: A 33-year follow-up study of university students. *Journal of Behavioral Medicine, 12,* 105–121.

Hecker, M. H. L., Chesney, M. A., Black, G. W., & Frautschi, N. (1988). Coronary-prone behaviors in the Western Collaborative Group Study. *Psychosomatic Medicine, 50,* 153–164.

Helmer, D. C., Ragland, D. R., & Syme, S. L. (1991). Hostility and coronary artery disease. *American Journal of Epidemiology, 133,* 112–122.

Hofstee, W. K. B., de Raad, B., & Goldberg, L. R. (1992). Integration of the big five and circumplex approaches to trait structure. *Journal of Personality and Social Psychology, 63,* 146–163.

Hokanson, J. E. (1970). Psychophysiological evaluation of the catharsis hypothesis. In E. L. Megargee & J. E. Hokanson (Eds.), *The dynamics of aggression* (pp. 74–86). New York: Harper & Row.

Holroyd, K. A., & Coyne, J. (1987). Personality and health in the 1980s: Psychosomatic medicine revisited? *Journal of Personality, 55,* 359–375.

Jenkins, C. D., Zyzanski, S. J., & Rosenman, R. H. (1971). Progress toward validation of a computer-scored test for the Type A coronary-prone behavior pattern. *New England Journal of Medicine, 284,* 244–255.

John, O. P. (1990). The "big five" factor taxonomy: Dimensions of personality in the natural language and in questionnaires. In L. A. Pervin (Ed.), *Handbook of personality: Theory and research* (pp. 66–100). New York: Guilford.

Krantz, D. S., Contrada, R. J., Hill, R. O., & Friedler, E. (1988). Environmental stress and biobehavioral antecedents of coronary heart disease. *Journal of Consulting and Clinical Psychology, 56,* 333–341.

Krantz, D. S., & Durel, L. A. (1983). Psychobiological substrates of the Type A behavior pattern. *Health Psychology, 2,* 393–411.

Krantz, D. S., & Hedges, S. M. (1987). Some cautions for research on personality and health. *Journal of Personality, 55,* 351–357.

Lazarus, R. S. (1991). *Emotion and adaptation.* New York: Oxford University Press.

Leary, T. (1957). *Interpersonal diagnosis of personality.* New York: Ronald Press.

Lee, D., Mendes de Leon, C. F., Jenkins, C. D., Croog, S. H., Levine, S., & Sudilovsky, A. (1992). Relation of hostility to medication adherence, symptom complaints, and blood pressure reduction in a clinical field trial of antihypertensive medication. *Journal of Psychosomatic Research, 36,* 181–190.

Leiker, M., & Hailey, B. J. (1988). A link between hostility and disease: Poor health habits? *Behavioral Medicine, 3,* 129–133.

Manuck, S. B., Kaplan, J. R., Muldoon, M. F., Adams, M. R., & Clarkson, T. B. (1991). The behavioral exacerbation of atherosclerosis and its inhibition by propranolol. In P. M. McCabe, N. Schneiderman, T. M. Field, & J. S. Skyler (Eds.), *Stress, coping, and disease* (pp. 51–72). Hillsdale, NJ: Lawrence Erlbaum Associates.

Matthews, K. A. (1988). CHD and Type A behaviors: Update on and alternative to the Booth–Kewley and Friedmann quantitative review. *Psychological Bulletin, 104,* 373–380.

Matthews, K. A. (1989). Are sociodemographic variables markers for psychological determinants of health? *Health Psychology, 8,* 641–648.

McCrae, R. R., & Costa, P. T., Jr. (1989). The structure of interpersonal traits: Wiggins' circumplex and the five-factor model. *Journal of Personality and Social Psychology, 56,* 586–595.

McCranie, E. W., Watkins, L. O., Brandsma, J. M., & Sisson, B. D. (1986). Hostility, coronary heart disease (CHD), incidence, and total mortality: Lack of association in a 25-year follow-up study of 478 physicians. *Journal of Behavioral Medicine, 9,* 119–125.

Meehl, P. E. (1978). Theoretical risks and tabular asterisks: Sir Karl, Sir Ronald, and the slow progress of soft psychology. *Journal of Consulting and Clinical Psychology, 46,* 806–834.

Megargee, E. I. (1985). The dynamics of aggression and their application to cardiovascular disorders. In M. A. Chesney & R. H. Rosenman (Eds.), *Anger and hostility in cardiovascular and behavioral disorders* (pp. 31–57). Washington, DC: Hemisphere.

Menninger, K. A., & Menninger, W. C. (1936). Psychoanalytic observations in cardiac disorders. *American Heart Journal, 11*, 10.

Plomin, R., Chipuer, H. M., & Loehlin, J. C. (1990). Behavioral genetics and personality. In L. A. Pervin (Ed.), *Handbook of personality: Theory and research* (pp 225–243). New York: Guilford.

Plutchik, R. (1980). *Emotion: A psychoevolutionary synthesis.* New York: Harper & Row.

Pope, M. K., Smith, T. W., & Rhodewalt, F. (1990). Cognitive, behavioral, and affective correlates of the Cook and Medley Hostility scale. *Journal of Personality Assessment, 54*, 501–514.

Reiss, D., Plomin, R., & Hetherington, E. M. (1991). Genetics and psychiatry: An unheralded window on the environment. *American Journal of Psychiatry, 148*, 283–291.

Shaver, P., Schwartz, J., Kirson, D., & O'Connor, C. (1987). Emotion knowledge: Further exploration of a prototype approach. *Journal of Personality and Social Psychology, 52*, 1061–1086.

Shekelle, R. B., Gale, M., Ostfeld, A. M., & Paul, O. (1983). Hostility, risk of coronary heart disease, and mortality. *Psychosomatic Medicine, 45*, 109–114.

Siegler, I. C., Zonderman, A. B., Barefoot, J. C., Williams, R. B., Jr., Costa, P. T., Jr., & McCrae, R. R. (1990). Predicting personality in adulthood from college MMPI scores: Implications for follow-up studies in psychosomatic medicine. *Psychosomatic Medicine, 52*, 644–652.

Siegman, A. W., Dembroski, T. M., & Ringel, N. (1987). Components of hostility and the severity of coronary artery disease. *Psychosomatic Medicine, 48*, 127–135.

Smith, T. W. (1992). Hostility and health: Current status of a psychosomatic hypothesis. *Health Psychology, 11*, 139–150.

Smith, T. W., Allred, K. D., Morrison, C., & Carlson, S. (1989). Cardiovascular reactivity and interpersonal influence: Active coping in a social context. *Journal of Personality and Social Psychology, 56*, 209–218.

Smith, T. W., Baldwin, M., & Christensen, A. J. (1990). Interpersonal influence as active coping: Effects of task difficulty on cardiovascular reactivity. *Psychophysiology, 27*, 429–437.

Smith, T. W., & Brown, P. C. (1991). Cynical hostility, attempts to exert social control, and cardiovascular reactivity in married couples. *Journal of Behavioral Medicine, 14*, 579–590.

Smith, T. W., & Christensen, A. J. (1992a). Hostility, health, and social contexts. In H. S. Friedman (Ed.), *Hostility, coping, and health* (pp. 33–48). Washington, DC: American Psychological Association.

Smith, T. W., & Christensen, A. J. (1992b). Cardiovascular reactivity and interpersonal relations: Psychosomatic processes in social context. *Journal of Social and Clinical Psychology, 11*, 279–301.

Smith, T. W., & Frohm, K. D. (1985). What's so unhealthy about hostility? Construct validity and psychosocial correlates of the Cook and Medley Ho scale. *Health Psychology, 4*, 503–520.

Smith, T. W., & Pope, M. K. (1990). Cynical hostility as a health risk: Current status and future directions. *Journal of Social Behavior and Personality, 5*, 77–88.

Smith, T. W., Pope, M. K., Sanders, J. D., Allred, K. D., & O'Keeffe, J. L. (1988). Cynical hostility at home and work: Psychosocial vulnerability across domains. *Journal of Research in Personality, 22*, 525–548.

Smith, T. W., Sanders, J. D., & Alexander, J. F. (1990). What does the Cook and Medley Hostility Scale measure? Affect, behavior, and attributions in the marital context. *Journal of Personality and Social Psychology, 58*, 699–708.

Smith, T. W., & Williams, P. G. (1992). Personality and health: Advantages and limitations of the five-factor model. *Journal of Personality, 60*, 395–423.

Spielberger, C. D., Johnson, E. H., Russell, S. F., Crane, R. J., Jacobs, G. A., & Worden, T. J. (1985). The experience and expression of anger. Construction and validation of an anger expression scale. In M. A. Chesney & R. H. Rosenman (Eds.), *Anger and hostility in cardiovascular and behavioral disorders* (pp. 5–30). Washington, DC: Hemisphere.

Stone, S. V., & Costa, P. T., Jr. (1990). Disease-prone personality or distress-prone personality? The role of neuroticism in coronary heart disease. In H. S. Friedman (Ed.), *Personality and disease* (pp. 178–200). New York: Wiley.

Suls, J., & Rittenhouse, J. D. (1990). Models of linkages between personality and disease. In H. S. Friedman (Ed.), *Personality and disease* (pp. 38–64). New York: Wiley.

Syme, S. L. (1987). Coronary artery disease: A sociocultural perspective. *Circulation, 76,* 1112–1116.

Thoresen, C. E., & Powell, L. H. (1992). Type A behavior pattern: New perspectives on theory, assessment and intervention. *Journal of Consulting and Clinical Psychology, 60,* 595–604.

Verrier, R. L., Hagestad, E. L., & Lown, B. (1987). Delayed myocardial ischemia induced by anger. *Circulation, 75,* 249–254.

Wiggins, J. S., & Broughton, R. (1985). The interpersonal circle: A structural model for the integration of personality research. In R. Hogan & W. H. Jones (Eds.), *Perspective in personality* (Vol. 1, pp. 1–47). Greenwich, CT: JAI.

Williams, R. B., Jr. (1987). Psychological factors in coronary artery disease: Epidemiological evidence. *Circulation, 76*(Suppl. 1), 1177–1123.

Williams, R. B., Jr., Barefoot, J. C., & Shekelle, R. B. (1985). The health consequences of hostility. In M. A. Chesney & R. H. Rosenman (Eds.), *Anger and hostility in cardiovascular and behavioral disorders* (pp. 173–185). Washington, DC: Hemisphere.

3

THE ASSESSMENT OF ANGER AND HOSTILITY

John C. Barefoot
Isaac M. Lipkus
Behavioral Medicine Research Center
Duke University Medical Center

Measurement issues are a critical part of the study of anger, hostility, and health. Poorly designed instruments may lead to studies that fail to find effects because of measurement error. Conversely, researchers may erroneously find and interpret associations if their measures are confounded with other psychological attributes. Most important, decisions about measurement are inextricably linked to theory, for the way that we conceptualize hostility has direct implications for the operationalization of the construct.

There are special problems in the measurement of anger and hostility, partially because there are numerous definitions of these constructs, and theorists disagree over terminology. However, it is apparent that we are dealing with a multifaceted phenomenon that includes cognitive, affective, and behavioral manifestations (Barefoot, 1992; Novaco, 1985; Spielberger, Johnson, Russell, Crane, Jacobs, & Worden, 1985). Cognitive aspects of hostility include negative beliefs about others, such as cynical attitudes and suspiciousness. Affective components not only include anger, but also related negative feelings, such as disgust and contempt. Behaviorally, the expression of anger and hostility can take many forms. Overt aggression is the clearest behavioral expression, but it occurs only rarely in normal daily living (Averill, 1982). More subtle and socially acceptable ways of expressing anger and hostility are available and can be more frequently observed in the course of normal interaction. If measures target different aspects of anger and hostility (e.g., affects, cognitions, behaviors) they may be only moderately intercorrelated as a result. This can lead to confusion and miscommunication if researchers assume that all instruments are designed to assess the same monolithic construct (Barefoot, 1992).

Another source of disagreement between measures stems from the large amount of method variance associated with different measurement strategies. Popular techniques for the assessment of anger and hostility can be divided into two general types: self-report and interview-based. These two measurement strategies have very different premises and different sets of strengths and weaknesses. In this chapter we review the major issues involved with the use of these measurement strategies and provide examples of measures that have been prominent in past research on hostility and health. We also discuss peer reports, a measurement strategy that has not been frequently used, but deserves consideration for future research.

SELF-REPORT MEASURES

Measurement Issues

The most obvious, easiest, and, therefore, the most popular way to assess anger and hostility is through self-report. In Allport's (1942) words, "If we want to know how people feel, what they experience and what they remember, what their emotions and motives are like, and their reasons for acting as they do— why not ask them?" (p. 37). This straightforward approach has many advantages; however, it rests on three assumptions: (a) the respondent can accurately comprehend the researcher's questions; (b) the respondent knows the answers to those questions; and (c) the respondent will honestly answer the questions. The researcher must consider the validity of these assumptions in order to evaluate the adequacy of a particular self-report measure.

Does the Respondent Understand the Question? It may seem superfluous to raise the issue of the respondent's comprehension because almost all items used in standard scales have been tested to ensure that they are understandable. However, it must be remembered that psychologists often develop their instruments on samples of college students or other highly educated respondents. The resulting questions may be inappropriate for less well-educated groups. This practice is unfortunate in light of the need to understand the impact that anger and hostility have on health in all segments of society without assuming that the phenomena that are true for the upper middle class are also true for other groups (Barefoot et al., 1991).

We are a part of a research program that has been gathering data on hostility from coronary patients at Duke University Medical Center for the past 17 years. We have found that we can not administer many promising self-report scales because the patients have difficulty completing them. Questions that require more than a sixth-grade level of reading ability will cause problems for some patients. In addition, instruments often pose complex hypothetical questions or require responses in formats that are unfamiliar to many people (e.g., sophisticated comparisons, rankings, or rating procedures). It is our impression that these difficulties are not simply due to low intelligence or inadequate education. Many intelligent respondents have problems because they are not used to completing questionnaires that inquire about their opinions or responses to hypothetical situations. Despite instructions to the contrary, they often approach the task as if the questions had factual answers and the scale is a test of their ability. Needless to say, questions such as "Would most people lie to get ahead?" pose formidable problems under such a test-taking set.

The issue of comprehension is not confined to the patient setting. We observed a similar phenomenon in a recent study that used students, patients, and volunteers from community civic groups (Barefoot & Beckham, 1992). Students, whether from college or from an educational program for retired persons, had less difficulty with the questionnaires than either cardiac patients or civic group volunteers. In support of our impressions, the correlations between scores on self-report hostility scales and observations of actual hostile behavior during an interview also tended to be higher in the student groups. Clearly, researchers must carefully consider the appropriateness of their instruments for the respondents.

Does the Respondent Know the Answer?   Higher levels of self-awareness are thought to improve the accuracy of self-reports, as judged by the congruence between self-reports and overt behavior. Manipulations designed to enhance self-awareness were shown to lead to more congruence (Duval & Wicklund, 1972). Several researchers (e.g., Fenigstein, Scheier, & Buss, 1975; Snyder, 1979) proposed that there are sizable individual differences in the degree of self-awareness. In one study, Scheier, Buss, and Buss (1978) found that students who had higher levels of self-awareness, as indicated by their scores on a scale of "private self-consciousness," also gave self-reports of their aggressiveness that were more predictive of their actual level of aggression during a laboratory task.

Self-awareness may be another aspect of the differences between student and nonstudent samples. Although admittedly anecdotal, our experience suggests that students tend to be much more introspective and, therefore, more able to report their anger and hostility accurately. The higher correlations between self-reports and overt hostile behavior in students compared to nonstudents support this conjecture (Barefoot & Beckham, 1992).

To complicate this issue, it appears that differences in self-awareness are affected by psychological processes other than the tendency to be introspective. Because anger and hostility are negatively valued dispositions, individuals may be motivated to deny or fail to recognize their own antagonistic tendencies (Paulhus, 1984; Weinberger, 1990). This phenomenon is of interest aside from its implications for measurement, because it has been suggested that those who are defensive about their hostility are placed in psychological conflict that results in higher levels of cardiovascular reactivity (Jamner, Shapiro, Goldstein, & Hug, 1991).

Will the Respondent Answer with Complete Honesty?   There are a number of response sets that can affect the validity of psychological measures (Robinson, Shaver, & Wrightsman, 1991). The tendency for the respondents to present themselves in the most socially desirable light is especially important for the measurement of anger and hostility. Because anger and hostility are not positively valued characteristics, it is understandable that respondents might be reluctant to admit to them. One indication of the influence of socially desirable response sets is the finding that studies conducted in evaluative test-taking situations report much lower hostility scores than studies conducted in settings that minimize the pressures to present oneself positively (Barefoot, 1992).

The question of how to minimize the impact of social desirability biases has been widely debated (Paulhus, 1991). One proposed solution is to administer scales specifically designed to detect socially desirable responding and use scores on these scales to eliminate subjects or statistically adjust scores on the measure of hostility. However, this strategy has been challenged as too simplistic, because it fails to distinguish between responses that are distorted in a socially desirable direction and socially desirable responses that the respondent believes to be true. The respondent who answers in a socially desirable direction may actually have more positive qualities than most people, or they may be processing information in a self-deceptive fashion that leads them to believe that they have these positive qualities (Paulhus, 1986). In either case, indicators of socially desirable responding can be considered substantively meaningful rather than reflections of mere response bias. In support of this viewpoint, it has been shown that controlling for socially desirable responding actually *decreases* the criterion-related validity of personality measures (McCrae & Costa, 1983; McCrae et al., 1989).

Summary.   There are potential pitfalls in the measurement of anger and hostility with self-reports. The exposition of these problems is not meant to present a pessimistic picture of the utility of self-report measures. In most cases, the assumptions underlying Allport's dictum are probably valid. However, an awareness of the potential threats to valid measurement should allow the careful researcher to minimize or eliminate their impact.

Self-Report Measures and Health

There are numerous self-report measures of anger and hostility (see Matthews, Jamison, & Cottington, 1985, for a review). Rather than attempting a comprehensive treatment of the available measures, discussion here is limited to those instruments that have been shown to be associated with coronary heart disease (CHD) outcomes in empirical studies.

Cook–Medley Ho Scale.   The Ho scale, which is part of the MMPI, is the most widely used hostility questionnaire in health psychology research. It was empirically derived to differentiate between teachers with good versus bad rapport with their students (Cook & Medley, 1954). The popularity of the Ho scale stems from empirical demonstrations of its associations with a number of health outcomes, including coronary artery disease, CHD events, peripheral artery disease, cardiovascular reactivity, hypertension, risk factor status, and premature mortality from all causes. This research has been conducted with both cross-sectional and prospective data. Not all studies have been positive, but the preponderance of evidence suggests that the Ho scale is measuring something that is important for health (see Barefoot, 1992 and Smith, 1992, for reviews).

Although the Ho scale is used as an indicator of general hostility, the question of what it is actually measuring has been the subject of debate. For example, Megargee (1985) questioned the status of the Ho scale as a measure of hostility because it was not associated with suicidal behavior, ratings of hostility in psychiatric patients, or tendencies to commit criminally violent acts. Rosenman, Swan, and Carmelli (1988) suggested that the scale was a measure of psychopathology rather than hostility. On the other hand, Smith and his colleagues amassed evidence in several studies that supports the convergent and discriminant validity of the scale as a measure of hostility (Smith, 1992).

To complicate matters, the Ho scale does not appear to have an internal structure that is invariant across samples and analytic procedures. Using factor analysis, two studies (Greenglass & Julkunen, 1989; Smith & Frohm, 1985) found one stable factor called cynical mistrust, but Costa, Zonderman, McCrae, and Williams (1986) reported two factors labeled cynicism and paranoid alienation. In yet another approach, Lipkus, Barefoot, Beckham, and Haney (1993) used multidimensional scaling techniques to derive three dimensions: (a) social withdrawal/paranoia versus proactive aggression; (b) rigidity of moral standards; and (c) aggression versus cynicism.

The source of these ambiguities about the psychometric properties of the Ho scale lies in its origin as a scale that was empirically derived to correlate with teacher attitudes. It should not be surprising if such a scale construction technique resulted in the inclusion of items that measured psychological factors other than hostility, because there are behavioral characteristics other than hostility that are important for student/teacher rapport. The heterogeneity of item content in the scale was illustrated by Barefoot, Dodge, Peterson, Haney, and Williams (1989), who conducted a rational analysis of the content of the scale based on the face validity of the items. They identified three subsets of items (a total of 27 items) that appeared to reflect the cognitive, affective, and behavioral manifestations of hostility. Another subset of 12 items was judged to represent a tendency to attribute hostile intent to other people's behavior, including aspects of paranoia. The remaining 11 items were judged to measure psychological constructs other than hostility. Correlations of these item subsets with the NEO Personality Inventory (Costa & McCrae, 1985) in three samples tended to support their convergent and discriminant validity.

Despite its psychometric problems, there is general agreement that the core of the Ho scale is comprised of items reflecting cynical beliefs and mistrust of others. The ability of Ho scores to predict health outcomes despite its imperfections argues for the importance of these psychological dimensions.

Factor L. Like the Ho scale, Factor L is also a subscale of a more general personality inventory, in this case Cattell's 16 P.F. (Cattell, Eber, & Tatsuoka, 1970). It is described as a measure of suspiciousness versus trust, which is conceptually related to the psychological domain measured by the Ho scale. Correlations between Factor L scores and Ho scores have been found to range from .41 to .51 depending on the form of the 16 P.F. that was administered (Barefoot, 1992).

Three studies demonstrated relationships between Factor L scores and health outcomes. Highly suspicious participants in the Western Electric Study had a higher 10-year incidence of CHD events than did their more trusting counterparts (Ostfeld, Lebovitz, Shekelle, & Paul, 1964). Factor L scores were also shown to predict all-cause mortality among participants in the Boston Normative Aging Study (Aldwin, Workman-Daniels, Spiro, Levenson, & Bosse, 1989). In another study of older individuals, Factor L scores predicted total mortality among participants in the Second Duke Longitudinal Study, even after controlling for age, sex, smoking, cholesterol, reported alcohol use, and physician's ratings of functional health at the time of testing (Barefoot et al., 1987). In cross-sectional analyses, Factor L scores were also correlated with physician's ratings of health in the Duke study.

Buss–Durkee Hostility Inventory (BDHI). The BDHI (Buss & Durkee, 1957) is one of the most comprehensive instruments to measure hostility, with seven subscales: Assault, Indirect Hostility, Irritability, Negativity, Resentment, Suspicion, and Verbal Hostility. Factor analyses of these scales yield two factors, overt expression and a second dimension that represents experiential aspects of hostility. Most of the work on the relation of BDHI scores to health variables has been done by Siegman and his colleagues (see Siegman, this volume). That work found scores on the expression factor, but not the experience factor, to be positively related to CHD-related outcomes, including severity of coronary artery disease (Siegman, Dembroski, & Ringel, 1987).

Other Factors Affecting the Use of Self-Report Scales

The choice of hostility measures is determined as much by matters of convenience as by theoretical and psychometric considerations. Much of the popularity of the Ho scale stems from demonstrations of its ability to predict health outcomes in longitudinal data. These demonstrations were possible because the Ho scale is part of the MMPI, and there are large archives of MMPI data from the 1950s onward, making it relatively easy to conduct follow-up studies. The same is true for the Factor L measure, which is part of a larger personality inventory that was administered for other purposes in several longitudinal studies of health. Newer measures are more difficult to link to health outcomes in prospective studies, even though they may be more desirable on the basis of theoretical or psychometric considerations. However, the process of collecting the necessary data is now underway. For example, the NEO Personality Inventory (Costa & McCrae, 1985) is based on the five-factor theory of personality and contains scales to measure hostility and antagonism. It has been administered in two large ongoing studies, the Baltimore Longitudinal Study of Aging and the UNC Alumni Heart Study (Siegler et al., 1990). It is hoped that other instruments that have been shown to be promising in cross-sectional studies, such as the Multidimensional Anger Inventory (Siegel, 1986) and the Anger Expression scale (Spielberger et al., 1985) will be used more widely in follow-up studies of health.

Another matter of convenience that influences the choice of instruments for large-scale studies of health is simply the length of the scale. Typically, such projects have lengthy protocols, which preclude the administration of extensive questionnaires because of respondent burden. Thus, the researcher is caught between the opposing forces of the need for more comprehensive measurement and the necessity for brevity. Brief scales may have good predictive ability, however, even though their psychometric properties may be less than ideal. For example, a study of 3,750 twins in Finland (Koskenvuo et al., 1988) found an association between CHD and a scale of anger, irritability, and argumentativeness that contained only three items. Even though compromises in psychometric qualities may have to be made, it is important to have the questions included in large-scale epidemiologic studies, because the evidence emerging from those studies is often very convincing.

INTERVIEW-BASED ASSESSMENTS

Measurement Issues

The most prominent alternative to self-report measures is to have trained assessors make judgments of hostility based on the respondent's behavior during a standardized interview. This approach was popularized by the Western Collaborative Group Study (WCGS; Rosenman et al., 1975), where it was used to assess Type A behavior. Subsequent studies (e.g., Matthews, Glass, Rosenman, & Bortner, 1977) made separate ratings of each of the behavioral components that make up the Type A pattern, including hostility. Most interview assessment procedures have been devised to measure a number of Type A components, but newer techniques have evolved that place more emphasis on hostility.

A significant development in the evolution of interview-assessment techniques is the recognition of a distinction between hostility as judged from the content of the respondent's answers and hostility as judged on the basis of the respondent's manner of interacting with the interviewer. In early scoring systems, the assessor took both aspects of interview behavior into account, but the distinction was introduced in an attempt to make scoring criteria more explicit. Initial research comparing ratings based on speech content to those based on interactional style showed that ratings of hostile interaction style have better predictive validity (Dembroski, MacDougall, Costa, & Grandits, 1989).

One implication of these findings is the possibility that valid hostility assessments can be made from interview behavior regardless of the content of the questions. Traditionally, research on interview-assessed hostility uses the WCGS Structured Interview (SI), a set of questions concerning competitiveness, time urgency, and anger expression that lasts approximately 15 minutes. However, the finding that the most critical judgments are not based on answers to specific questions may mean that the nature of the interview questions is of secondary importance. In support of this position, an analysis of behavior during the SI on a question-by-question basis found that some questions elicited more anger and hostile behavior than others, but behavior during anger-eliciting questions did not have more validity (as judged by its relationship to CAD severity) than did behavior during noneliciting questions (Haney, Barefoot, Houseworth, Harlan, Williams, & Scherwitz, 1992). This finding suggests that it may be possible to extend work on interview-assessed hostility to other settings and to expand the content of the interview to other topics.

Judgments of the respondent's interaction style also have the advantage of minimizing the problems with self-report that we noted previously. Because the respondent's answers to the questions are of secondary interest, inability to understand the question and lack of self-awareness are not major threats to validity. Social desirability remains a factor, because social norms dictate that it is inappropriate to behave in an overtly hostile fashion in settings such as the SI. It is rare for respondents to openly confront the interviewer, and it is, therefore, necessary to train assessors to detect more subtle hostile acts that are less easily disguised (see following paragraphs).

The major drawbacks to interview assessments are the significant practical problems in administering and scoring interviews. The logistics of administering individual face-to-face interviews, the need to have skilled interviewers, and the need to train assessors pose formidable obstacles to the widespread adoption of the interview-based assessment strategy. These problems would be especially serious in the type of large-scale longitudinal studies that provide the most convincing evidence concerning the precursors of disease.

The task of training assessors is particularly important and difficult. Because of the variety and complexity of behaviors that occur during an interview, it is impossible to catalog all of the specific acts that are to be counted as hostility. It is also impossible to communicate the scoring rules comprehensively in written form, partially because so much relies on vocal stylistics and the context of a response. Interview-based assessments rely on the ability of the assessors to make attributions about the respondent's intent. It should not be surprising that these complex perceptual and logical processes cannot be easily codified. Nevertheless, it is critical that assessors use standard principles of scoring. Otherwise, the literature would quickly become filled with conflicting findings from researchers who were unwittingly using different scoring rules. Therefore, the best currently available solution is to describe the principles of scoring as best as possible in print, but rely on face-to-face training sessions to ensure that assessors are making their judgments in a reliable manner. Furthermore, the necessity of such training sessions should not cause us to question the scientific validity of interview-based measures because many accepted assessment procedures (e.g., reading an X-ray or an EKG) also require skills that can only be taught on a face-to-face basis.

One aspect of interview-based measures that has been relatively neglected is the construct validity of the assessments. Attempts to correlate interview-based assessments with established self-report measures of hostility have produced moderate associations (Barefoot & Beckham, 1992; Dembroski, MacDougall, Williams, Haney, & Blumenthal, 1985; Musante, MacDougall, Dembroski, & Costa, 1989). However, it is not clear that one should expect high correlations between measures obtained with the two strategies because they differ so dramatically in procedures and underlying assumptions. More attention is needed to the documentation of the convergent and discriminant validity of interview-based assessments using behavioral criteria.

Interview-Based Measures and Health

As with self-report measures, we will not attempt to be comprehensive in our description of interview-based assessment techniques, but we have limited our discussion to the most recent versions of those techniques that have been clearly related to CHD outcomes. In so doing, we have not been able to review some well-developed assessment systems (e.g., Friedman & Powell, 1984; Johnson, 1991) that can play important roles in research on anger, hostility, and health.

Hostility Facet Scoring System.   Dembroski et al. (1989) recently extended the system for rating components of Type A behavior that had been used successfully in previous research (Dembroski et al., 1985; MacDougall, Dembroski, Dimsdale, & Hackett, 1985; Matthews et al., 1977). In addition to a rating of Total Potential for Hostility, the new scoring system makes separate assessments of three facets of hostility: Content, Intensity, and Style. Although the system was not given a specific name by Dembroski et al., we named it the Hostility Facet Scoring System (HFSS) to facilitate our discussion.

Potential for Hostility is conceptualized as "a stable predisposition to respond to a relatively broad range of frustrating circumstances with varying degrees and combinations of anger, irritation, disgust, arrogance, contempt, resentment, and the like, which may or may not be associated with overt behavior directed against the source of the frustration" (MacDougall et al., 1985, pp. 140–141). In practice, the rating is based on the presence or absence of antagonistic behaviors such as verbal admissions of anger, harsh generalizations, emotionally laden ways of expressing negative feelings, and rudeness toward the interviewer (MacDougall et al., 1985). One judgment of Potential for Hostility based on the entire interview is made on a five-point scale.

Dembroski et al. (1989) subdivided the Potential for Hostility construct into three facets. Hostile Content is a rating based on the manifest content of the answers, the degree to which the respondent reports annoyance or anger. As implied by the name, Intensity of Hostility is a judgment of intensity with which the respondent expresses negative feelings toward others. Stylistic Hostility is a rating based on the respondent's mode of interaction with the interviewer. Uncooperative, rude, or condescending behavior contributes to a higher score. As with Total Potential for Hostility, one rating that is based on the entire interview is made for each facet. Interrater reliabilities for these hostility ratings ranged between .73 and .81 (Dembroski et al., 1989).

The predictive validity of HFSS ratings was evaluated in a case-control study of participants in the prospective Multiple Risk Factor Intervention Trial (MRFIT; Shekelle et al., 1985). Interviews with 192 participants who later developed CHD were compared with 384 controls who did not. Both Total

Potential for Hostility and Stylistic Hostility were found to discriminate between cases and controls in univariate analyses, but results were weakened in multivariate analyses controlling for traditional risk factors. When analyses were conducted separately for participants above and below the median age in the sample, Stylistic Hostility was found to significantly discriminate between cases and controls in the data of younger patients, even in multivariate analyses. None of the ratings were successful predictors in the data of older patients, a pattern of findings consistent with a body of research showing that a number of risk factors have diminishing impact with age (Williams et al., 1988).

These results testify to the importance of the distinction between self-reported hostility and the actual manner of a person's interaction in a standardized setting. Ratings of Hostile Content failed to be associated with disease outcomes, perhaps because of some of the problems with self-reports that were discussed previously. Ratings of interaction style had better predictive validity.

Component Scoring System (CSS).   The CSS (Chesney, Hecker, & Black, 1989; Hecker, Chesney, Black, & Frautschi, 1988) also grew out of research on Type A behavior. Fourteen separate dimensions of the Type A behavior pattern are scored, with hostility as one of those dimensions. Improved scoring mechanics and more specific operational definitions are innovative aspects of the CSS. Whereas the assessors using the HFSS make one rating based on a gestalt of the entire interview, the CSS divides the interview into small units associated with specific questions. This makes the task of the assessor much easier because there is no need to recall behaviors across the entire span of the interview and integrate them into one overall impression. The CSS also specifies the criteria for making ratings in more detail than previous scoring systems do, improving our ability to communicate exactly what behaviors are being rated. These features make it easier to achieve adequate reliabilities and should help researchers establish the construct validity of interview-based assessments.

The hostility index of the CSS is based on the observation of four types of behaviors, which are differentially weighted to obtain an overall score for each unit of the interview. One point is scored if the respondent is evasive and uncooperative in replying to the question. A hostile tone of voice merits two points. Challenging or deprecating the interviewer in an indirect fashion (e.g., answering in a way that implies the question was pointless) is scored as three points. Four points are given if the respondent openly and directly challenges the interviewer. A maximum of four points can be awarded for each unit of the interview. The summary Hostility Index is obtained by summing across units.

The predictive validity of the CSS was demonstrated in a reanalysis of interviews (250 cases and 500 controls) from the WCGS (Hecker, Chesney, Black, & Frautschi, 1988). Cases were drawn from those who had a CHD event within the 8½ year period following the interviews. The Hostility Index was found to be the component that best discriminated between cases and controls, and remained significant in multivariate analyses controlling for other Type A components. Another reanalysis of the WCGS data found that the CSS Hostility Index predicted total mortality over a 22-year follow-up period (Carmelli, Swan, Rosenman, Hecker, & Ragland, 1989).

One failure to find an association between CSS ratings and health outcomes was recently reported. Helmer, Ragland, and Syme (1991) found no relationship between the Hostility Index and CAD severity in a sample of 152 coronary angiography patients. However, Barefoot, Haney, Harper, Chesney, Siegler, and Williams (1992) applied CSS ratings to interviews with 124 angiography patients and observed a strong association with an index of CAD severity. Barefoot et al. noted that the Hostility Index scores in the Helmer et al. study were comparatively low and suggested that their negative results could have been due to an atypical sample or a tendency to score only the most obvious instances of hostile behavior. Since the more subtle manifestations of hostility are perhaps the best correlates of disease (Barefoot, 1992), Helmer et al. may have missed some of the more important instances of hostility in their patients. Future studies will be needed to test the validity of this explanation.

Interpersonal Hostility Assessment Technique (IHAT).   The IHAT (Barefoot, 1992; Haney et al., 1992) is an extension and blend of the HFSS and the CSS. The scoring mechanics are very similar to those of the CSS, although only hostility is scored and the differential weighting of the four types of hostile behaviors has been eliminated. The IHAT incorporates the HFSS distinction between Stylistic Hostility and Hostile Content, placing more emphasis on the respondent's manner of interpersonal interaction than on self-reports.

The operational definitions of hostile behavior are similar to those of the CSS, but special effort is made to be attentive to subtle indicators of hostility. Overt rudeness and confrontation are rare during the SI, so respondents tend to express their antagonism in more indirect ways. Voice stylistics are crucial to the identification of such hostile acts. For example, the response, "Of course," can be said in a friendly and non-hostile fashion, or it can be said in a way that implies that the question was pointless and the interviewer incompetent. IHAT assessors pay special attention to voice stylistics, not only to detect the implications of the answer, but also to identify instances in which the respondent appears to be getting emotionally aroused in a negative way. Therefore, the admission of a past angry event would not be scored if it were described in an unemotional tone, but would be scored as a hostile act if voice stylistics indicated that the respondent was experiencing arousal by actually reliving that anger.

The emphasis on subtle manifestations of hostility presents special problems for the training of assessors and the communication of the system to interested researchers. However, interrater reliabilities as high as .90 have been achieved. A training program was devised to make it easier for assessors to become proficient in IHAT scoring (Haney et al., 1992), and efforts are being made to make IHAT operational definitions even more explicit. The ultimate goal of the IHAT is to get the assessors away from making subjective ratings of the respondent's hostility to a process of counting specific types of hostile acts.

The criterion-related validity of IHAT ratings was examined in a series of coronary angiography studies. For example, scores on the IHAT hostility scores were found to correlate .57 with an index of CAD severity in a sample of 135 male angiography patients less than 50 years old, a finding that remained highly significant after controlling for traditional risk factors. Similar associations were observed in samples of women and older patients (Barefoot & Haney, 1992).

There are methodological issues that must be taken into account when interpreting angiographic studies such as the one by Haney, et al. as demonstrations of the criterion-related validity of IHAT scores. Although studies of angiography samples have unique advantages, they also have significant methodological problems (Cohen & Matthews, 1987; Pearson, 1984). First, angiography patients are not truly representative of those who develop coronary disease because those with silent CHD events and those who die suddenly do not undergo angiography. Furthermore, a number of referral biases affect selection into angiography samples. For example, angiography patients who are found to have little or no disease also have relatively high scores on indicators of somatic preoccupation (Barefoot, Beckham, Peterson, Haney, & Williams, 1992). It is thought that the tendency of these people to report high levels of symptomatology and to seek health care frequently results in a high likelihood that they will be selected into angiography. Finally, the most important problem with angiography studies in the context of the present discussion is their cross-sectional nature. Because patients are interviewed after the onset of disease, one does not know if the observed hostility is a precursor or a product of their illness. One might speculate that the pain and discomfort associated with CHD might make these patients irritable and short-tempered, resulting in high hostility scores. Whereas the opposite (that those with CHD might become more passive) is just as plausible, there is no way for studies such as Haney et al. to definitively eliminate this problem.

These methodological problems were addressed in a study of an unusual angiography sample, asymptomatic Air Force personnel who were referred for the procedure because of their results on routine noninvasive tests

(Barefoot, Patterson, Haney, & Williams, 1991). Because these men were in the early stages of coronary artery disease, had no symptoms, and were referred for angiography through the same structured process, the biases and methodological problems of the traditional angiography design were not operative. Comparisons were made between 24 cases, defined as those having any evidence of CAD and 25 controls with no detectable occlusion. Cases had low levels of CAD, with only 4 cases having enough disease considered to be clinically significant. Despite the small sample size, IHAT ratings successfully discriminated between cases and controls ($p = .03$). These data support the criterion-related validity of IHAT ratings by showing that their association with CAD is probably not due to the artifacts of the typical angiographic study.

New Directions in Interview-Based Assessments

The strategy of using interview behavior to assess anger and hostility has the potential to be extended in a number of ways. That potential comes from the richness of behavior displayed by respondents during the interview. Whereas questionnaires constrain behavior to a set of responses predetermined by the researcher, the interview setting permits the respondents a good deal of freedom to express their antagonism (or lack of it) in their own characteristic way. It is this variety of behavior that makes it difficult to describe the operational definitions of hostility, and makes training necessary to achieve satisfactory interrater reliabilities. However, the richness of interview behavior also presents the opportunity to devise rating systems that could describe the respondent's actions in much more detail. Thus, a more fine-grained analysis of interview behavior could take assessment beyond the production of one summary score to the study of the variety of ways that anger and hostility are expressed.

It is likely that the most consequential phenomena in the study of anger, hostility, and health take place in the course of social encounters (see Smith, this volume). Therefore, another way to capitalize on the richness of the interview setting is to use it to study the interaction between personality and the social environment. Manipulations of variables such as interviewer style and status could be easily done within the SI (see Siegman, Feldstein, Tomasso, Ringel, & Lating, 1987, for an example), and that would broaden the scope of the assessment procedure to a conceptualization which takes the social context into account more explicitly.

Yet another way to extend current interview-based procedures would be to incorporate facial expression and other aspects of nonverbal behavior into the assessment process. Whereas the hostility assessment procedures we discussed here relied exclusively on vocal stylistics obtained from audiotape,

Friedman and Powell (1984) have long recognized the advantages of video-tapes for scoring components of Type A behavior, including hostility. Chesney, Ekman, Friesen, Black, and Hecker (1990) also conducted research into facial expressions that are associated with hostile behavior during the SI. They found that those who scored high on the Hostility Index of the CSS showed more facial expression indicative of disgust than the less hostile respondents did. Interestingly, the frequency of angry facial expressions was not associated with CSS scores, perhaps because of the nonprovocative nature of the SI. These findings illustrate the potential for facial expression data to help establish the construct validity of interview-based assessment techniques. However, it should be noted that no study has yet provided an empirical demonstration that the inclusion of facial and nonverbal cues into the assessment procedures measurably improves the validity of the existing hostility measures.

Finally, researchers can take advantage of sophisticated speech analysis techniques (e.g., Swingle, 1984) using computer technology to augment interview-assessment procedures with more objectively defined indicators of speech patterns. Although it is doubtful that speech analysis can detect all of the nuances in behavior that can be observed by a human assessor, this approach could aid assessments to the extent that anger and hostility are reliably associated with specific vocal cues. Siegman et al. (1987; Siegman, this volume) have already produced some very promising findings showing strong associations between objectively measured speech patterns and CAD levels in angiography patients.

PEER REPORTS

Peer reports represent an alternative strategy for the assessment of anger and hostility that has rarely been used in previous research, but has a number of potential advantages. Peer reports avoid the major problems of interview assessments because they are almost as easy to obtain as self-reports, and data collection can be done with standard scales. At the same time, peer reports may not be as affected by the biases and problems with self-awareness that are issues in self-reports. Because there is not an extensive past literature on the use of peer reports in health psychology, the goal of this section is to alert researchers to the possible strengths and weaknesses of this methodology. The majority of research on peer reports has dealt with the extent of their agreement with self-reports. Although it can be argued that self-reports are not an adequate criterion for the evaluation of the validity of peer reports, this literature illustrates many of the measurement issues that will be encountered by researchers using this assessment strategy.

Congruence Between Self- and Peer Reports

The interest in whether a person's self-view is congruent with others' perceptions of him or her has a long history in psychology. Symbolic interactionism (e.g., Mead, 1925) proposed the idea of a "looking glass self," which emphasizes the social origins of one's self-concept. In Mead's (1925) words, "We are in possession of selves only insofar as we can and do take the attitudes of others toward ourselves and respond to those attitudes" (p. 273). Consequently, perceptions of self and others should be very similar (Cooley, 1902). Empirical attempts to verify the idea of a "looking glass self" blossomed in the late 1930s through mid 1950s in the area of person perception accuracy (e.g., Taft, 1966). However, research on accuracy came to a near standstill after Cronbach's (1955) devastating criticisms of the statistical methods and interpretation of accuracy scores (Cook, 1984; Kenny & Albright, 1987). Overall, the evidence provided bleak support for the symbolic interactionist position (Schrauger & Schoeneman, 1979). However, the emergence of new methodologies (e.g., Funder, 1980; Kenny & La Voie, 1984; Wright, 1989), now provide substantial evidence indicating that peer and self-ratings are significantly correlated, and progress has been made toward identifying factors that affect the size of that association.

One established finding is that correlations between self–peer ratings are higher when the parties are more closely acquainted (e.g., Cloyd, 1977; Edwards & Klockar, 1981; Funder, 1980; Funder & Colvin, 1988; Funder & Dobroth, 1987; Norman & Goldberg, 1966). It is not too surprising that agreement should increase the longer people are acquainted for several reasons: (a) there are more mutual exchanges of ideas that can provide important cues concerning how the other person thinks and feels; (b) long-term acquaintances are probably more aware of subtle unobservable factors (Paunonen, 1989); (c) the parties have more opportunities to influence each other so that others' perceptions become congruent with self-perceptions (Swann, 1984); (d) there are more occasions to observe the other person's behaviors in different situations; and (e) each member has the opportunity to test his/her impression about the other person (e.g., Snyder & Swann, 1978). It is also possible that these findings are partially due to the tendency for close acquaintances to be similar to each other and the tendency for people to assume that others are similar to themselves, resulting in artifactual inflation of the correlation between peer and self-reports (Cronbach, 1955; DePaulo, Kenny, Hoover, Webb, Oliver, 1987; Paunonen, 1989).

Another factor influencing self–other agreement is the public visibility of the trait being assessed. According to Funder and Dobroth (1987), a trait seems most easily visible when: (a) it is easy to imagine behaviors that can confirm or disconfirm it; (b) its manifestation is possible across occasions; (c) few confirming behaviors are needed to establish the trait; and (d) the trait is easy to evaluate. Ratings on traits that are highly observable were shown to have relatively high levels of self–other agreement (e.g., Albright, Kenny, & Malloy, 1988; Cheek, 1982; Funder & Colvin, 1988; Kenrick & Springfield, 1980; Norman & Goldberg, 1966; Paunonen, 1989, 1991), especially for unacquainted individuals (Paunonen, 1989).

Self–peer correlations are also enhanced as the number of raters increases (Watson, 1989) and as the traits are averaged (i.e., aggregated) across raters and situations (Cheek, 1982; Epstein, 1979, 1983). In part, these aggregation techniques serve to increase self–other agreement because they reduce the impact of the idiosyncrasies of the observer on the ratings. Because individuals differ in social sensitivity, attributional styles, and other information-processing characteristics, peer ratings are a product of the qualities of the observer, as well as the characteristics of the person being observed. Averaging across multiple observers reduces the influence of any individual observer, thereby reducing this "observer variance."

Biases in Peer Reports

Thus far, we have portrayed a rather favorable picture of peer reports. However, it should also be noted that self–other correlations are remarkably high in pairs of unacquainted individuals (e.g., Albright, Kenny, & Malloy, 1988; Colvin & Funder, 1991; Paunonen, 1989). This finding suggests that there may be biases that artifactually inflate the levels of self–other agreement.

The problems of socially desirable responding apply to peer reports, as well as to self-reports. Funder (1980) found high self–peer correlations on traits that were socially desirable. This result may be due to a general positivity bias (e.g., Bruner & Taguiri, 1954), an inclination to see others in a positive light (cf. Matlin & Stang, 1978). There also may be a reluctance to express disapproval of a spouse or peer to a researcher. In addition, Cloyd (1977) argued that the tendency for respondents to rate others as similar to themselves may lead them to rate the target as an attractive, likeable person. Thus, we can expect peer reports to be somewhat biased in a positive direction.

The use of stereotypes also may present problems in peer assessments. Shared stereotypes may spuriously inflate correlations between raters (Bourne, 1977; Cronbach, 1955). The halo effect (Cooper, 1981) is related to the use of stereotypes. It occurs when a person's standing on one important or visible characteristic influences the perceiver's estimate that the person also has other characteristics. Both of these phenomena are due to the use of implicit personality theories (Schneider, 1973), lay notions about how traits are intercorrelated. Peer reports can be biased to the extent that the raters rely on these implicit personality theories rather than actual observation of the individuating characteristics of the target.

Stereotypes and halo effects are likely to have more impact on peer reports when the rater and the target are not well acquainted (Cooper, 1981). Therefore, the use of raters who are highly familiar with the target is one way to minimize this type of bias. There are also various statistical and methodological techniques that can control for the use of stereotypes (Cronbach, 1955; Kenny & Albright, 1988). For example, the researcher may ask the observer to rate the "typical" person of the target's age, sex, and occupation on the attributes of interest, essentially gathering base-rate information, prior to obtaining ratings of the actual target. The base-rate information can then be used to adjust or interpret the peer ratings of the target (e.g., Anderson, 1984; Watson, 1989).

The Potential Role of Peer Reports in Studies of Hostility

Peer reports have appealing features that make them attractive for use in studies of anger, hostility, and health. Even if the person is not fully aware of their own antagonistic tendencies because of the lack of introspection or the presence of denial, a close friend or spouse is likely to recognize those tendencies during their daily interaction with the person. Furthermore, peers and spouses typically observe the individual in a wide range of situations, not just in the standardized settings that are the basis of interview assessments. The promise of this measurement strategy is illustrated by one study that evaluated the ability of spouse and self-reports of anger to discriminate thallium scan patients with CHD from those found to have no evidence of disease (Kneip et al., in press). Patient self-reports were not associated with disease status, but spouse reports of the patient's anger and hostility were higher for those patients with CHD.

A number of precautions designed to enhance the validity of peer reports should increase the usefulness of this methodology. Peer reports should be obtained from individuals who are well acquainted with the person being evaluated. Researchers should gather information about the extent and nature of the relationship between the peer and the target. If possible, obtain ratings of each target from multiple observers. Multiple raters alleviate some potential biases (see aforementioned), but the amount of agreement between raters could itself be a variable of interest. Researchers should pay as much attention to the psychometric properties of the instrument used to obtain peer reports as they would when selecting a self-report instrument. Finally, researchers should expect that peer reports will measure some aspects of anger and hostility better than other aspects. In particular, the more overt expressions of antagonism are more likely to be easily detected by peers. Therefore, the ideal research strategy would combine peer reports with other measures designed to assess some of the more covert and cognitive aspects of the constructs.

CONCLUSIONS

The most obvious need for further research pertaining to anger and hostility assessment is in the area of construct validity. The phenomena being assessed are complex, multifaceted, and have been conceptualized in a variety of ways (see Smith, this volume). There are also large differences between measures, both in the measurement strategies and in the aspects of the constructs that they assess. Consequently, complications arise in communicating and in comparing results across studies. Work on construct validity is necessary to reduce these obstacles and to allow better evaluation of each instrument as a reflection of particular theoretical approaches to anger and hostility.

Although a complete solution to the measurement problems in this area is unattainable, there are a number of positive steps that can be taken that will improve future studies. Foremost is the adoption of a comprehensive measurement strategy. When new instruments are developed, they should be designed to assess a broad range of the phenomena associated with anger and hostility. Another way to achieve more comprehensiveness is through the use of multiple measures. Even if practical problems (e.g., respondent burden) prevent the researcher from administering a broadly based battery of measures, many potential problems can be avoided simply through an awareness and discussion of construct validity issues.

The outcomes of a comprehensive measurement strategy are illustrated by a recent study designed to investigate age differences in anger and hostility (Barefoot, Beckham, Haney, Siegler, & Lipkus, in press). Middle-aged and older adults were administered a broadly based battery of measures, including six self-report scales and the SI, which was scored using the IHAT. Principal components analysis of the self-report scales revealed three factors (a) Overt Hostility, reflecting open expressiveness; (b) Covert Hostility, reflecting resentment and a tendency not to openly express; and (c) a cognitive factor reflecting cynicism and suspicion that was called Hostile Beliefs. Scores on Overt Hostility factor were *negatively* related to age, but scores on the Hostile Beliefs factor and IHAT scores were *positively* related to age. Covert Hostility scores were not correlated with age. This study demonstrates that different aspects of anger and hostility can have different relationships to other variables, and that a comprehensive measurement strategy can enhance our understanding of these complexities.

Finally, we wish to summarize this review by noting that each strategy we discussed has it own strengths and weaknesses. We considered some of the criteria that could be used to evaluate a measure: predictive validity, ease of administration, susceptibility to bias, and psychometric properties. Other criteria (e.g., theoretical coherence) are relevant as well. No one approach to the assessment of anger and hostility can be considered to be superior to others. The choice of an instrument should be based on the specific needs of the study in which it is to be applied and the appropriateness of the measure for those needs.

ACKNOWLEDGMENTS

Preparation of this chapter was supported by grants AG-09276 from the National Institute on Aging, HL-36587 from the National Heart, Lung, and Blood Institute, and 5T32-Mh19109 from the National Institute of Mental Health. The authors wish to thank Jean C. Beckham, PhD, for her comments on an earlier draft.

REFERENCES

Albright, L., Kenny, D. A., & Malloy, T. E. (1988). Consensus in personality judgements at zero acquaintance. *Journal of Personality and Social Psychology, 55,* 387–395.

Aldwin, C. M., Workman-Daniels, K., Spiro, A., III, Levenson, M. R., & Bosse, R. (1989, November). *Suspiciousness and mortality: Findings from the Normative Aging Study.* Paper presented at the meeting of the Gerontological Society of America, Minneapolis, MN.

Allport, G. W. (1942). The use of personal documents in psychological science (Social Science Research Council, Bulletin 49). Ann Arbor, MI: Edwards Borthers.

Anderson, S. (1984). Self-Knowledge and social inference: II. The diagnosticity of cognitive and behavioral data. *Journal of Personality and Social Psychology, 46,* 294–307.

Averill, J. R. (1982). *Anger and aggression: An essay on emotion.* New York: Springer-Verlag.

Barefoot, J. C. (1993). Developments in the measurement of hostility. In H. Friedman (Ed.), *Hostility, coping, and health* (pp. 13–31). Washington, DC: American Psychological Association.

Barefoot, J. C. (1992). [Personality measures of angiography patients]. Unpublished raw data.

Barefoot, J. C., & Beckham, J. C. (1992). [Relationships between self-report and interview-based measures of hostility]. Unpublished raw data.

Barefoot, J. C., Beckham, J. C., Haney, T. L., Siegler, I. C., & Lipkus, I. M. (1993). Age differences in hostility among middle-aged and older adults. *Psychology and Aging, 8,* 3–9.

Barefoot, J. C., Beckham, J. C., Peterson, B. L., Haney, T. L., & Williams, R. B. (1992). Measures of neuroticism and disease status in coronary angiography patients. *Journal of Consulting and Clinical Psychology, 60,* 127–132.

Barefoot, J. C., Dodge, K. A., Peterson, B. L., Dahlstrom, W. G., & Williams, R. B. (1989). The Cook–Medley hostility scale: Item content and ability to predict survival. *Psychosomatic Medicine, 51,* 46–57.

Barefoot, J. C., & Haney, T. L. (1992). [Interview-assessed hostility and coronary artery disease: Further studies]. Unpublished raw data.

Barefoot, J. C., Haney, T. L., Harper, R. R., Chesney, M. A., Siegler, I. C., & Williams, R. B. (1992). *Interview-assessed hostility and coronary artery disease in angiography patients.* Manuscript submitted for publication.

Barefoot, J. C., Patterson, J., Haney, T. L., & Williams, R. B. (1991). Hostility and early stage coronary artery disease (CAD). *Psychosomatic Medicine, 53,* 234.

Barefoot, J. C., Peterson, B. L., Dahlstrom, W. G., Siegler, I. C., Anderson, N. B., & Williams, R. B. (1991). Hostility patterns and health implications: Correlates of Cook–Medley hostility scale scores in a national survey. *Health Psychology, 10*, 18–24.

Barefoot, J. C., Siegler, I. C., Nowlin, J. B., Peterson, B. L., Haney, T. L., & Williams, R. B. (1987). Suspiciousness, health, and mortality: A follow-up study of 500 older adults. *Psychosomatic Medicine, 49*, 450–457.

Bourne, E. (1977). Can we describe an individual's personality? Agreement on stereotype versus individual attributes. *Journal of Personality and Social Psychology, 35*, 863–872.

Bruner, J. S., & Taguiri, R. (1954). Person perception. In G. Lindzey (Ed.), *Handbook of social psychology* (Vol. 2, pp. 634–654). Reading, MA: Addison-Wesley.

Buss, A. H., & Durkee, A. (1957). An inventory for assessing different kinds of hostility. *Journal of Consulting Psychology, 42*, 155–162.

Carmelli, D., Swan, G. E., Rosenman, R. H., Hecker, M. H., & Ragland, D. R. (1989). *Behavioral components and total mortality in the WCGS*. Paper presented at the Society of Behavioral Medicine Meetings, San Francisco.

Cattell, R. B., Eber, H. W., & Tatsuoka, M. M. (1970) *Handbook for the Sixteen Personality Factor Questionnaire (16PF)*. Champaign, IL: Institute for Personality and Ability Testing.

Cheek, J. M. (1982). Aggregation, moderator variables, and the validity of personality tests: A peer-rating study. *Journal of Personality and Social Psychology, 43*, 1254–1269.

Chesney, M. A., Ekman, P., Friesen, W. V., Black, G. W., & Hecker, M. (1990). Type A behavior pattern: Facial behavior and speech components. *Psychosomatic Medicine, 52*, 307–319.

Chesney, M. A., Hecker, M., & Black, G. W. (1989). Coronary-prone components of Type A behavior in the WCGS: A new methodology. In B. K. Houston & C. R. Snyder (Eds.), *Type A behavior pattern: Research, theory and intervention* (pp. 168–188). New York: Wiley.

Cloyd, L. (1977). Effects of acquaintanceship on accuracy of person perception. *Perceptual and Motor Skills, 44*, 819–826.

Cohen, S., & Matthews, K. A. (1987). Social support, Type A behavior, and coronary artery disease. *Psychosomatic Medicine, 49*, 325–330.

Colvin, C. R., & Funder, D. C. (1991). Predicting personality and behavior: A boundary on the acquaintanceship effect. *Journal of Personality and Social Psychology, 60*, 884–894.

Cook, M. (1984). *Issues in person perception*. London: Methuen.

Cook, W. W., & Medley, D. M. (1954). Proposed hostility and pharasaic-virtue scales for the MMPI. *Journal of Applied Psychology, 38*, 414–418.

Cooley, C. H. (1902). *Human nature and the social order*. New York: Scribner.

Cooper, W. H. (1981). Ubiquitous Halo. *Psychological Bulletin, 90*, 218–244.

Costa, P. T., & McCrae, R. R. (1985). *The NEO Personality Inventory Manual*. Odessa, FL: Psychological Assessment Resources.

Costa, P. T., Zonderman, A. B., McCrae, R. R., & Williams, R. B. (1986). Cynicism and paranoid alienation in the Cook and Medley hostility scale. *Psychosomatic Medicine, 48*, 283–285.

Cronbach, L. J. (1955). Processes affecting scores on "understanding others" and "assumed similarity." *Psychological Bulletin, 52*, 177–193.

Dembroski, T. M., MacDougall, J. M., Costa, P. T., & Grandits, G. A. (1989). Components of hostility as predictors of sudden death and myocardial infarction in the Multiple Risk Factor Intervention Trial. *Psychosomatic Medicine, 51*, 514–522.

Dembroski, T. M., MacDougall, J. M., Williams, R. B., Haney, T. L., & Blumenthal, J. A. (1985). Components of Type A, hostility, and anger-in: Relationship to angiographic findings. *Psychosomatic Medicine, 47*, 219–233.

DePaulo, B. M., Kenny, D. A., Hoover, C. W., Webb, W., & Oliver, P. V. (1987). Accuracy of person perception. Do people know what kind of impression they convey? *Journal of Personality and Social Psychology, 52*, 303–315.

Duval, S., & Wicklund, R. A. (1972). *A theory of objective self-awareness*. New York: Academic Press.

Edwards, A. L., & Klockars, A. J. (1981). Significant others and self-evaluation between perceived and actual evaluations. *Personality and Social Psychology Bulletin, 7*, 244–251.

Epstein, S. (1979). The stability of behavior: I. On predicting most of the people most of the time. *Journal of Personality and Social Psychology, 37,* 1097–1126.

Epstein, S. (1983). Aggregation and beyond: Some basic issues on the prediction of behavior. *Journal of Personality, 51,* 360–392.

Fenigstein, A., Scheier, M. F., & Buss, A. H. (1975). Public and private self-consciousness: Assessment and theory. *Journal of Consulting and Clinical Psychology, 43,* 522–527.

Friedman, M., & Powell, L. H. (1984). The diagnosis and quantitative assessment of Type A behavior: Introduction and description of the videotaped structured interview. *Integrative Psychiatry, 2,* 123–131.

Funder, D. C. (1980). On seeing ourselves as others see us: Self–other agreement and discrepancy in personality ratings. *Journal of Personality, 48,* 473–493.

Funder, D. C., & Colvin, C. R. (1988). Friends and strangers: Acquaintanceship, agreement, and the accuracy of personality judgement. *Journal of Personality and Social Psychology, 55,* 149–158.

Funder, D. C., & Dobroth, K. M. (1987). Differences between traits: Properties associated with interjudge agreement. *Journal of Personality and Social Psychology, 52,* 409–418.

Greenglass, E. R., & Julkunen, J. (1989). Construct validity and sex differences in Cook–Medley hostility. *Personality and Individual Differences, 10,* 209–218.

Haney, T. L., Barefoot, J. C., Houseworth, S. J., Harlan, E., Williams, R. B., & Scherwitz, L. (1992). *The Interpersonal Hostility Assessment Technique.* Manuscript submitted for publication.

Hecker, M., Chesney, M. A., Black, G. W., & Frautschi, N. (1988). Coronary-prone behaviors in the Western Collaborative Group Study. *Psychosomatic Medicine, 50,* 153–164.

Helmer, D. C., Ragland, D. R., & Syme, S. L. (1991). Hostility and coronary artery disease. *American Journal of Epidemiology, 133,* 112–122.

Jamner, L. D., Shapiro, D., Goldstein, I., & Hug, R. (1991). Ambulatory blood pressure and heart rate in paramedics: Effects of cynical hostility and defensiveness. *Psychosomatic Medicine, 53,* 393–406.

Johnson, E. H. (1991, August). *Development and validation of the structured anger assessment interview.* Paper presented at the meetings of the American Psychological Association, San Francisco.

Kenny, D. A., & Albright, L. (1987). Accuracy in interpersonal perception: A social relations analysis. *Journal of Personality and Social Psychology, 52,* 390–402.

Kenny, D. A., & La Voie, L. (1984). The social relations model. In L. Berkowitz (Ed.), *Advances in experimental social psychology* (Vol. 18, pp. 142–182). Orlando, FL: Academic Press.

Kenrick, D. T., & Springfield, D. O. (1980). Personality traits and the eye of the beholder: Crossing some traditional philosophical boundaries in the search for consistency in all the people. *Psychological Review, 87,* 88–104.

Kneip, R., Delamater, A. M., Ismond, T., Milford, C., Salvia, L., & Schwartz, D. (in press). Self- and spouse ratings of anger and hostility as predictors of coronary heart disease. *Health Psychology.*

Koskenvuo, M., Kaprio, J., Rose, R. J., Kesaniemi, A., Heikkila, K., & Langinvainio, H. (1988). Hostility as a risk factor for mortality and ischemic heart disease in men. *Psychosomatic Medicine, 50,* 330–340.

Lipkus, I. M., Barefoot, J. C., Beckham, J. C., & Haney, T. L. (1993, March). *The structure of the Cook–Medley hostility scale as assessed by multidimensional scaling.* Paper presented at the meetings of the Society of Behavioral Medicine, San Francisco.

MacDougall, J. M., Dembroski, T. M., Dimsdale, J. E., & Hackett, T. P. (1985). Components of Type A, hostility, and anger-in: Further relationships to angiographic findings. *Health Psychology, 4,* 137–152.

Matlin, M. W., & Stang, D. J. (1978). *The pollyanna principle.* Cambridge, MA: Schenkman.

Matthews, K. A., Glass, D. C., Rosenman, R. H., & Bortner, R. W. (1977). Competitive drive, Pattern A, and coronary heart disease: A further analysis of some data from the Western Collaborative Group Study. *Journal of Chronic Diseases, 30,* 489–498.

Matthews, K. A., Jamison, J. W., & Cottington, E. M. (1985). Assessment of Type A, anger, and hostility: A review of scales through 1982. In A. M. Ostfeld & E. D. Eaker (Eds.), *Measuring psychosocial variables in epidemiologic studies of cardiovascular disease* (NIH Publication No. 85-2270, pp. 207–312). Washington, DC: U.S. Department of Health and Human Services.

McCrae, R. R., & Costa, P. T. (1983). Social desirability scales: More substance than style. *Journal of Consulting and Clinical Psychology, 51*, 882–888.

McCrae, R. R., Costa, P. T., Dahlstrom, W. G., Barefoot, J. C., Siegler, I. C., & Williams, R. B. (1989). A caution on the use of the MMPI K correction in research on psychosomatic medicine. *Psychosomatic Medicine, 51*, 58–61.

Mead, G. H. (1925). The genesis of the self- and social control. *International Journal of Ethics, 35*, 251–273.

Megargee, E. I. (1985). The dynamics of aggression and their application to cardiovascular disorders. In M. A. Chesney & R. H. Rosenman (Eds.), *Anger and hostility in cardiovascular and behavioral disorders* (pp. 31–57). New York: McGraw-Hill/Hemisphere.

Musante, L., MacDougall, J. M., Dembroski, T. M., & Costa, P. T., Jr. (1989). Potential for hostility and dimensions of anger. *Health Psychology, 8*, 343–354.

Norman, W. T., & Goldberg, I. R. (1966). Raters, ratees, and randomness in personality structure. *Journal of Personality and Social Psychology, 4*, 681–691.

Novaco, R. W. (1975). *Anger control: The development and evaluation of an experimental treatment.* Lexington, MA: Lexington Books.

Ostfeld, A. M., Lebovitz, B. L., Shekelle, R. B., & Paul, O. (1964). A prospective study of the relationship between personality and coronary heart disease. *Journal of Chronic Disease, 17*, 265–276.

Paulhus, D. L. (1984). Two-component models of socially desirable responding. *Journal of Personality and Social Psychology, 46*, 598–609.

Paulhus, D. L. (1986). Self-deception and impression management in test responses. In A. Angleitner & J. Wiggins (Eds.), *Personality assessment via questionnaire* (pp. 143–165). New York: Springer-Verlag.

Paulhus, D. L. (1991). Measurement and control of response bias. In J. P. Robinson, P. R. Shaver, & L. S. Wrightsman (Eds.), *Measures of personality and social psychological attitudes* (pp. 17–59). New York: Academic Press.

Paunonen, S. V. (1989). Consensus in personality judgements: Moderation of target-rater acquaintanceship and behavior observability. *Journal of Personality and Social Psychology, 56*, 823–833.

Paunonen, S. V. (1991). On the accuracy of ratings by strangers. *Journal of Personality and Social Psychology, 61*, 471–477.

Pearson, T. A. (1984). Coronary arteriography in the study of the epidemiology of coronary artery disease. *Epidemiologic Reviews, 6*, 140–166.

Robinson, J. P., Shaver, P. R., & Wrightsman, L. S. (1991). Criteria for scale selection and evaluation. In J. P. Robinson, P. R. Shaver, & L. S. Wrightsman (Eds.), *Measures of personality and social psychological attitudes* (pp. 1–16). New York: Academic Press.

Rosenman, R. H., Brand, R. J., Jenkins, D., Friedman, M., Straus, R., & Wurm, M. (1975). Coronary heart disease in the Western Collaborative Group Study: Final follow-up experience of 8½ years. *Journal of the American Medical Association, 233*, 872–877.

Rosenman, R. H., Swan, G. E., & Carmelli, D. (1988). Definition, assessment, and evolution of the Type A behavior pattern. In B. K. Houston & C. R. Snyder (Eds.), *Type A behavior pattern: Research, theory, and intervention* (pp. 8–31). New York: Wiley.

Scheier, M. F., Buss, A. H., & Buss, D. M. (1978). Self-consciousness, self-report of aggressiveness, and aggression. *Journal of Research in Personality, 12*, 133–140.

Schneider, D. J. (1973). Implicit personality theory: A review. *Psychological Bulletin, 79*, 294–309.

Schrauger, J. S., & Schoeneman, T. J. (1979). Symbolic interactionists view of self-concept: Through the looking glass darkly. *Psychological Bulletin, 86*, 549–573.

Shekelle, R. B., Hulley, S. B., Neaton, J. D., Billings, J. H., Borhani, N. O., Gerace, T. A., Jacobs, D. R., Lasser, N. L., Mittlemark, M. B., & Stamler, J. (1985). The MRFIT behavior pattern study: Type A behavior and incidence of coronary heart disease. *American Journal of Epidemiology, 122,* 559–570.

Siegel, J. M. (1986). The Multidimensional Anger Inventory. *Journal of Personality and Social Psychology, 51,* 191–200.

Siegler, I. C., Zonderman, A. B., Barefoot, J. C., Williams, R. B., Costa, P. T., & McCrae, R. R. (1990). Predicting personality in adulthood from college MMPI scores: Implications for follow-up studies in psychosomatic medicine. *Psychosomatic Medicine, 52,* 644–652.

Siegman, A. W., Dembroski, T. M., & Ringel, N. (1987). Components of hostility and the severity of coronary artery disease. *Psychosomatic Medicine, 49,* 127–135.

Siegman, A. W., Feldstein, S., Tommaso, C. T., Ringel, N., & Lating, J. (1987). Expressive vocal behavior and the severity of coronary artery disease. *Psychosomatic Medicine, 49,* 545–561.

Smith, T. W., & Frohm, K. D. (1985). What's so unhealthy about hostility? Construct validity and psychological correlates of the Cook and Medley Ho scale. *Health Psychology, 4,* 503–520.

Smith, T. W. (1992). Hostility and health: Current status of a psychosomatic hypothesis. *Health Psychology, 11,* 139–150.

Snyder, M., & Swann, W. B. (1978). Behavioral confirmation in social interaction: From social perception to social reality. *Journal of Experimental Social Psychology, 14,* 148–162.

Snyder, M. (1979). Self-monitoring processes. In L. Berkowitz (Ed.), *Advances in experimental social psychology* (Vol. 12, pp. 85–128). New York: Academic Press.

Spielberger, C. D., Johnson, E. H., Russell, S. F., Crane, R. J., Jacobs, G. A., & Worden, T. J. (1985). The experience and expression of anger: Construction and validation of an anger expression scale. In M. A. Chesney & R. H. Rosenman (Eds.), *Anger and hostility in cardiovascular and behavioral disorders* (pp. 5–30). New York: McGraw-Hill/Hemisphere.

Swann, W. B. (1984). Quest for accuracy in person perception: A matter of pragmatics. *Psychological Review, 91,* 457–477.

Swingle, P. G. (1984). Temporal measures of vocalization: Some methodological considerations. *Journal of Personality and Social Psychology, 47,* 1263–1280.

Taft, R. (1966). Accuracy and empathic judgements of acquaintances and strangers. *Journal of Personality and Social Psychology, 3,* 600–604.

Watson, D. (1989). Strangers' ratings of five robust personality factors: Evidence of a surprising convergence with self-reports. *Journal of Personality and Social Psychology, 57,* 120–128.

Weinberger, D. A. (1990). The construct validity of the repressive coping style. In J. L. Singer (Ed.), *Repression and dissociation: Implications for personality theory, psychopathology, and health* (pp. 337–386). Chicago: The University of Chicago Press.

Williams, R. B., Barefoot, J. C., Haney, T. L., Harrell, F. E., Blumenthal, J. A., Pryor, D. B., & Peterson, B. L. (1988). Type A behavior and angiographically documented coronary atherosclerosis in a sample of 2289 patients. *Psychosomatic Medicine, 50,* 139–152.

Wright, J. C. (1989). An alternative paradigm for studying the accuracy of person perception: Simulated personalities. In D. M. Buss & N. Cantor (Eds.), *Personality psychology: Recent trends and emerging directions* (pp. 61–81). New York: Springer-Verlag.

4

ASSOCIATIONS OF HOSTILITY AND CORONARY ARTERY DISEASE: A REVIEW OF STUDIES

Karin F. Helmers
Donna M. Posluszny
David S. Krantz
Uniformed Services University of the Health Sciences

The goal of this chapter is to evaluate studies that have examined the personality construct of hostility in relation to coronary artery disease (CAD) endpoints of myocardial infarction (MI), sudden cardiac death, and angiographic evidence of CAD. For purposes of this review, existing studies are first separated into cross-sectional and longitudinal studies. Second, within each of these categories we treat those studies that used a paper-and-pencil questionnaire (e.g., Cook–Medley Hostility Inventory) separately from those studies that used a behavioral measure of hostility (e.g., Type A Structured Interview).

Hostility, anger, and aggression are often used interchangeably in the literature. Whereas hostility is viewed as a negative attitudinal set (Williams, Barefoot, & Shekelle, 1985), anger is seen as an emotional state, or, as a trait, and is seen as a proneness to becoming angry (Spielberger et al., 1985), and aggression is seen as a behavioral response directed toward another individual or object (Spielberger et al., 1985). Although these constructs are all believed to be different, interrelationships exist among them. For example, a highly hostile individual experiences anger and may exert aggression more frequently than a person with low hostility (Williams, Barefoot, & Shekelle, 1985). For purposes of this review, these three constructs are examined separately, but are viewed as one construct, which, for simplicity's sake, is referred to as hostility. Before reviewing the relevant studies, the issues that are related to the measurement of hostility and CAD endpoints need to be considered, as well as the issues that are related to the methodological biases and limitations in these studies.

Measurement of Hostility

Hostility may be assessed through either a paper-and-pencil questionnaire or a Structured Interview (SI); see chapter by Barefoot in this volume. To characterize its construct, as measured by the Cook–Medley Hostility Inventory (Cook & Medley, 1954), several factor analyses of hostility were performed. Barefoot, Dodge, Peterson, Dahlstrom, and Williams (1989) performed a conceptual rational analysis of items to obtain descriptors of psychological dimensions, including Cynicism, Hostile Attribution, Aggressive Responding, Hostile Affect, and Social Avoidance. Based on correlations with other established psychological inventories, Blumenthal, Barefoot, Burg, and Williams (1987) suggested that the scale measures four general behavioral dimensions: Anger and Hostility, ineffective coping styles, Neuroticism, and social maladjustment. Similarly, Costa, Zonderman, McCrae, and Williams (1986) factor-analyzed items from the Cook–Medley Hostility Inventory revealing the components of Cynicism and Paranoid Alienation.

The Type A SI developed by Friedman and Rosenman (Rosenman, 1978) provided a more behavioral measure of hostility. More important than the actual content of the subject's answers are overt behaviors during the interview, including vigorous speech and motor mannerisms. The SI component scoring system yielded several stylistic dimensions, including the variable of interest, potential-for-hostility, as well as loud voice, explosive speech, rapid and accelerated speech, response latency, anger-in, and competition for control of interview (Dembroski, 1983; Matthews, Glass, Rosenman, & Bortner, 1977). SI-based assessments of potential for hostility show only a modest .37 correlation with the Cook–Medley Hostility Inventory (Dembroski, MacDougall, Williams, Haney, & Blumenthal, 1985). Thus, these two measures share 13.7% variance with each other, indicating they are similar but not identical. Similarly, Swan, Carmelli, and Rosenman (1990) found a .29 correlation between SI potential for hostility and the Cook–Medley Hostility Inventory. This relatively low concordance between the two measures may be due to differences in what aspects of hostility each measure taps (Smith, 1992). SI potential for hostility is more strongly related to expressive aspects, or overt behaviors, of hostility (Musante, MacDougall, Dembroski, & Costa, 1989), whereas the Cook–Medley Hostility Inventory is more closely correlated with experiential aspects, or cognitions, of hostility (Smith & Frohm, 1985).

Other measures of hostility have been used (e.g. the Aggression subscale from Cesarec–Marke Personality Schedule, the Dutch Hostility scale, Buss–Durkee Hostility Inventory, and the Hostility subscale from Jenkins Activity Survey) and are included in our review. However, the majority of studies in this area have used either the Cook–Medley Hostility Inventory or the SI derived hostility subcomponent.

Methodological Bias Deriving from Choice of Various Coronary Disease Endpoints

There are several endpoints that can be measured as indicative of CAD: angina, MI, sudden cardiac death, and the extent of occlusion in coronary arteries. A brief review of the methodological biases of these CAD endpoints follows.

Angina. The use of angina as a coronary disease endpoint has several limitations. Angina is a symptom of coronary disease, but it is not always accompanied by clinical evidence of coronary disease (e.g., severity of atherosclerosis, MI). Because angina is a self-report measure, one's memory can be biased, for example, approximately 20% of subjects who reported angina will claim five years later that they never have had angina (Medalie, Snyder, Groen, Neufeld, Goldbourt, & Riss, 1973). Furthermore, although increasing obstruction of the coronary arteries is hypothesized to be positively correlated to severity of angina, inconsistent results were found in that those patients with the least occlusion reported they had the most severe angina symptoms (Jenkins, Stanton, Klein, Savageau, & Harken, 1983). Finally, several studies demonstrated that Neuroticism, which includes the variables of anger, anxiety, and depression, is related to angina, but not to the clinical endpoints of MI or cardiac death (Belgian–French Pooling Project, 1984; Costa & McCrae, 1987). As a result of these methodological limitations, using angina as a marker of CAD can lead to spurious associations; consequently, we excluded any studies that solely used angina as an endpoint. Unfortunately, the majority of longitudinal studies include angina, as well as objective clinical outcomes of CAD, and group them together in the analyses. This methodological limitation may affect results from individual studies using angina and therefore, one needs to keep this in mind when reviewing the literature.

Extent of Atherosclerosis. Studies employing cardiac catheterizations evaluate the extent of atherosclerosis or obstruction of the coronary arteries. There is a marked patient selection bias inherent in cardiac catherization studies, because only patients who are at high risk for the development of coronary disease or who are already diagnosed with CAD are referred for coronary angiography. Therefore, the association between hostility and coronary disease may be more difficult to find because of the restricted range of variance in the extent of atherosclerosis. Furthermore, if there is a positive relationship between hostility and coronary disease, presumably patients who are at high risk of development of CAD would also be more hostile, which would then restrict the variance found for hostility. This restriction in range both for hostility and for disease severity may decrease the magnitude of the association between hostility and coronary disease (Miller, Turner, Tindale, Posavac, & Dugoni, 1991; Pickering, 1985).

Myocardial Infarction and Cardiac Death.   The hard, clinical endpoint of myocardial infarction is employed in cross-sectional studies. Cross-sectional studies involve comparing patients with known CAD to control subjects without CAD. These case-control studies necessarily suffer from a major methodological flaw: The personality trait is measured at some point after the occurrence of the CAD event (e.g., myocardial infarction). Thus, the results from this research are unclear as to whether increased hostility leads to the CAD event or whether the CAD event leads to increased hostility (reverse causality hypothesis). As evidence of this problem, Cleveland and Johnson (1962) evaluated hostility in patients hospitalized for coronary disease (e.g., MI), a serious life-threatening surgical procedure, or some minor surgical procedure. Results demonstrated greater hostility scores in coronary disease patients and in patients who underwent a life-threatening surgical procedure as compared to patients who underwent minor surgery. These findings suggest that serious life-threatening events could increase hostility. Despite this uncertainty in the direction of causality, cross-sectional studies provide a necessary first step in examining possible associations between hostility and coronary disease.

In a prospective study, one uses the hard endpoints of MI and cardiac death. In such studies, a sample of subjects is assessed for hostility and then followed over time for occurrence of disease (e.g., MI or cardiac death). The temporal measurement allows for a more discerning test of cause and effect investigations. However, determination of causality is influenced by ability to recognize disease onset, the stability of the environment prior to disease onset, and the permanence of the personality trait (Kasl, 1985). In particular, the development of coronary disease may take many years before the manifestation of any hard clinical endpoints, and these endpoints occur relatively infrequently (Rose, 1982). Thus, large samples of subjects are needed to obtain a large pool of subjects with hard clinical endpoints. In addition, some subjects may be lost at follow up because of attrition rates or because they have undergone CAD interventions, such as angioplasty. Thus, longitudinal studies are limited because of the time factor, which may allow for other confounding influences to occur. As such, the mechanism that links hostility and the gradual development of coronary disease is often difficult to determine.

Review Inclusion Criteria

We initially conducted a computer-based search of the existing literature on CAD association with measures of hostility. The majority of the relevant studies were published in *Psychosomatic Medicine, Journal of Behavioral Medicine, Journal of Chronic Diseases, Journal of Psychosomatic Research*, and *Health Psychology*. An additional search of these journals was undertaken for the years 1984–1991. The following criteria were used for inclusion/exclusion in the present review (a) exclusion of studies that used projective tests, because these studies lacked standardized scoring criteria; (b) exclusion of studies that used state measurements of hostility or anger because of limited temporal stability; and (c) exclusion of studies that solely used angina as an endpoint.

The relationship between hostility and CAD is examined separately in cross-sectional and longitudinal studies. The individual studies are reviewed and a summary for each section is provided. A general discussion follows.

CROSS-SECTIONAL STUDIES

Taken together, cross-sectional studies comparing patients with CAD to a control group of subjects without CAD, and cardiac catheterization studies evaluating subjects at high risk for coronary disease development, provide support for a positive association between hostility and coronary disease, although methodological problems occasionally hinder confident interpretation of these findings. In the following section, a selected review of case-control studies is provided, followed by a review of catheterization studies evaluating patients at high risk for CAD.

Selected Review of Case-Control Studies

A brief summary of nine cross-sectional studies evaluating hostility is provided in Table 4.1. Of these nine studies, three well-conducted studies are particularly noteworthy. Van Dijl (1982) compared male MI patients with a control sample matched for age, sex, and education in three independent samples of a Dutch population. Results indicated that male MI patients were significantly more hostile than the control samples, as measured by a nine item hostility/aggressiveness scale. Similarly, Bengtsson, Hallstrom, and Tibblin (1973) compared 42 women post MI (6–36 months) and a random subsample of 68 non-CAD females. Compared to controls, the MI females evidenced higher scores on the Aggression subscale of the Cesarec–Marke's Personality Schedule. A third study was unusual in that it extends the investigation of the hostility-coronary disease association to peripheral artery disease, which is presumed to involve many of the same pathophysiological mechanisms as coronary artery disease. Joesoef, Wetterhall, DeStefano, Stroup, and Fronek (1989) examined the prevalence of peripheral artery disease by ultrasound Doppler examination in a young population of 4,462 male Vietnam veterans. The Cook–Medley Hostility Inventory positively predicted the prevalence of peripheral artery disease, even after adjusting for standard risk factors in a multiple logistic regression.

In summary, seven out of nine case-control studies revealed positive relationships between hostility traits and the presence of coronary disease (see

TABLE 4.1
Cross-Sectional Studies of Hostility and CAD

Authors	Subjects	Hostility Variable	Result	Comments
Bengstton et al., 1973	42 female MI patients and 68 randomly selected control females.	Aggression from Cesarec–Marke's personality schedule.	+	
Croog et al., 1976	283 male MI patients, wives as controls.	Self-rating on how easily angered.	+	May merely reflect gender difference.
Joesoef et al., 1989	4,462 young male Vietnam veterans.	Cook–Medley Hostility Inventory.	+	Prevalence of peripheral artery disease.
Miles et al., 1954	46 young MI & 49 controls. Different for SES and education.	Aggression from psychiatric interview.	+	Interviewers not blind to group status. 50% attrition rate from original study.
Miller, 1965	34 MI & 34 controls. Matched on age, sex, and education.	Hostility from verbal analysis of interview.	ns +	Nonsignificant in total group. Positive in young age group. Interviewers not blind but raters blind to clinical status.
Theorell, 1973	62 male MI & 109 randomly selected control males.	One-item hostility question.	+	Questionable reliability of one item question.
Theorell et al., 1979	30 male pairs of twins. More healthy and less healthy twin.	Buss Aggression Inventory.	ns	Dropped 4 subjects from analysis. Questionable CAD rating.
V. Dijl, 1982	Male MI & control patients. Matched age and SES. 3 independent samples: 204, 196, 126 subjects.	Dutch hostility scale.	+	Nine item questionnaire.
Wardwell et al., 1963	32 male MI & 32 males hospitalized for acute condition. Age matched.	One-item hostility question.	ns	Questionable reliability of one item question.

Table 4.1). Unfortunately, the majority of these studies have methodological flaws such as (a) lack of blind ratings of hostility, or interviewers being aware of the patients' CAD status (Miles, Waldfoger, Barrabee, & Cobb, 1954; Miller, 1965); (b) large attrition rates when reexamining an existing study sample (Miles et al., 1954; Theorell, DeFaire, Schalling, Adams, & Askevold, 1979); (c) use of a single item hostility question, which may have limited reliability (Theorell, 1973; Wardwell, Bahnson, & Caron, 1963); and (d) use of an inappropriate control group, such as wives of the coronary patients (Croog, Koslowsky, & Levine, 1976; Theorell et al., 1979). As noted, three of these nine studies appeared to be methodologically sound (Bengstton et al., 1973; Joesoef et al., 1989; Van Dijl, 1982), and these three studies revealed positive relationships in both males and females. Thus, although problems exist, case-control studies do suggest a relationship between hostility and CAD and provide a basis for undertaking more elaborate and costly longitudinal studies.

Coronary Angiography Studies

Studies evaluating patients referred for coronary angiography are separated into those which used paper-and-pencil questionnaires and those which employed a behavioral measure of hostility (studies are summarized in Table 4.2).

Cook–Medley Hostility Inventory. Three studies used high risk patients to examine relationships between hostility and angiographic evidence of severity of atherosclerosis. In one of the first studies in this area, Williams, Haney, Lee, Kong, Blumenthal, and Whalen (1980) demonstrated that hostility was significantly related to coronary occlusion at cardiac catheterization in 424 angiography patients, including 117 women. Forty-eight % of patients with a low level of hostility (scores below 10) had significant occlusion in comparison to 70% of the patients with a high level of hostility (scores greater than or equal to 10). This relationship was not linear, but instead appeared to involve a threshold effect: Subjects with hostility scores greater than 10 (ranging from 11 to a possible 50) were at approximately equal risk for obstruction. Because both men and women were analyzed together, this study could be confounded by gender. Specifically, as women are found to be less hostile (Barefoot, Peterson, Dahlstrom, Siegler, Anderson, & Williams, 1991; Blumenthal et al., 1987), and because they develop CAD at a later age than men (Johansson, 1989), these results may be due to gender differences.

A recent study by Helmer, Ragland, and Syme (1991) evaluated both the Cook–Medley Hostility Inventory and an SI-derived measure of hostility in 118 men and 40 women who underwent diagnostic cardiac catheterization. Cook–Medley hostility scores were analyzed as continuous scores, as a dichotomous score, and by several different cutpoints similar to those used

TABLE 4.2
Cross-Sectional Studies of Hostility in High Risk and CAD Populations

Authors	Subjects	Hostility Variable	CAD Endpoint	Result
Arrowood et al., 1982	76 patients referred for coronary angiography.	SI hostility	Degree of obstruction	+
Dembroski et al., 1985	98 men & 33 women referred for coronary angiography.	SI hostility	# of obstructed arteries	+
			Severity of obstruction	+
		anger-in	# of obstructed arteries	+
			Severity of obstruction	+
	Subsample of 80 patients.	Cook-Medley hostility	# of obstructed arteries	ns
			Severity of obstruction	ns
Helmer, Ragland, & Syme, 1991	118 men & 40 women referred for coronary angiography.	Cook-Medley hostility	≥ 75% obstruction	ns
		SI hostility	≥ 75% obstruction	ns
Helmers et al., 1991	63 CAD men & 17 CAD women referred for thallium stress testing.	Cook-Medley full-scale composite score	Severity of ischemia	ns
			Severity of ischemia	+
Kneip et al., 1991	112 men & 73 women referred for thallium stress testing.	Multidimensional Anger Inventory		
		self-rating	Abnormal scan	ns
		spouse-rating	Abnormal scan	+
MacDougall et al., 1985	126 men referred for coronary angiography.	SI hostility	# of obstructed arteries	+
		anger-in		+
Siegman, Dembroski, & Ringel, 1987	51 men & 21 women referred for coronary angiography.	Buss-Durkee neurotic hostility	# of obstructed arteries	ns
			Atherosclerotic severity	−
		reactive hostility	# of obstructed arteries	+
			Atherosclerotic severity	+
Stevens et al., 1984	21 men & 23 women referred for carotid artery angiography.	Jenkins Activity Survey hostility	Obstruction: None / Moderate / Severe	curvi-linear
Williams et al., 1980	307 men & 117 women referred for coronary angiography.	Cook-Medley hostility	Obstruction: Nonsignificant / Significant	+

in previous research. No significant relationships were found between Cook–Medley hostility and the presence or absence of significant coronary occlusion ($<$ 75%), or for mean occlusion in the four coronary arteries. Furthermore, coronary occlusion data was also analyzed for a gender by hostility interaction and an age (younger versus older) by hostility interaction; no significant interactions were demonstrated. These results suggest that, in this sample, hostility was not associated with angiographic evidence of coronary disease, regardless of age and gender. These analyses were repeated using the SI-derived hostility, with no significant relationships emerging from these analyses.

In summary, research demonstrated an inconsistent relationship between Cook–Medley Hostility Inventory and coronary angiographic evidence of CAD. Only one of the three studies found a positive relationship (Williams et al., 1980), whereas the two remaining studies found nonsignificant relationships (Dembroski et al., 1985; Helmer et al., 1991).

Other Self-Report Questionnaires. Research conducted in other countries and in the United States employed other measures of hostility to examine associations with CAD endpoints. Three studies evaluated patients referred for cardiac catheterization. Siegman, Dembroski, and Ringel (1987) evaluated two hostility components from the Buss–Durkee Hostility Inventory—Neurotic Hostility and Reactive Hostility—in 51 males and 21 females referred for diagnostic coronary angiography. Neuroticism has been found to be related to angina, but not to clinical CAD endpoints (Costa & McCrae, 1987). Neurotic Hostility is characterized by resentment, suspicion, and the experience of anger and irritability, whereas Reactive Hostility refers to self-reports of the display of anger and annoyance. The dependent measures in this study were the number of vessels with obstruction greater than 75% and a severity of atherosclerosis measurement that incorporated both the amount of occlusion and the location of the occluded artery. In subjects below 60 years of age, Neurotic Hostility was inversely related to the severity of atherosclerosis, whereas Reactive Hostility was positively related to the number of obstructed vessels and severity of atherosclerosis, even when gender was statistically controlled. There were no significant relationships found among the older patients. This study underscores the importance of separating out the neurotic component from hostility, because the neurotic component can lead to nonsignificant or negative associations. These findings also suggest that the relationship between hostility and CAD is limited to younger populations.

In an unusual study, Stevens, Turner, Rhodewalt, and Talbot (1984) examined severity of carotid atherosclerosis—which results in cerebral vascular disease rather than CAD—as an endpoint. The presumption was that the same pathophysiological mechanisms for coronary atherosclerosis would also result in carotid atherosclerosis. Twenty-one males and 23 female subjects were categorized into severe (>75%; $n = 10$), moderate (25%–75%; $n = 17$) or no stenosis (<25%; $n = 17$) groups based on estimates of blockage. Response on a 3-item, hostility questionnaire from the Jenkins Activity Survey revealed that hostility was marginally significantly related to severity of stenosis categories. However, inspection of the means revealed that the most severe stenosis group had the least hostility, the moderate stenosis group had the greatest hostility, and the no stenosis group had intermediate hostility scores. Although contrary to the initial hypothesis, this curvilinear relationship was also found in the prospective study by Shekelle, Gale, Ostfeld, and Oglesby (1983) using the Cook–Medley Hostility Inventory, which we review in a subsequent section. However, gender was not considered in the analyses and may have confounded these results if women had less severe disease.

In a more recent study, Kneip et al. (in press) evaluated both spouse and self-ratings of anger as predictors of either normal or abnormal thallium exercise stress tests in 112 men and 73 women referred for the evaluation of chest pain. The Multidimension Anger Inventory was used to assess Hostile Outlook and Anger Suppression. The self-rating for Hostile Outlook and Anger Suppression was not associated with abnormal thallium stress tests, but spouses ratings of patients' Hostile Outlook and Anger Suppression were significantly associated with the presence of abnormal thallium scans. Spouse ratings of Hostile Outlook remained significant, even after adjusting for standard risk factors. The nonsignificant self-ratings of Hostile Outlook and Anger Suppression may have been due to the inverse relationship between self-reports of Hostile Outlook and Anger Suppression and social desirability, indicating that patients may not have accurately self-reported. These results suggest that a spouse rating of patient hostility could be used in behavioral cardiology research, and may be less influenced by social desirability factors.

To summarize briefly, two of the three high risk studies that used other paper-and-pencil measures of hostility found positive relationships to disease endpoints (Kneip et al., 1992; Siegman et al., 1987). Siegman's study underscores the importance of evaluating younger populations and obtaining a hostility measure that does not measure neuroticism. The study by Kneip et al. (1992) suggested that a spouse rating of patient hostility may more accurately reflect components that are associated with coronary disease.

Structured Interview. Four studies employed hostility derived from the SI in evaluating angiographic evidence of CAD. Arrowood, Uhrich, Gomillion, Popio, and Raft (1982) examined 76 patients admitted for diagnostic coronary angiography. The hostility component of the SI was significantly correlated with the degree of CAD obstruction. These data are presented in a short research abstract form, so no information on the population's age or gender was provided; therefore, caution is warranted when interpreting this study.

Dembroski, MacDougall, and colleagues conducted two separate studies that analyzed relationships among both SI Potential for Hostility and Anger-in (suppression of anger), and cardiac catheterization results (Dembroski et al., 1985; MacDougall, Dembroski, Dimsdale, & Hackett, 1985). Dembroski et al. (1985) evaluated 131 patients (including 33 females) who were referred for diagnostic coronary angiography at Duke University. Patients were selected from a sample who had 0, 2, or 3 diseased vessels. The outcome measures in the study were the number of vessels with significant stenosis, and a stenosis severity score summing extent of disease in all four coronary arteries. Study results indicated that the characteristics of Potential for Hostility and Anger-in added significantly to standard risk factors in predicting both the number and severity of stenosis in obstructed vessels. Furthermore, there was a significant interaction between Potential for Hostility and Anger-in; that is, high-hostile patients who were also high on Anger-in had the greatest number of obstructed vessels and the most severe vessel stenosis, even after statistically adjusting for standard risk factors. As reviewed previously, Cook–Medley hostility scores were obtained on 80 of these 131 high-risk patients, but no significant association between Cook–Medley hostility and the number or severity of obstructed vessels was found.

A second study evaluated 126 male patients from Massachusetts General Hospital who were referred for diagnostic coronary angiography (MacDougall et al., 1985). Potential for Hostility and Anger-in significantly predicted the number of obstructed vessels, even after controlling for standard risk factors. Unlike the previous study, no significant interaction between Hostility and Anger-in was found.

A fourth study in this category was already reviewed in the Cook–Medley section (Helmer et al., 1991). The results indicated no significant relationship between the SI based hostility and significant occlusion in 118 men and 40 women referred for coronary angiography.

In conclusion, three out of four high-risk studies using the SI derived hostility found positive associations with extent of coronary occlusion (Arrowood et al., 1982; Dembroski et al., 1985; MacDougall et al., 1985), and one recent study did not find a significant association (Helmer et al., 1991).

Studies of Coronary Patients

Recently, Helmers, Krantz, Howell, Klein, Bairey, and Rozanski (1993) evaluated Cook–Medley association with extent of exercise induced myocardial ischemia in patients with a high probability of CAD. Exercise tomographic thallium testing is a sensitive technique for detecting the severity of exercise-induced ischemia. In this study, a Composite Hostility score (obtained from Barefoot et al.'s, 1989, scoring criteria of the Cook–Medley) was found to be predictive of exercise-induced ischemia in CAD patients. The full-scale Cook–

Medley hostility score was marginally predictive of exercise-induced ischemia in 80 CAD patients, but no significant relationship was found when males
and females were analyzed separately: in a subsample of men (N = 63), in
a subsample of females (N = 17), and in middle-aged males below the age
of 60 (N = 17). However, Composite Hostility was predictive of severity of
exercise thallium ischemia in the full sample of 80 patients, and was predictive of ischemia in women (N = 17) and in men below the age of 60 (N =
17). There was no significant relationship between Composite Hostility and
thallium exercise ischemia for the total subsample of men. These results suggest that the relationship between hostility and exercise ischemia may only
be exhibited in middle-aged male populations; this would imply that factors
associated with aging may have obscured this relationship in the total male
subsample. Factors associated with aging may not have had as much influence
on the women in this sample, because women develop coronary disease at
a later age than men develop it (Johansson, 1989). Though being slightly older
than the men, these women may be at an earlier stage in CAD development,
which allows for a positive association between hostility and severity of ischemia. To summarize, Composite Hostility, rather than the full-scale hostility
score was significantly related to thallium exercise-induced ischemia. Thus,
the Composite Hostility may be a more sensitive measure of hostility than
the full-scale score for CAD endpoints. These results underscore the need
to separately evaluate men versus women, as well as old versus young patient populations.

Summary

Seven out of nine studies using high risk patients and one study on patients
with probable coronary disease found a positive association between hostility and the measured CAD endpoint. Using paper-and-pencil questionnaires,
Williams et al. (1980) found a positive threshold relationship between hostility and significant coronary obstruction, Kneip et al. (1992) demonstrated that
a spouse rating is associated with abnormal thallium scans, and Siegman et
al. (1987) and Helmers et al. (1993) demonstrated a positive association between hostility and CAD in young populations, but not in older populations.
Using the SI derived hostility, a positive association was demonstrated in three
studies (Arrowood et al., 1982; Dembroski et al., 1985; MacDougall, 1985)
and one study did not find an association (Helmer et al., 1991). Stevens et
al. evaluated carotid atherosclerosis rather than coronary atherosclerosis and
demonstrated a curvilinear relationship between hostility and carotid atherosclerosis. Finally two studies used both the Cook–Medley Hostility Inventory
and the SI-derived hostility: Dembroski et al. (1985) found a positive association with the SI hostility but not Cook–Medley hostility, whereas Helmer et al.
(1991) did not find an association using either one of the measures of hostility.

LONGITUDINAL STUDIES

In the following section, we first review studies that examined initially healthy subjects and then review prospective studies on coronary patients. We first review those studies that utilized the Cook–Medley Hostility Inventory, followed by those studies that used other paper-and-pencil questionnaires, and, lastly, review studies that implemented the SI.

Studies of Initially Healthy Subjects

Cook–Medley Hostility Inventory. There are currently six longitudinal studies of initially healthy subjects that were published using the Cook–Medley Hostility Inventory. Barefoot, Dahlstrom, and Williams (1983) analyzed hostility in a 22-year follow-up study of 225 male medical students from the University of North Carolina. There were significantly fewer CAD events for those subjects with hostility scores below the median of Cook–Medley scores (< 13) in comparison to those subjects with hostility scores above the median (> 13). In a second study, Barefoot et al. (1989) evaluated 118 law students in a 29-year follow-up and found a positive association between hostility scores and total mortality. This analysis could not be done solely for CAD mortality because only 6 out of the 13 deaths were attributed to CAD. Furthermore, a Composite Hostility score was a better predictor of mortality than the full-scale hostility score. The Composite Hostility score was obtained from the summation of three factor analytically derived components of the Cook–Medley Hostility Inventory described as Cynicism, Hostile Affect, and Aggressive Responding. Gender was not reported and it is unclear if this could have affected results. This study used the objective endpoint of mortality, which is in contrast to the previous study by Barefoot et al. (1983), which mixed self-report endpoint data (MI and angina) from the subjects with CAD deaths. Unfortunately, both studies used relatively small samples of subjects (118 and 225), which precluded obtaining a large number of patients with coronary disease over the course of the studies.

A larger sample of 656 young physicians with an average age of 47 at follow-up was evaluated by McCranie, Watkins, Brandsma, and Sisson (1986). The MMPI was administered some 22 years earlier during subjects' medical school admission interviews. At follow-up, self-report data were obtained regarding angina history and MI status. Results indicate that no significant relationship was demonstrated between hostility and CAD development. This study, however, may be confounded by factors related to social desirability because the Cook–Medley Hostility Inventory was administered during an admission interview. The students may have presented themselves in a more favorable manner, thus explaining the markedly lower hostility scores obtained in this study when compared to other studies. Therefore, the lack of a relationship between hostility and the development of CAD may have been due to biased self-reports of hostility.

A social desirability bias may also explain the lack of a significant relationship between hostility and subsequent development of CAD in another study using 280 middle-aged men (Leon, Finn, Murray, & Bailey, 1987). Subjects were businessmen and professionals from Minnesota, average age 45, who were followed for 30 years. There were no significant differences in hostility scores in men who developed heart disease versus those who remained healthy; as such, hostility did not predict future CHD, either before or after adjustment for standard risk factors. However, the authors indicated that the mean hostility score was low for this particular group in comparison to similar groups of men. This may reflect social desirability factors, and could possibly account for the nonsignificant results.

Factors associated with social desirability do not appear to explain the lack of significant results reported by Hearn, Murray, and Luepker (1989). This 33-year follow-up of 1,399 men (mean age 52) who had taken the MMPI as part of their freshmen orientation at the University of Minnesota indicated that there was no relationship between Cook–Medley hostility and CAD mortality and CAD morbidity. An extensive range of positive results found in other studies were considered in this data set, including linear, threshold, and curvilinear relationships, but no significant relationships were found. These null findings may be attributed to the subjects' young age at assessment. Subjects were on average 19 years old when the Cook–Medley was administered, considerably younger than subjects in other studies, and personality traits may not be fully formed at this age. Thus, the reliability between hostility scores at age 19 and at some later age may be low, resulting in a nonsignificant relationship.

The final study that used the Cook–Medley Hostility Inventory reanalyzed data from the Western Electric Study for 10-year and 20-year incidence of MI and CAD death in 1,877 men (Shekelle et al., 1983). Using a logistic regression analysis, these authors specifically tested the hypothesis that a low hostility score (< 10), would be associated with a decreased risk of CAD death. Dichotomized hostility scores were significant predictors of CAD death at the 10-year follow-up, even after controlling for standard CAD risk factors (equivalent to a lowered risk of .68 for low hostiles). At the 20-year follow-up, hostility scores were subdivided into quintiles, and hostility was marginally related to CAD mortality, after adjusting for standard risk factors. Results indicated a nonlinear relationship, which is difficult to interpret. The highest incidence of CAD mortality was in the middle quintile for both the 10-year and 20-year follow-up. Thus, these results demonstrate an inverse U-shaped curve, rather than a linear or threshold relationship, between hostility and CAD mortality, yet this study is frequently cited as support for the hostility–CAD mortality hypothesis.

In summary, longitudinal studies of initially healthy subjects involving the Cook–Medley Hostility Inventory yielded inconsistent findings. Of the studies, two were positive (Barefoot et al., 1983; 1989), one found an inverse U-shaped relationship (Shekelle et al., 1983) and three were negative (Hearn et al., 1989; Leon et al., 1987; McCranie et al., 1986). These studies were confounded by issues related to social desirability (McCranie et al., 1986; Leon et al., 1987), stability of hostility trait (Hearn et al., 1989) and use of small sample sizes (Barefoot et al., 1983; 1989).

Other Self-Report Questionnaires.   There are three longitudinal studies that have used other paper-and-pencil questionnaires to evaluate the hostility–coronary disease association. Hallstrom, Lapidus, Bengtsson, and Edstrom (1986) conducted the only study that evaluated the development of CAD solely in women. In a 12-year prospective study, 795 middle-aged women were administered the Cesarec–Marke Personality Schedule, which has an aggression subscale. The authors compared the data separately for the 11 MI and control patients, and the 33 coronary death patients and control patients. Aggression was not significantly different in either of these analyses. By contrast, in the initial cross-sectional study of this project examining the same sample of women, aggression was greater in the MI patients when compared to control subjects (Bengtsson et al., 1973). These results suggest that the level of aggression may change once the diagnosis of CAD is made.

Haynes, Feinleib, and Kannel (1980) analyzed 1,674 subjects from the Framingham Heart Study for development of CAD over an 8-year period. CAD cases were of a mixed profile, which included MI, sudden death, and angina with or without any EKG abnormalities. The variables of interest here are Anger-in (suppression of anger), Anger-out (the expression of anger), and Anger-discuss (a problem-solving approach to feelings of anger). Men and women were evaluated separately, as well as in three age groups for each sex: 45–54, 55–64, 65+. In males, Anger-out was significantly higher in the 55–64 year-old male controls than among CAD patients. Coronary females in the 55–64 age had significantly higher Anger-in, and lower Anger-out, and Anger-discuss than did the control females. In this study, results suggested that suppression of anger was related to development of coronary disease. This study made a number of statistical comparisons, and few comparisons were found to be significantly different.

The final study discussed used a 3-item, hostility questionnaire to predict CAD death in Finnish men (age 40–59) over the course of 3 years (Koskenvuo et al., 1988). In initially healthy men ($N = 2,885$), there was no relationship between hostility and future CAD mortality. It is possible that a longer time period of follow-up was needed to find a significant association between hostility and coronary disease.

In summary, similar to the findings with the Cook–Medley Hostility Inventory, studies utilizing other paper-and-pencil measures have varied results. Koskenvuo et al. (1988) found no relationship between hostility and CAD death in healthy, middle-aged men, Hallstrom et al. (1986) found no relationship between aggression and incidence of CAD in healthy, middle-aged women, and Haynes et al. (1980) found that anger suppression rather than expression was linked to CAD development in both men and women.

Structured Interview.   This section reviews two studies that employed the SI to assess hostility. Matthews and colleagues were among the first to perform a component analysis of the SI to separate out factors, including hostility, that may predict CAD (Matthews et al., 1977). In this study, a subsample from the prospective Western Collaborative Group Study (WCGS) was analyzed. The subject sample consisted of 62 men who developed a mixed profile of CAD (49 MIs, 11 angina, and 2 with an unavailable specific diagnosis) over the course of 4.5 years and before age 50, and an age-matched control sample of 124 healthy men. The SI was administered prior to occurrence of disease symptomatology, was blindly rated, and resulted in five hostility-related items. Four of these five hostility items were significantly higher for the CAD patients: "potential for hostility," "irritation at waiting in lines," "anger directed outward," and reported "anger more than once per week." There was no difference between the groups on reported "irritation when others are late for an appointment." Since single item comparisons were made without any adjustment in significance levels in this study, caution in the interpretation of the results is suggested.

Hecker, Chesney, Black, and Frautschi (1988) extended Matthews et al.'s (1977) research on WCGS by comparing 250 men who developed CAD (CAD death, MI, and angina) to 500 male controls who were matched by age and the company where they worked. The mean age for the two groups was 48.5, and these men were followed for 8.5 years. Hostility was significantly higher in the CAD patients, even after controlling for the standard risk factors. These positive results on middle-aged men are in contrast to inconsistent results found in studies of middle-aged subject populations that used paper-and-pencil questionnaires on hostility (Hallstrom et al., 1986; Koskenvuo et al., 1988; Leon et al., 1987).

In conclusion, both longitudinal studies of initially healthy subjects using the SI had positive findings (Matthews et al., 1977; Hecker et al., 1988). However, these studies are not independent samples because they both used subjects from the WCGS; thus, they should be considered one study.

Studies of Coronary Patients and Those at High Risk for CAD

Three studies investigated prospectively the associations between hostility and occurrence of CAD events in either coronary patients or subjects at high risk for the development of CAD. These studies employed either a paper-and-pencil measure of hostility other than the Cook–Medley or the SI.

Other Self-Report Questionnaires. Koskenvuo et al. (1988) evaluated a subgroup of men ($N = 104$) who self-reported CAD and/or hypertension, in addition to the previously reported initially healthy men. The 3-item, hostility questionnaire was predictive of future CAD mortality at three years of follow-up, even after adjusting for standard risk factors.

Structured Interview. Dembroski, MacDougall, Costa, and Grandits (1989) compared 192 high-risk men who developed CAD to 384 men who remained free of disease in a 7.1 year follow-up of the MRFIT study. These men were matched for clinical center, but not specifically for age and SES, although known risk factors such as age were adjusted in all analyses. Multiple regression analyses were done using a full range of scores and median splits into high/low hostility scores to predict MI or coronary death. Results indicated that dichotomized hostility scores (high/low hostility) added significantly to known risk factors in predicting MI or cardiac death, whereas the full-scale scores did not predict CAD endpoints. These analyses were repeated for patients who were 47 years of age or younger (median), versus those who were older than 47 years of age. In the younger patients, the dichotomous hostility score was significantly related to MI or coronary death, but the full-scale hostility score was not a significant predictor of disease. Neither the full-scale nor the dichotomized hostility scores was predictive in the older patients. These results suggest that there is a threshold effect rather than a linear effect for hostility scores in high-risk populations, because there were no significant linear relationships. Furthermore, the relationship between hostility and CAD is manifested in younger populations, even after adjusting for known risk factors.

In the final longitudinal study reviewed, Powell and Thoresen (1985) utilized a subsample from the Recurrent Coronary Prevention Project, which followed 118 men with a previously diagnosed MI for the recurrence of a cardiac event (MI, CAD death, or congestive heart failure). By the end of a two-year follow-up period, 44 of the 118 men experienced a second cardiac event. Hostility was found to be significantly higher in those men with a second MI; however, those men with recurrent cardiac events also experienced significantly more severe initial heart attacks, the latter not being controlled for statistically. Thus, the two groups differed on level of hostility, and on the severity of heart damage because of initial MI.

Three studies of CAD patients or patients at high risk for the development of CAD found that hostility predicted future occurrence of a cardiac event. Koskenvuo et al. (1988) demonstrated that hostility was predictive of CAD mortality in self-reported CAD or hypertensive patients. Powell and Thoresen (1985) found that SI derived hostility predicted a recurrent cardiac event in cardiac patients and Dembroski et al. (1989) demonstrated that the SI hostility predicted MI or cardiac death in high-risk patients.

Summary

Of the 13 longitudinal studies reviewed, nine had positive findings and four had negative findings (see Table 4.3). In studies that used paper-and-pencil measures with initially healthy subjects, the findings are split. In studies using the Cook–Medley Hostility Inventory, Barefoot et al. (1983, 1989) found a positive relationship between hostility and CAD, and Shekelle et al. (1983) found an inverse U-shaped relationship. However, no relationship was found in the remaining three studies with the Cook–Medley Hostility Inventory (Hearn et al., 1989; Leon et al., 1987; McCranie et al., 1986). Of the three studies that utiltized other paper-and-pencil hostility measures in initially healthy subjects, Koskenvuo et al. (1988) found no relationship between hostility and CAD death, Hallstrom et al. (1986) found no relationship between aggression and CAD incidence in a sample of women, and Haynes et al. (1980) found that anger suppression was related to CAD development in men and women. Both of the studies of initially healthy subjects that employed the SI found a positive relationship between hostility and CAD, although the two samples are related (Matthews et al., 1977; Hecker et al., 1988).

In the three studies that used patients already diagnosed with CAD or patients at high risk for CAD, a significant relationship was found between hostility and CAD. Koskenvou et al. (1988) demonstrated that a paper-and-pencil hostility measure predicted CAD mortality. Powell and Thoresen (1985) found that SI-derived hostility predicted a recurrent cardiac event and Dembroski et al.'s (1989) findings indicated that the SI-derived hostility predicted MI or cardiac death.

GENERAL DISCUSSION

From the preceding review, the hostility measurements used clearly indicate the strength and consistency of association of hostility with CAD endpoints. All except one of the studies that utilized the SI yielded positive results, whereas studies using paper-and-pencil measures of hostility appeared to be equally split with conflicting results, some positive and some nonsignificant. A brief summary of studies using different measures of hostility follows.

TABLE 4.3
Longitudinal Studies of Hostility and CAD

Authors	Subjects	Hostility Variable	Result	Comments
Barefoot, Dahlstrom, & Williams, 1983	225 male medical students from NC. 22-year follow-up.	Cook-Medley Low vs. High scores	+	CAD of mixed profile.
Barefoot et al., 1989	118 law students. 29-year follow-up.	Cook-Medley Full-scale score Composite score	+ +	Used total mortality. Only 6 out of 13 deaths were related to CAD. Composite hostility score better predictor.
Dembroski et al., 1989	MRFIT—192 high risk men who developed CAD, 384 high risk controls. Not matched. 7-year follow-up.	SI Hostility Low vs. High scores Full-scale score	+ ns	Relationship found in total population and in younger coronary patients, not in older coronary patients.
Haynes, Feinleib, & Kannel, 1980	1,674 subjects from Framingham heart study. 8-year follow-up.	Males: 55–64 years old anger symptoms anger-out anger-in anger-discuss Females: 55–64 years old anger symptoms anger-out anger-in anger-discuss	ns – ns ns ns – + –	Significance found only in 55–64 age group. Measuring coping mechanism or state anger rather than trait anger. CAD of mixed profile.
Hallstrom et al., 1986	795 females. 12-year follow-up.	Aggression from Cesarec-Mark Personality Sched.	ns	Positive relationship found in case-control study (Bengstton et al., 1973).
Hearn, Murray, & Luepker, 1989	1,399 male freshman college students. 33-year follow-up.	Cook-Medley	ns	Subjects younger than any previous longitudinal study.
Hecker et al., 1988	WCGS—250 males who developed CAD, 500 controls. Matched age. 8.5-year follow-up.	SI Hostility	+	CAD includes patients with angina. Significant relationship even after controlling for risk factors.
Koskenvuo et al., 1988	3,750 men, 2,885 healthy & 104 CAD. 3-year follow-up.	3-item hostility questionnaire.	+ ns	Positive relationship found in CAD patients. Nonsignificant relationship in healthy men.
Leon et al., 1987	280 middle-aged business men. 30-year follow-up.	Cook-Medley	ns	Hostility scores were low.

(Continued)

TABLE 4.3
(Continued)

Authors	Subjects	Hostility Variable	Result	Comments
Matthews et al., 1977	WCGS—62 young males who developed CAD, 124 controls. Matched age. 4.5-year follow-up.	SI–5 items measuring hostility	+	4 out of 5 items significant. CAD of mixed profile—MI, angina, and uncertain.
McCranie et al., 1986	656 medical students. 22-year follow-up.	Cook-Medley	ns	MMPI taken during medical school admission interview.
Powell & Thoresen, 1985	44 males with 2nd cardiac event, 78 males without 2nd cardiac event. 2-year follow-up.	SI Hostility	+	Males with 2nd cardiac event had more severe 1st cardiac event.
Shekelle et al., 1983	1877 males. 10- and 20-year follow-up.	Cook-Medley Low vs. high scores Scores divided into quintiles.	+ curvi-linear	After adjusting for standard risk factors, Middle scores associated with highest mortality.

Studies Using the Cook–Medley Hostility Inventory

Of ten studies employing the Cook–Medley Hostility Inventory, four were found to show a positive relationship with CAD. Two longitudinal studies demonstrated a positive relationship (Barefoot et al., 1983; 1989), one cardiac catheterization study was positive for a high-risk population (Williams et al., 1980), and one study was positive in patients with coronary disease (Helmers et al., 1993). Four of the six longitudinal studies that did not demonstrate a positive relationship (Leon et al., 1987; Hearn et al., 1989; McCranie et al., 1986; Shekelle et al., 1983) were criticized on issues related to social desirability factors, and age at entry into the study. Finally, two cardiac catheterization studies found no relationship between Cook–Medley hostility scores and severity of obstruction (Dembroski et al., 1985; Helmer et al., 1991). In general, the Cook–Medley Hostility Inventory does not demonstrate consistent results between hostility and development of CAD, nor is it associated with increasing angiographic evidence of CAD in high risk patients. Other methodological issues that have not been satisfactorily addressed in most of these studies are related to use of gender, use of small sample sizes, and use of self-report data rather than objective data for CAD.

Two of the positive studies used the Cook–Medley composite score proposed by Barefoot and colleagues (1989). Through content analysis, the components of Cynicism, Hostile Affect, and Aggressive Responding were isolated. When grouped together, they appear to be related to survival and extent of myocardial ischemia. Both studies that utilized the Composite Hostility score found positive results, whereas the full-scale score did not have as strong of an association to CAD endpoints (Barefoot et al., 1989; Helmers et al., 1993). Perhaps the Composite Hostility score, in comparison to the full-scale score, more accurately captures the critical elements of the Cook–Medley Hostility Inventory that are predictive of disease.

Studies Using Other Self-Report Questionnaires

Out of six studies employing other paper-and-pencil measures, three found a positive relationship to coronary disease. Siegman et al. (1987) found a positive relationship between Reactive Hostility and angiographic evidence of coronary disease in a young patient population. Kneip et al. (1992) found a positive relationship between cardiac ischemia indexed by abnormal thallium scans and spouse ratings of Hostile Outlook in high-risk patients. Koskenvuo et al. (1988) found a positive relationship of hostility in coronary patients for future CAD mortality, but no relationship in intially healthy men. A fourth study demonstrated that anger suppression rather than anger expression was related to CAD development, however multiple analyses were done without adjusting significance values (Haynes et al., 1980). Two other studies found nonsignificant results (Stevens et al., 1984; Hallstrom et al., 1986) but have limitations of using a questionnaire with relatively few items. A large multi-item hostility questionnaire may be more sensitive and reliable for detecting individual differences in hostility. Furthermore, as seen in Siegman et al.'s (1987) study, hostility questionnaires may also be measuring other factors that are not strictly associated with hostility, but are associated with neuroticism. Clearly, the components of hostility that are predictive of CAD need to be established; thus, allowing for a more definitive test of the hostility–coronary disease relationship.

Studies Using Structured Interview Potential-for-Hostility

In summary, all but one of the eight studies that have used the SI to assess hostility demonstrated a positive relationship between hostility and coronary disease. Positive associations were found in cross-sectional studies evaluating high-risk patients, in longitudinal studies of initially healthy men, and in coronary patients for recurrence of a cardiac event. The greater predictive ability of the SI-derived hostility may derive from the measurement of overt behavioral hostility rather than from self-report hostility. In an interview situation, it is possible not only to obtain content answers, but more important, to assess behaviors. An individual's behavior may more closely reflect his or her personality, and reflect how that individual interacts with the environment on a day-to-day basis. This behavioral component is lacking in the Cook–Medley Hostility Inventory, as well as in the other paper-and-pencil measures.

Summary of Measurement Differences

In conclusion, the SI potential for hostility appears more consistently to measure the aspect of hostility that is related to coronary disease. However, paper-and-pencil questionnaires are clearly needed; they are cost efficient, easy to administer, and less time consuming than an interview. Further research needs to be done on paper-and-pencil questionnaires to determine their specific disease-relavent hostility components. The Composite Hostility score obtained from Barefoot et al.'s (1989) study may reflect such a component.

What is Hostility Measuring?

Inconsistent results obtained with the Cook–Medley Hostility Inventory and other paper-and-pencil measures indicate that, for a variety of reasons, they may not capture the personality aspects that are linked to heart disease. The Composite Hostility score obtained from the Cook–Medley scale suggests that certain dimensions within hostility may have a stronger association with heart disease than other dimensions. To identify and gain a better understanding of these dimensions, studies have correlated Cook–Medley Hostility scores with a variety of other personality dimensions and social variables. The Cook–Medley Hostility Inventory shows a positive correlation with trait anger, frequency of angry episodes, and a negative association with social support (Hardy & Smith, 1988; Smith & Frohm, 1985). Fontana et al. (1989) demonstrated a positive association between hostility and dependency on others, feelings of self-worth, and self-criticism that were interpreted as suggesting that hostile individuals are conflicted about the desire to oppose others. Both suppression of anger and expression of anger obtained from the Anger Expression Scale have positive associations with the Cook–Medley Hostility Inventory (Suarez & Williams, 1990; Smith & Houston, 1987). Finally, the Cook–Medley Hostility Inventory also shows a positive association to Neuroticism (Suarez & Williams, 1990). Neuroticism appears to measure anger, depression, and anxiety as a personality dimension. Neuroticism is related to angina, but not to hard clinical endpoints of CAD (Belgian–French Pooling Project, 1984; Costa & McCrae, 1987). The Cook–Medley Hostility Inventory is measuring many different dimensions that may or may not be related to CAD disease. Thus, inconsistent results with the Cook–Medley Hostility Inventory may be a result of differences in how various subject samples score on specific dimensions of the scale. For example, one sample of subjects may score high on the neurotic component of the Cook–Medley scale, and thus have no association with hard clinical endpoints, whereas another sample of subjects may score high on Anger-out, which may be the component of the Cook–Medley scale that is associated with coronary disease endpoints. Future research needs to more fully address what specific elements comprise hostility, which elements are associated with disease, and how these elements can be measured.

The Expression of Hostility and Anger

Hostility coping styles may provide further insight into the relationship between hostility and coronary disease. In the previous section, it was noted that the Cook–Medley Hostility Inventory is associated with both anger expression and anger suppression. Very few studies have evaluated both hostility and anger/hostility expression. Dembroski et al.'s (1985) study evaluated both anger suppression and hostility and demonstrated that those who were hostile and suppressed their anger had the most severe coronary artery disease, although this was not replicated by MacDougall et al. (1985). Similarly, Haynes et al. (1980) demonstrated that suppression of anger in both men and women was related to future development of CAD. Furthermore, Miles et al. (1954) found in a cross-sectional study that coronary patients either expressed or repressed their anger more frequently than controls. These results suggest that extremes in anger coping styles may be associated with the development of coronary disease.

The Stability of Hostility Traits

The stability of hostility is another issue that needs to be considered. Personality traits are considered to be stable psychological characteristics (Epstein, 1980), yet it is unclear at what age level they become fully developed, or the extent to which they change over the life span. Prospective studies can span 20 or more years, during which time personality traits are presumed to be stable enough for initial assessments to reflect chronic characteristics. Some evidence for the stability of hostility comes from research that assessed hostility twice, finding that the Cook–Medley Hostility Inventory had a reliability coefficient of .85 for one year (Barefoot et al., 1983) and .84 for 4 years (Shekelle et al., 1983). However, the 24 year test–retest correlation of the Cook–Medley Hostility Inventory was moderate ($r = .39$) in 1,635 subjects aged 17–21 in 1964 (Siegler et al., 1990). This study concluded that personality traits may not be stable until after the age of 21 and perhaps not until age 30. In future research, hostility needs to be assessed periodically throughout the study in the same way that presence and extent of disease is periodically measured.

Issues Related to Social Desirability

The inconsistent results obtained using self-report questionnaires of hostility raise the important issue of accuracy of self-reports in comparison to external evaluations of overt behavior. At several points in this review, we noted that the issue of social desirability was a possible confounding variable in studies that utilized paper-and-pencil measures of hostility. It is unclear to what extent individuals will make conscious efforts to describe themselves favorably on the questionnaire, or to what extent they are unaware of their behavior and are incapable of making objective self-assessments. The SI is an unbiased observation of an individual using both content of answer and quantifiable behavior to assess hostility, which may account for the significant associations found between SI-derived hostility and CAD.

Demographic Issues

Age and gender are known to have an influence on the development of CAD (Johansson, 1989). However, age and gender have not been extensively studied with respect to the hostility and coronary disease relationship.

Age. It has been hypothesized that hostility primarily exerts a pathogenic influence in younger patients rather than in older patients (Williams et al., 1988). The influence of hostility may only be evidenced in the early stages of clinical CAD, and would be overshadowed during later stages by the chronic disease process or factors associated with aging. Therefore, younger patients who are hostile may not survive to the later stages, and those hostile individuals who do survive may be more biologically hardy. This selection would essentially result in an older population of nonhostile and very hardy hostiles; thus, possibly explaining the lack of significant findings in the older populations (Williams et al., 1988). Furthermore, young hostile subjects with CAD may be selected out of studies on middle-aged populations and may explain nonsignificant results demonstrated in these longitudinal studies on initially healthy middle-aged populations (Leon et al., 1987; Hallstrom et al., 1986; Koskenvuo et al., 1988). In our review, we found positive relationships between hostility and CAD endpoints in young subjects at high risk for the development of CAD (Siegman et al., 1987) and in CAD patients (Helmers et al., 1993). Longitudinal studies also demonstrated the development of CAD in young hostile subjects (Matthews et al., 1977; Dembroski et al., 1989), although nonsignificant results were found in young populations (McCranie et al., 1986). Nevertheless, the hypothesis that the relationship between hostility and coronary disease would manifest itself in younger populations appears to be substantiated. Therefore hostility may be a risk factor for premature development of CAD.

Gender.   Studies on CAD patients predominantly involved men, and only three studies evaluated women (Haynes et al., 1980; Hallstrom et al., 1986; Helmers et al., 1993). Two of these were longitudinal studies on women: in one, aggression was not predictive of the development of coronary disease (Hallstrom et al., 1986) and in another, suppression of anger rather than expression of anger was predictive of CAD development (Haynes et al., 1980). A third study evaluated women with CAD and found a positive relationship between a Composite Hostility score obtained from the Cook–Medley scale and severity of thallium exercise ischemia (Helmers et al., 1993). From these studies it is not clear whether the association between hostility and coronary disease found in men holds for women, and further research needs to evaluate this issue.

A common methodological problem in most studies is the failure to control for gender. Because women develop CAD at a later age and are also less hostile than men (Barefoot et al., 1991; Johansson, 1989), differences between men and women could result in spurious positive findings for hostility and CAD. For example, a positive relationship for hostility may be due to women having less hostility and coronary artery obstruction than men; thus, reflecting gender differences. Future studies that use both men and women need to adjust for gender before any statement can be made about the influence of hostility on CAD.

Socioeconomic Status.   Another demographic variable that has rarely been evaluated is the socioeconomic status (SES) of subjects. Very little is known about the interrelationships between SES, hostility, and CAD. Most longitudinal studies involve populations of higher educational levels (e.g. college freshmen, medical school students, businessmen); thus, the positive associations found between hostility and development of CAD have been limited to studies of high SES groups. In cardiac catheterization studies, the SES status of the subjects is rarely reported; thus, it is unknown if lower SES groups have been evaluated. In one cross-sectional study, hostility scores were inversely related to the SES markers of education and occupation (Barefoot et al., 1991). Although CAD is more prevalent in lower SES groups (Pincus, Callahan, & Burkhauser, 1987), it is unknown how hostility would impact lower SES groups in CAD development. Recommendations for future studies are to include lower SES individuals because CAD is more prevalent in this particular SES, and to evaluate for a differential effect of SES on the hostility–CAD relationship.

Concluding Remarks

The personality trait of hostility holds promise for future studies involving (a) patients referred for cardiac catheterization; (b) CAD patients experiencing a second cardiac event; and (c) subjects who develop CAD at a young age in longitudinal studies. Gender of subjects must be controlled in analyses, but more important, research needs to evaluate whether the hostility–coronary disease association is similar in men and women. In addition, studies on low SES groups need to be conducted. If a hostility–coronary disease association is to be found in longitudinal studies, hostility needs to be measured periodically throughout the study, and larger sample sizes must be evaluated in order to obtain a pool of young coronary patients. Finally, although previous research indicates that a behavioral hostility measure may be more accurate, future research needs to distinguish which hostility components are related to coronary disease and how these components can be measured in a standardized manner.

ACKNOWLEDGMENT

This research was supported by grants from the John D. and Catherine T. MacArthur Foundation, USUHS protocol R07233, and NIH grant HL47337. The opinions and assertions expressed herein are those of the authors and should not be construed as representing the views of the USUHS or the Department of Defense.

REFERENCES

Arrowood, M. E., Uhrich, K., Gomillion, C., Popio, K. A., & Raft, D. (1982). New markers of coronary-prone behavior in a rural population. *Psychosomatic Medicine, 44,* 119.

Barefoot, J. C., Dahlstrom, W. G., & Williams, R. B. (1983). Hostility, CHD incidence and total mortality: A 25-year follow-up study of 255 physicians. *Psychosomatic Medicine, 45,* 59–64.

Barefoot, J., Dodge, K., Peterson, B., Dahlstrom, G., & Williams, R. (1989). The Cook–Medley hostility scale: Item content and ability to predict survival. *Psychosomatic Medicine, 51,* 46–57.

Barefoot, J., Peterson, B., Dahlstrom, W. G., Siegler, I., Anderson, N., & Williams, R. (1991). Hostility patterns and health implications: Correlates of Cook–Medley Hostility Scale scores in a national survey. *Health Psychology, 10,* 18–24.

Belgian-French Pooling Project (1984). Assessment of Type-A behaviour by the Bortner scale and ischemic heart disease. *European Heart Journal, 5,* 440–446.

Bengtsson, C., Hallstrom, T., & Tibblin, G. (1973). Social factors, stress experience, and personality traits in women with ischemic heart disease, compared to a population sample of women. *Acta Medica Scandinavica, 549*(Suppl.), 82–92.

Blumenthal, J., Barefoot, J., Burg, M., & Williams, R. (1987). Psychological correlates of hostility among patients undergoing coronary angiography. *British Journal of Medical Psychology, 60,* 349–355.

Blumenthal, J. A., Thompson, L. W., Williams, R. B., & Kong, Y. (1979). Anxiety-proneness and coronary heart disease. *Journal of Psychosomatic Research, 23,* 17–21.

Cleveland, S. E., & Johnson, D. L. (1962). Personality patterns in young males with coronary disease. *Psychosomatic Medicine, 24,* 600–611.

Cook, W., & Medley, D. (1954). Proposed hostility and pharasaic-virtue scales for the MMPI. *Journal of Applied Psychology, 38,* 414–418.

Costa, P. T., & McCrae, R. R. (1987). Neuroticism, somatic complaints and disease: Is the bark worse than the bite? *Journal of Personality, 55,* 299–316.

Costa, P. T., Zonderman, A. B., McCrae, R. R., & Williams, R. B. (1986). Cynicism and paranoid alienation in the Cook and Medley HO-scale. *Psychosomatic Medicine, 48,* 283–285.

Croog, S. H., Koslowsky, J., & Levine, S. (1976). Personality self-perception of male heart patients and their wives: Issues of congruence and "coronary personality". *Perceptual and Motor Skills, 43,* 927–937.

Dembroski, T. M. (1983). Reliability and validity of procedures used to assess coronary-prone behavior. In T. M. Dembroski, S. Weiss, J. Shields, S. Haynes, & M. Feinleib (Eds.), *Coronary-prone Behavior.* New York: Springer-Verlag.

Dembroski, T. M., MacDougall, J. M., Williams, R. B., Haney, T. L. & Blumenthal, J. A. (1985). Components of Type-A, hostility, and anger-in: Relationship to angiographic findings. *Psychosomatic Medicine, 47,* 219–233.

Dembroski, T., MacDougall, J., Costa, P., & Grandits, G. (1989). Components of hostility as predictors of sudden death and myocardial infarction in the multiple risk factor intervention trial. *Psychosomatic Medicine, 51,* 514–522.

Dimsdale, J. E., Hutter, A. M., Hackett, T. P., & Block, P. (1981). Predicting extensive coronary artery disease. *Journal of Chronic Diseases, 34,* 513–517.

Epstein, S. (1980). The stability of behavior. *American Psychologist, 35,* 790–806.

Fontana, A., Kerns, R., Blatt, S., Rosenberg, R., Burg, M., & Colonese, K. (1989). Cynical mistrust and the search for self-worth. *Psychosomatic Research, 33,* 449–456.

Friedman, M. & Rosenman, R. H. (1959). Association of specific overt behavior pattern with blood and cardiovascular findings. Blood cholesterol, blood clotting time, incidence of arcus senilis and clinical coronary artery disease. *Journal of American Medical Association, 169,* 1286–1296.

Hackett, T. P. & Cassem, N. H. (1973). Psychological adaptation to convalescence in myocardial infarction patients. In J. P. Naughton, H. K. Hellerstein, & I. Mohler (Eds.), *Exercise testing and exercise training in coronary heart disease.* New York: Academic Press.

Hallstrom, T., Lapidus, L., Bengtsson, C., & Edstrom, K. (1986). Psychosocial factors and risk of ischemic heart disease and death in women: A twelve-year follow-up of participants in the population study of women in Gothenburg, Sweden. *Journal of Psychosomatic Research, 30,* 451–459.

Hardy, J., & Smith, T. (1988). Cynical hostility and vulnerability to disease: Social support, life stress, and physiological response to conflict. *Health Psychology, 7,* 447–459.

Haynes, S. G., Feinleib, M., & Kannel, W. B. (1980). The relationship of psychosocial factors to coronary heart disease in the Framingham study: III. Eight-year incidence of coronary heart disease. *American Journal of Epidemiology, 111,* 37–58.

Hearn, M., Murray, D., & Luepker, R. (1989). Hostility, coronary heart disease, and total mortality: A 33-year follow-up study of university students. *Journal of Behavioral Medicine, 12,* 105–121.

Hecker, M., Chesney, M., Black, G., & Frautschi, N. (1988). Coronary-prone behaviors in the Western Collaborative Group Study. *Psychosomatic Medicine, 50,* 153–164.

Helmer, D. C., Ragland, D. R., & Syme, S. L. (1991). Hostility and coronary artery disease. *American Journal of Epidemiology, 133,* 112–122.

Helmers, K., Krantz, D., Howell, R., Klein, J., Bairey, N., & Rozanski, A. (1993). Hostility and myocardial ischemia in coronary artery disease patients: Evaluation by gender and ischemic index. *Psychosomatic Medicine, 50,* 29–36.

Jenkins, C. D., Stanton, B., Klein, M. D., Savageau, J. A., & Harken, D. E. (1983). Correlates of angina pectoris among men awaiting coronary bypass surgery. *Psychosomatic Medicine, 45,* 141–153.

Joesoef, R., Wetterhall, S., DeStefano, F., Stroup, N., & Fronek, A. (1989). The association of peripheral arterial disease with hostility in a young, healthy veteran population. *Psychosomatic Medicine, 51,* 285–289.

Johansson, S. (1989). Longevity in women. In P. Douglas & A. Brest (Eds.), *Heart disease in women.* Philadelphia: F. A. Davis Co.

Kannel, W. B., Sorlie, P., & McNamara, P. M. (1979). Prognosis after initial myocardial infarction: The Framingham study. *American Journal of Cardiology, 44,* 53–59.

Kasl, S. V. (1985). Environmental exposure and disease: An epidemiological perspective on some methodological issues in Health Psychology and Behavioral Medicine. In J. E. Singer and A. Baum (Eds.) *Advances in environmental psychology: Methods and environmental psychology* (Vol. 5, pp. 119–146). Hillsdale, NJ: Lawrence Erlbaum Associates.

Kneip, R., Delamater, A., Ismond, T., Milford, C., Salvia, L., & Schwartz, D. (in press). Self- and spouse ratings of anger and hostility as predictors of coronary heart disease. *Health Psychology.*

Koskenvuo, M., Kaprio, J., Rose, R., Kesaniemi, A., Sarna, S., Heikkila, K., & Langinvainio, H. (1988). Hostility as a risk factor for mortality and ischemic heart disease in men. *Psychosomatic Medicine, 50,* 330–340.

Leon, G., Finn, S., Bailey, J., & Murray, D. (1987). The inability to predict cardiovascular disease from MMPI special scales related to Type-A patterns. *Psychosomatic Medicine, 49,* 205 (Abstract).

MacDougall, J. M., Dembroski, T. M., Dimsdale, J. E., & Hackett, T. P. (1985). Components of Type-A, hostility, and anger-in: Further relationships to angiographic findings. *Health Psychology, 4,* 137–152.

Matthews, K. A. (1988). Coronary heart disease and Type-A behaviors: Update on an alternative to the Booth–Kewley & Friedman (1987) quantitative review. *Psychological Bulletin, 104,* 373–380.

Matthews, K. A., Glass, D. C., Rosenman, R. H., & Bortner, R. W. (1977). Competititve drive, Pattern-A and coronary heart disease: A further analysis of some data from the Western Collaborative Group Study. *Journal of Chronic Diseases, 30,* 489–498.

McCranie, E., Watkins, L., Brandsma, J., & Sisson, B. (1986). Hostility, coronary heart disease (CHD) incidence, and total mortality: Lack of association in a 25-year follow-up study of 478 physicians. *Journal of Behavioral Medicine, 9,* 119–125.

Medalie, J. H. Snyder, M., Groen, J. J., Neufeld, H. N., Goldbourt, U., & Riss, E. (1973). Angina pectoris among 10,000 men: 5-year incidence and univariate analysis. *American Journal of Medicine, 55,* 583–594.

Medalie, J., Kahn, H., Groen, J., Neufeld, H., & Riss, E. (1968). The prevalence of ischemic heart disease in relation to selected variables. *Israel Journal of Medical Science, 4,* 789–800.

Miles, H., Waldfoger, S., Barrabee, E., & Cobb, S. (1954). Psychosomatic study of 46 young men with coronary artery disease. *Psychosomatic Medicine, 16,* 455–477.

Miller, C. K. (1965). Psychological correlates of coronary artery disease. *Psychosomatic Medicine, 27,* 257–265.

Miller, T., Turner, C., Tindale, S., Posavac, E., & Dugoni, B. (1991). Reasons for the trend toward null findings in research on Type A-Behavior. *Psychological Bulletin, 110,* 469–485.

Musante, L., MacDougall, J. M., Dembroski, T. M., & Costa, P. T. (1989). Potential for hostility and dimensions of anger. *Health Psychology, 8,* 343–354.

Ostfeld, A. M. Lebovitz, B. Z., Shekelle, R. B. & Paul, O. (1964). A prospective study of the relationship between personality and coronary heart disease. *Journal of Chronic Diseases, 17,* 265–276.

Pickering, T. G. (1985). Should studies of patients undergoing coronary angiography be used to evaluate the role of behavioral risk factors for coronary heart disease? *Journal of Behavioral Medicine, 8,* 203–213.

Pincus, T., Callahan, L. F., & Burkhauser, R. V. (1987). Most chronic diseases are reported more frequently by individuals with fewer than 12 years of formal education in the age 18–64 U.S. population. *Journal of Chronic Diseases, 9,* 865–874.

Powell, L. H., & Thoresen, C. E. (1985). Behavioral and physiologic determinants of long-term prognosis after myocardial infarction. *Journal of Chronic Diseases, 38,* 253–263.

Rose, G. (1982). Incubation period for coronary heart disease. *British Medical Journal, 284*, 1600–1601.

Rosenman, R. H. (1978). The interview method of assessment of the coronary-prone behavior pattern. In T. M. Dembroski, S. M. Weiss, J. L. Shields, S. G. Haynes, & M. Feinleib (Eds.), *Coronary-prone behavior.* New York: Springer-Verlag.

Shekelle, R. B., Gale, M., Ostfeld, A. M., & Oglesby, P. (1983). Hostility, risk of coronary heart disease, and mortality. *Psychosomatic Medicine, 45*, 109–114.

Shekelle, R. B., Hulley, S. B., Neaton, J. (1985). The MRFIT behavioral pattern study: II. Type-A behavior pattern and risk of coronary death in MRFIT. *American Journal of Epidemiology*, 559–570.

Siegler, I., Zonderman, A., Barefoot, J., Williams, R., Costa, P., & McCrae, R. (1990). Predicting personality in adulthood from college MMPI scores: Implications for follow-up studies in psychosomatic medicine. *Psychosomatic Medicine, 52*, 644–652.

Siegman, A., Dembroski, T., & Ringel, N. (1987). Components of hostility and the severity of coronary artery disease. *Psychosomatic Medicine, 49*, 127–135.

Smith, T. W. (1992). Hostility and health: Current status of a psychosomatic hypothesis. *Health Psychology, 11*, 139–150.

Smith, T. W., & Frohm, K. (1985). What's so unhealthy about hostility? Construct validity and psychosocial correlates of the Cook & Medley Ho-scale. *Health Psychology, 4*, 503–520.

Smith, M., & Houston, K. (1987). Hostility, anger expression, cardiovascular responsivity, and social support. *Biological Psychology, 24*, 39–48.

Spielberger, C., Johnson, E., Russell, S., Crane, R., Jacobs, G., & Worden, T. (1985). The experience and expression of anger: Construction and validation of an Anger Expression Scale. In M. Chesney & R. Rosenman (Eds.), *Anger and hostility in cardiovascular and behavioral disorders.* New York: Hemisphere.

Stevens, J. H., Turner, C., Rhodewalt, F., & Talbot, S. (1984). The TABP and carotid artery atherosclerosis. *Psychosomatic Medicine, 46*, 105–113.

Suarez, E., & Williams, R. (1990). The relationships between dimensions of hostility and cardiovascular reactivity as a function of task characteristics. *Psychosomatic Medicine, 52*, 558–570.

Swan, G., Carmelli, D., & Rosenman, R. (1990). Cook & Medley hostility and the Type-A behavior pattern: Psychological correlates of two coronary-prone behaviors. *Journal of Social Behavior and Personality, 5*, 89–106.

Theorell, T. (1973). Psychosocial factors and myocardial infarction—why and how? *Advances in Cardiology, 8*, 117–131.

Theorell, T., DeFaire, U., Schalling, D., Adamson, U., & Askevold, F. (1979). Personality traits and psychophysiological reactions to a stressful interview in twins with varying degrees of coronary heart disease. *Journal of Psychosomatic Research, 23*, 89–99.

Thomas, C. B., Ross, D., & Duszynski, K. R. (1975). Youthful hypercholesterremia: Its associated characteristics and role in premature myocardial infarctions. *The Johns Hopkins Medical Journal, 136*, 193–208.

U.S. Department of Health, Education, and Welfare (1979). Healthy people: Surgeon General's report on health promotion and disease prevention (DHEW Publication No. 79-55071). Washington, D.C.: U.S. Government Printing Office.

Van Dijl, H. (1982). Myocardial infarction patients and heightened aggressiveness/hostility. *Journal of Psychosomatic Research, 26*, 203–208.

Wardwell, W., Bahnson, C., & Caron, H. (1963). Social and psychological factors in coronary heart disease. *Journal of Health and Social Behavior, 4*, 154–165.

Williams, R., Barefoot, J. C., Haney, T. L., Harrell, F. E., Blumenthal, J. A., Pryor, D. B., & Peterson, B. L. (1988). Type-A behavior and angiographically documented coronary atherosclerosis in a sample of 2,289 patients. *Psychosomatic Medicine, 50*, 139–152.

Williams, R., Barefoot, J., & Shekelle, R. (1985). The health consequences of hostility. In M. Chesney & R. Rosenman (Eds.), *Anger and hostility in cardiovascular and behavioral disorders*. New York: Hemisphere.

Williams, R. B., Haney, T. L., Lee, K. L., Kong, Y., Blumenthal, J. A., & Whalen, R. E. (1980). Type-A behavior, hostility, and coronary atherosclerosis. *Psychosomatic Medicine, 42*, 539–549.

5

ANGER, HOSTILITY, AND PSYCHOPHYSIOLOGICAL REACTIVITY

B. Kent Houston
University of Kansas

Psychophysiological reactivity has been hypothesized to contribute to the link between cardiovascular disease (CVD) and anger, hostility, and related behaviors (see Williams, chapter 6). An important question, then, is what evidence is there that anger, hostility, and related behaviors are associated with psychophysiological reactivity?

Before this question can be adequately addressed, consideration should be given to issues of conceptualization and assessment of these variables. (See Smith, chapter 2, for a more detailed discussion of conceptualization, and Barefoot and Lipkus, chapter 3, for a more detailed discussion of assessment.)

Anger generally is regarded as an emotional state that involves displeasure, ranging in intensity from mild irritation to rage (Buss, 1961); thus, anger is an affective psychological feature. In regard to affect, anger-related feelings such as contempt, disgust, resentment, and so forth, have appeared in the literature concerning cardiovascular disease and should not be overlooked. Recently, anger-related feelings have been subsumed under the more general term *neurotic hostility* because they have been found to correlate with measures of anxiety and neuroticism (Dembroski & Costa, 1977).

Hostility has been defined as an enduring attitude of ill will and a negative view of others (Buss, 1961) and as such is a cognitive psychological feature. Anger-related feelings and hostility are frequently associated with behaviors that are aversive or harmful to others. Specifically, the term *aggression* has been used to refer to behaviors that result in harm to people or objects (Buss, 1961). Further, behaviors that are aversive or harmful to others recently have been subsumed under the more general term *expressive hostility* (Dembroski & Costa, 1987). Thus, aggression and expressive hostility are behavioral features.

Conceptually, then, these variables can be differentiated into those that are cognitive (viz. hostility), affective (e.g., anger, neurotic hostility, etc.), and behavioral (e.g., aggression, expressive hostility, etc.). In considering the role that these variables may play in the development of CVD, attention has focused on enduring or dispositional variables. The process by which CVD develops takes time, and if psychological or behavioral variables contribute to this process, they must persist in time rather than be transient. (This, however, does not deny the possibility that transient episodes of anger or aggression may contribute to precipitating a clinical event.)

Although distinctions can be made between the conceptual definitions of anger, hostility, aggression, and neurotic and expressive hostility, with the exception of anger, the measures that are typically used in psychophysiological and epidemiological studies have not been derived in a rational, a priori fashion to assess these constructs, and thus do not provide operational definitions that clearly assess or distinguish between them. Thus, most of the ostensible measures of the aforementioned concepts are heterogeneous in regard to the constructs actually assessed. Ultimately, this state of affairs obscures the conclusions that can be drawn concerning the extent to which particular variables, namely, hostility, aggression, and so forth, are associated with psychophysiological reactivity and/or cardiovascular disease.

In addition to the aforementioned variables, there has also been interest in the relation between CVD, psychophysiological reactivity, and measures which reflect inhibited or uninhibited modes of dealing with anger-related feelings and behaviors. The extent to which people deny the experience of anger-related feelings and/or inhibit overtly expressing such feelings can be construed as attempts to cope in a manner that involves inhibiting thought processes (e.g., awareness of provocation, the feelings themselves, etc.) and/or anger-related behaviors. This mode of dealing with anger-related feelings and behaviors frequently is referred to as *Anger-in*, though the use of the same term to refer to the inhibition of both the *experience* and the overt *expression* of anger-related feelings obscures a distinction that may be theoretically and practically important. In any event, this mode has been contrasted with the extent to which people overtly express anger-related feelings, which could be construed either as coping, in terms of ventilating these feelings, or as failing to cope in the sense of being unable to inhibit overtly expressing them. This mode of dealing with anger-related feelings frequently is referred to as *Anger-out*.

In terms of measurement, the extent to which people overtly express anger-related feelings has, for the most part, been measured by scales labeled as *Anger-out* that were designed to directly assess this mode of dealing with anger-related feelings. In contrast, people who deny the experience of anger-related feelings and/or inhibit overtly expressing such feelings have been identified in two ways. One way is from high scores on scales labeled as *Anger-in* that were designed to directly assess this manner of dealing with anger-related feelings. The second way, almost always post hoc, is from low scores on measures of anger-related feelings, hostility, aggressive behavior, and Anger-out by assuming that some of the people who obtain low scores on these measures are denying experiencing or expressing anger-related feelings. The second approach to assessing Anger-in creates interpretive problems. For instance, how does a person know a priori whether low scores on measures of anger-related feelings, hostility, aggressive behavior, and Anger-out simply reflect low levels of these constructs, or whether low scores on these measures reflect the denial of experiencing or expressing anger-related feelings?

Conceptually, mode of dealing with anger-related feelings may best be viewed as a moderating variable. That is, from a theoretical point of view (see also Engebretson, Matthews, & Scheier, 1989), the manner in which individuals deal with anger-related feelings may be important primarily or only for those individuals who chronically experience such feelings by virtue of enduring characteristics of their personalities (e.g., anger-proneness, hostility, etc.), and/or their environments (e.g., frequent or pervasive exposure to interpersonal stressors). In terms of study design, this point is most clearly seen in those investigations in which interactions are examined between a measure that may be interpreted as assessing the manner in which individuals deal with anger-related feelings and a measure of anger, hostility, and so forth, or levels of interpersonal stress.

It should be noted though that scales created to measure Anger-in and Anger-out also tend to be correlated with measures of anger-proneness (Spielberger et al., 1985), and neurotic and expressive hostility and antagonism (Suarez & Williams, 1990).[1] Perhaps these associations come about because of how frequently and/or intensely people inhibit or express anger-related feelings depends on how frequently and/or intensely they experience these feelings. The reason aside, the relations occasionally found between measures of Anger-in and Anger-out and psychophysiological reactivity and CVD may be due to the combination of Anger-in or Anger-out and the dispositions to experience anger-related feelings and express anger-related behaviors with which they are correlated. However, these correlations are

---

[1]As noted later, compared with Anger-in, Anger-out tends to be more related to antagonism and expressive hostility and less related to neurotic hostility (see Suarez & Williams, 1990).

not sufficiently strong to result in consistent or robust relations with reactivity by themselves. Thus, both conceptually and practically, measures of Anger-in and Anger-out are probably best employed as moderators of relations between reactivity, environmental events, and/or measures of dispositions to experience anger-related feelings or express anger-related behaviors.

Having addressed issues of conceptualization and operationalization of the variables, we now turn to the two major objectives of the present chapter. One objective is to survey studies that investigated relations between psychophysiological reactivity, and (a) measures that have been regarded as assessing anger, neurotic hostility, hostility, aggression, and expressive hostility; and (b) measures that have been interpreted as reflecting inhibition of the experience of anger, inhibition of the expression of anger-related feelings, and uninhibited expression of anger-related feelings.

The second objective is to call attention to some of the issues that need to be considered by researchers who investigate possible associations between these variables and reactivity. In this regard, an important encompassing consideration is that anger-related characteristics operate within a framework of other variables and processes to potentially affect reactivity. In other words, an anger-related characteristic does not influence reactivity separately or directly, but it does in the context of other variables and processes, which include, but are not confined to, other personality characteristics, individual differences, the nature of the situation that the individual encounters, and so forth. It is important to look at certain aspects of the study that the subjects encounter, including the investigator, the assessment devices, and so forth. In this regard, a "negativistic subject role" (see Kazdin, 1980) may be more likely to occur in research that deals with anger-related variables than other variables. Such a role is associated with behaving in a manner that will be of no use to the experimenter and/or is opposite to what the experimenter intends. This role has been suggested as resulting from subjects' concerns over being controlled, or being placed in a position where they are forced to respond.

Various personality characteristics are now considered under three headings that correspond to the labels ascribed to the measures employed: (a) anger and anger-related feelings such as neurotic hostility; (b) hostility; (c) aggression and aggression-related behaviors such as expressive hostility; and (d) Anger-in and Anger-out.

The research reviewed here is intended to be representative of an area, rather than comprehensive. Further, the review is confined to studies in which reactivity was investigated in adult humans and was elicited in identifiable situations. Thus, studies in which children or animals were investigated are not included here.

ANGER/NEUROTIC HOSTILITY

The relationship between reactivity and anger as an enduring characteristic or neurotic hostility has had very little investigation. In a study of males, Holroyd and Gorkin (1983) found that scores on an anger scale by Novaco were related to cardiovascular reactivity during role-played social interactions that were either neutral in nature or assertive in nature. It was found that, across the role-played situations, low-scoring subjects, on the Novaco scale, manifested greater systolic blood pressure (SBP) and heart rate (HR), but not diastolic blood pressure (DBP) responses as compared to high-scoring subjects. These results were interpreted in terms of subjects who cope with the experience of anger with suppression or denial and exhibit greater reactivity.

In a study of males by Suarez and Williams (1990), a factor analysis of measures from Spielberger's Anger Expression Scale, the NEO Personality Inventory, and the Buss–Durkee Hostility Inventory (BDHI) was performed. One factor that emerged was labeled neurotic hostility. Factor scores for neurotic hostility were found to be significantly, positively related to increases in subjects' forearm blood flow (FBF) while they performed an anagrams task and were harassed, but were not related while they performed the task without harassment.

The following explanation may account for the apparent inconsistency in the results of the aforementioned studies. In the absence of interpersonal stress, as when performing an anagrams tasks without harassment in the Suarez and Williams study, individuals with high, in contrast to low anger/neurotic hostility, may not be differentially engaged by the situation, and thus, do not differ in reactivity. In reaction to some interpersonal stress (e.g., being called on to role-play social situations in the Holroyd and Gorkin study), individuals with high, in contrast to low anger/neurotic hostility, may psychologically disengage from the situation either to avoid unpleasant feelings of arousal or to express opposition toward the experiment(er); and thus exhibit substantially less physiological arousal. However, in the face of a high level of interpersonal stress (e.g., harassment, as in the Suarez and Williams' study), individuals with high, in contrast to low anger/neurotic hostility, may no longer be able to inhibit their feelings; and thus exhibit somewhat greater arousal.

Whether or not this interpretation is correct, the findings of the study by Suarez and Williams bring up an important issue, namely, person by situation interaction. The nature of the situation in which the people find themselves, whether experimentally or naturally created, may influence whether the personality characteristic under study will be engaged, and thus its effect on physiological arousal. We return later to emphasize that a person by situation interaction is involved in every study of the relation between anger-related characteristics and reactivity. Generally, this notion highlights the point made in the introduction that anger-related characteristics influence reactivity in the context of other variables and processes, in this instance, the nature of the situation with which the individual is presented.

HOSTILITY

As noted in earlier chapters in this volume, two of the most prominent measures to which the label of hostility has been ascribed are the Cook and Medley Hostility scale (Cook & Medley, 1954) and hostility as rated from the Structured Interview (SI), originally developed to assess Type A.

Cook–Medley Hostility Scale

The Cook and Medley Hostility (Ho) scale was empirically derived from the MMPI; thus, its items are heterogeneous in content. A number of studies conducted attempting to explicate the constructs measured by the Ho scale suggested that although the scale measures the construct of hostility as defined previously, it also measures a variety of other personality facets that are associated, in varying degrees, with hostility. (See Smith, 1992, for a review.) Consequently, the short descriptive label of "cynical hostility" was given to the scale (Smith & Frohm, 1985).

A number of studies were conducted to investigate the association between the Ho scale and reactivity. Generally, in studies in which subjects are confronted with interpersonally stressful situations, relations between Ho scale scores and reactivity are found. In a study by Hardy and Smith (1988), male subjects with high Ho scale scores compared to low Ho scale scores evidenced greater DBP responses during a role-play task involving interpersonal conflict. Reactivity was not related to subjects' Ho scale scores during low conflict interactions. Male subjects performed an anagram task during a study by Suarez and Williams (1989) in which they were either harassed or not harassed. Compared to low Ho subjects, high Ho subjects manifested greater DBP and FBF responses when they were harassed but not when they were not harassed. In a study by Smith and Allred (1989), male subjects took turns debating current events. High Ho subjects, as compared to low Ho subjects, exhibited greater SBP and DBP responses while debating than while not debating. Smith and Brown (1991) found that, when compared to low Ho score husbands, high Ho score husbands exhibited greater SBP while trying to influence their wives' opinion on a topic, but exhibited less SBP when just discussing the topic. Additionally, across conditions, husbands' Ho scores were positively related to HR reactivity. Interestingly, wives' Ho scale scores were unrelated to cardiovascular reactivity whether or not they were trying to influence their husbands' opinion or discuss the topic with them.

Because hostile individuals are suspicious and mistrustful of others (Smith, 1992), and because they have been hypothesized to be insecure (see Houston & Vavak, 1991), self-disclosure to others could be interpersonally stressful for them. Evidence of this was found in a study by Christensen and Smith (1993), in which, when compared to male subjects with low Ho scores, subjects with high Ho scores exhibited greater SBP and DBP responses in reaction to high levels of self-disclosure yet did not differ in reactivity during nondisclosive interaction. Employing ambulatory monitoring in a study of male paramedics, Jamner, Shapiro, Goldstein, and Hug (1991) found that the greatest DBP response manifested by subjects to various work settings was exhibited by high Ho scale subjects to a conflictual work setting (interactions at the hospital). Further, it was found that the greatest HR response exhibited by subjects was that to the conflictual work setting by high Ho scale score subjects who also were high in defensiveness (as measured by the Marlowe–Crowne scale), which was reflected in a significant hostility by defensiveness by work setting interaction. An interpretation of the latter finding is that individuals who try to inhibit experiencing and/or expressing their characteristically negative feelings toward others are particularly responsive to potentially provoking situations. The interpretation of the study by Jamner et al. raises another important issue, namely, the interaction of personality characteristics, as well as the situation in affecting reactivity. This issue underscores the point made earlier that anger-related characteristics influence reactivity in the context of other variables and processes, in this instance, another personality characteristic, as well as the nature of the situation with which the individual is presented.

In an investigation potentially relevant to the influence of interpersonal stressors, high Ho males and females, as compared to low Ho subjects, evidenced greater SBP and DBP responses to an anagrams task perhaps because they became suspicious of deception in the instructions delivered by the laboratory assistant (Weidner, Friend, Ficarrotto, & Mendell, 1989). Another potentially relevant study is that by Pope and Smith (1991) in which as compared to low Ho score males, high Ho score subjects were found to display significantly higher levels of urinary cortisol during the daytime but not on awakening or in the evening. The difference in cortisol secretion between high and low Ho subjects during the daytime, but not during the other two times, may in part have been due to subjects' encountering more interpersonal stressors during the daytime. Similar results were reported by Jamner et al. (1991) in the study of male paramedics mentioned previously. Overall, recordings of SBP during waking hours were significantly higher for high Ho than low Ho scale score subjects. However, recordings of SBP during periods of sleep were also higher for high than low Ho scale score subjects. These results for SBP are at variance with the findings by Pope and Smith (1991) for cortisol and Ho scale scores at more quiescent times of the day. Although, it is possible that ambulatory monitoring and being awakened by the device every two hours during the period of sleep in the Jamner et al. study may have been more disturbing to high than low Ho scale score subjects.

Ho scale scores have not been found to be related to reactivity in all studies in which subjects encountered interpersonal stressors. Ho scale scores were not found to be related to cardiovascular responses to the SI in a study of female subjects by Kamarck, Manuck, and Jennings (1990). Additionally, in a study by Allred and Smith (1991) high and low Ho male subjects were not found to differ in their cardiovascular responses to a task involving discussion of current events issues (e.g., changing abortion laws, capital punishment, etc.) on which subjects had strongly held beliefs. The reasons for these inconsistent results are unclear.

Ho scale scores have not been found to be related in a simple fashion to psychophysiological responses to laboratory tasks that are not associated with interpersonal stress. Ho scale scores were not found to be related to cardiovascular responses to the Stroop color-word interference task or to a mental arithmetic task in a study of males by Smith and Houston (1987). Similarly, Sallis, Johnson, Trevorrow, Kaplan, and Hovell (1987) did not find Ho scores to be related to cardiovascular responses to mental arithmetic or to the cold pressor in a sample of males and females. Moreover, in the study by Kamarck, Manuck, and Jennings (1990) mentioned previously, Ho scale scores of female subjects were not found to be related to cardiovascular responses to either mental arithmetic or concept formation tasks. Additionally, Ho scale scores were not found to be related to cardiovascular or neuroendocrine responses to a mental subtraction task or word identification task in a study of males by Williams, Suarez, Kuhn, Zimmerman, and Schanberg (1991).

In two studies, however, Ho scale scores have been found to be related in a more complex fashion to psychophysiological responses to laboratory tasks, even if they were not associated with interpersonal stress. Employing cluster analysis to identify male subjects who varied in their responses to Ho scale items, Houston, Smith, and Cates (1989) found that subjects who appeared to suppress anger and aggression responded with greater SBP to the Stroop color-word interference task and a mental arithmetic task. Additionally, in a study by Suarez, Williams, Kuhn, Zimmerman, and Schanberg (1991), interactions were found between Ho scale scores and male subjects' resting cholesterol levels for changes in epinephrine, norepinephrine, and HR in response to a mental subtraction task, although not for a word recognition task. The combination of high Ho scales scores and high levels of cholesterol were associated with greater increases in epinephrine, norepinephrine, and HR. Perhaps a disposition for hyperresponsivity in the high Ho subjects was responsible for both chronic high cholesterol levels and acute exaggerated psychophysiological responses to the mental subtraction task. The Suarez et al. findings suggested that consideration should be given more broadly to an interaction between personality characteristics and other individual differences, whether they are nonpersonality attributes or other personality characteristics.

In summary, research findings regarding relations between Ho scale scores and reactivity are most consistent and compelling in suggesting that high Ho scale score subjects exhibit greater psychophysiological responses than low Ho subjects to situations that are high but not low in interpersonal stress. Further, preliminary evidence suggests that other individual differences may moderate relations between Ho scale scores and reactivity to situations high, as well as low, in interpersonal stress. These preliminary findings should encourage further exploration of interactions between Ho scale scores, other individual differences, and situational factors.

Potential for Hostility

A number of studies were conducted on the relation between reactivity and potential for hostility, a variable that is a composite of expressing antagonistic behavior and the frequency and intensity of experiencing anger-related feelings (Dembroski & Costa, 1987). Potential for hostility is assessed via the SI in terms of the content and intensity of an interviewee's responses, as well as the interviewee's style of interacting with the interviewer (Dembroski & Costa, 1987).

The results of the studies concerning a relation between potential for hostility and reactivity have been mixed. Regarding males, Dembroski, MacDougall, Shields, Petitto, & Lushene (1978) found potential for hostility to be positively related to SBP and HR responses across three tasks, namely, a reaction time task, a video pong game, and performance of anagrams. However, potential for hostility was not found to be related to reactivity in males to the SI in a study by Chesney, Ekman, Friesen, Black, and Hecker (1990) or to a pong game under competition, frustration, or harassment conditions by Diamond, Schneiderman, Schwartz, Smith, Vorp, and Pasin (1984). Further, Glass, Lake, Contrada, Kehoe, and Erlanger (1983) found a negative relation in a sample of males between potential for hostility and SBP and DBP responses to a mental arithmetic task and a modified Stroop color-word interference task. Also relevant to this area of research, a measure of hostility derived from the Videotaped Structured Interview (VSI) was found for Swedish males to be related to SBP reactivity and tended to be related to epinephrine and norepinephrine responses to a variety of tasks (star-tracing, mental arithmetic, cold pressor, etc.) in a study by Lundberg, Hedman, Medlin, and Frankenhaeuser (1989). Additionally, Lundberg et al. found that VSI-derived hostility ratings were positively related to HR and tended to be positively related to SBP and cortisol responses at work relative to at home.

Regarding studies on females, in a set of studies by MacDougall, Dembroski, and Krantz (1981), potential for hostility was found to be positively related to SBP responses to the SI and negatively related to HR responses to a reaction-time task in a first study, but positively related to HR and SBP responses to a reaction-time task and unrelated to reactivity to the cold pressor task in a second study. In another study of females (Anderson et al., 1986), potential for hostility was not found to be related to reactivity to either the SI or a mental arithmetic task. In the study by Lundberg and colleagues (1989) mentioned previously, unlike the findings for males, the measure of hostility derived from the VSI was not found for females to be related to psychophysiological responses at work or to reactivity to the variety of laboratory tasks (star-tracing, mental arithmetic, cold pressor, etc.).

The reasons for the inconsistencies in the results concerning potential for hostility and reactivity are unclear. Unlike the studies of cynical hostility, few studies of potential for hostility have involved interpersonal stressors. Potential for hostility and responses to (a) the SI have been investigated in two studies of females, namely, the second study by MacDougall et al. (1981), which yielded expected results, and the study by Anderson et al. (1986), which produced null results; and (b) provocation while performing a task was investigated in a study of males by Diamond et al. (1984), although the study produced null results. More studies need to be conducted in which levels of interpersonal stress are experimentally or naturally manipulated. The process by which ratings of potential for hostility are made may have contributed to the inconsistent findings. Ratings of potential for hostility from SI audiotapes are a complex, subjective procedure (Dembroski, 1978). Ratings of hostility from the VSI are relatively unexplored, although they may be promising by virtue of the availability of both visual as well as auditory cues. The multidimensional nature of ratings for potential for hostility, that is, the combination of judgments concerning antagonistic behavior and frequency and intensity of anger-related feelings, may also contribute to inconsistent findings. It is interesting to note that in the study by Anderson et al. (1986) in which overall ratings of potential for hostility were not found to be related to cardiovascular reasponses to the SI, ratings of all three separate components, in particular antagonistic behavior, were found to be related to SBP and DBP responses to the SI. Thus, separation of ratings of the behavioral component from the affective components in the assessment of potential for hostility may be as fruitful for predicting psychophysiological reactivity as it has been for predicting CHD (cf. Dembroski, MacDougall, Costa, & Grandits, 1989).

AGGRESSION/EXPRESSIVE HOSTILITY

In a study by Jorgensen and Houston (1988), SBP, DBP, and HR were recorded while male subjects performed a mental arithmetic task, during which they were urged to perform more quickly and accurately, and a shock avoidance task. Assessed via scales from the BDHI, a disposition for physical aggression was found to be negatively related to SBP and DBP responses, and verbal aggression was found to be negatively related to DBP responses. These results were interpreted in terms of subjects who suppress aggressive tendencies manifesting greater reactivity.

In the study by Suarez and Williams (1990) mentioned previously, one of two factors found in the factor analysis of measures from Spielberger's Anger Expression scale, the NEO Personality Inventory, and the BDHI was considered to reflect expressive hostility. Factor scores for expressive hostility were found to be positively related to male subjects' SBP and FBF responses while they performed an anagrams task and were harassed but not while they performed the task without harassment.

The following explanation, which is similar to that given for studies of anger/neurotic hostility, may account for the apparent inconsistency in the results of the aforementioned studies. In the absence of interpersonal stress, as when performing an anagrams task without harassment in the Suarez and Williams' study (1990), individuals high in contrast to low aggressiveness/expressive hostility may not be differentially engaged by the situation; thus, they do not differ in physiological reactivity. In reaction to some interpersonal stress (e.g., being urged to perform a task more quickly and accurately and being threatened with shock, as in the study by Jorgensen and Houston, 1988), individuals high in contrast to low aggressiveness/expressive hostility may psychologically disengage from the situation either to avoid unpleasant feelings of arousal or to express opposition toward the experiment(er); and thus, exhibit substantially less physiological arousal. However, in the face of a high level of interpersonal stress (e.g., harassment as in the Suarez and Williams' study), individuals high in contrast to low aggressiveness/expressive hostility may no longer be able to inhibit their aggressive feelings; and thus, exhibit greater arousal. In any event, the results of the Suarez and Williams and Jorgensen and Houston studies again point out the importance of considering a person by situation interactive model in research on reactivity.

ANGER-IN AND ANGER-OUT

There have been relatively few studies on the relation between psychophysiological reactivity and measures that are interpreted as reflecting Anger-in and Anger-out modes of dealing with anger-related feelings and behaviors.

Smith and Houston (1987) did not find relations between cardiovascular responses of male subjects to two experimental tasks and measures, which were employed in the Framingham study (Haynes, Levine, Scotch, Feinleib, & Kannel, 1978), of either expressing anger outwardly or inhibiting anger-related feelings.

In a study by Mills, Schneider, and Dimsdale (1989), males' HR reactivity to a mental subtraction task was found to be significantly, negatively related to two measures of expressing anger outwardly, namely, the Anger-out subscale of Spielberger's Anger Expression scale and a component scoring for Anger-out from the SI. These results were interpreted in terms of subjects who suppress the expression of anger and exhibit greater reactivity. Surprisingly, however, reactivity was not found to be related to an ostensibly more direct measure of suppressing the expression of anger viz. the Anger-in portion of Spielberger's Anger Expression scale. The correlates of the measures of Anger-in and Anger-out employed by Mills et al. may assist in interpreting the conceptually incongruent results. The Anger-out subscale of Spielberger's Anger Expression scale has been found to correlate more highly with measures of antagonism and expressive hostility than the Anger-in subscale (Suarez & Williams, 1990). Thus, in the absence of provocation, high Anger-out individuals may have expressed their antagonism toward the experiment(er) by psychologically disengaging from the situation, which, in turn, eventuated in the negative association between HR reactivity and Anger-out. However, since high Anger-in individuals are less prone to expressive hostility and antagonism and they were not provoked, they did not differentially respond emotionally or physiologically to either the experimental task or the experiment itself; therefore, no association emerged between Anger-in and reactivity.

Several intriguing findings emerged from an elaborate study conducted by Engebretson, Matthews, and Scheier (1989) in an attempt to conceptually reconcile inconsistent findings in this area. First, it was found that the extent to which male subjects express anger outwardly or inhibit expression of anger tended to be associated with greater SBP and HR reactivity when subjects were provoked than when they were not provoked. This notion is congruent with the assertion made earlier that mode of anger expression may best be conceptualized as a moderating variable. Second, it was found that when provoked, but not in the absence of provocation, SBP reactivity tended to be higher when subjects were unable to employ their preferred manner of dealing with anger (i.e., Anger-out individuals were not able to express displeasure and Anger-in subjects were induced to express displeasure). Thus, Engebretson et al. suggested that whether mode of dealing with anger-related feelings is related to psychophysiological responses is influenced by the extent to which individuals are provoked and have or do not have the opportunity to behave in a fashion congruent with their preferred mode. These are intriguing notions that deserve further investigation.

CONCLUSIONS

With the possible exception of research on hostility as operationally defined by the Ho scale, inconsistent results characterize the findings of studies conducted to investigate relations between psycholophysiological reactivity and measures considered to assess dispositions for anger/neurotic hosility, hostility, aggression/expressive hostility, inhibiting the experience of anger, inhibiting expression of anger-related feelings, and uninhibited expression of anger-related feelings.

Research findings regarding relations between the Ho scale and reactivity have been fairly consistent. They suggest that Ho scale scores may be related to exaggerated psychophysiological responses in conjunction with interpersonal stress and/or additional personality characteristics and individual differences.

The findings of studies relating reactivity to both anger/neurotic hostility and aggression/expressive hostility are about equally inconsistent, although, perhaps for the same reasons. Relations between these variables and psychophysiological responses appear to be influenced by degree of interpersonal stress, success or lack of success in coping with anger-related feelings, as well as possible oppositional reactions to the study or investigator(s).

The inconsistency in results concerning potential for hostility may be due to psychometric problems as well as methodological issues. Thus, questions concerning the reliability of ratings of potential for hostility and how to deal with the multidimensional nature of ratings of potential for hostility need to be addressed. Additionally, because few studies of potential for hostility have involved interpersonal stressors, more investigations need to be conducted in which levels of interpersonal stress are experimentally or naturally manipulated.

The results of research on the association between reactivity and mode of dealing with anger-related feelings are also inconsistent. The degree of interpersonal stress which subjects experience, as well as possible oppositional reactions to the study or investigator(s), were discussed as possible reasons for the inconsistent findings.

ISSUES IN CONDUCTING RESEARCH ON ANGER, HOSTILITY, AND REACTIVITY

Although several issues in conducting research in this area have been mentioned in the course of the previous review, they are worth repeating, and others deserve to be highlighted. For the most part, these issues follow from the notion mentioned earlier that an anger-related characteristic does not influence reactivity separately or directly but in the context of other variables and processes, which include, but are not confined to other personality characteristics and individual differences, the nature of the situation with which the individual is presented, and aspects of being in a study, which include reactions to the experimenter, the assessment devices, and so forth.

Personality by Situation Interaction

The studies reviewed here aid in emphasizing that a subject's thoughts, emotions, and behaviors are influenced by a person by situation interaction that is implicitly involved in all reactivity research. Thus, consideration needs to be given to whether the research setting in which subjects find themselves would be expected to engage the anger-related characteristic under study and thus, contribute to physiological arousal.

The concept of a person by situation interaction is obvious when some aspect of an experimental arrangement is manipulated with the intention of investigating differences in relations between the anger-related characteristic and reactivity as a function of levels of the manipulated variable. Examples of this, mentioned previously, were the studies in which interpersonal stress was manipulated and relations between anger-related variables and reactivity were found in the interpersonal stress conditions but not in the control conditions (e.g., Engebretson et al., 1989; Hardy & Smith, 1988; Smith & Allred, 1989; Suarez & Williams, 1989, 1990).

A person by situation interaction, however, applies to the choice of experimental arrangements to which to expose subjects, even in the absence of experimental manipulations. Although the conceptualization of hostility would lead one to expect that experimental arrangements that created suspicion (see Weidner et al., 1988), and so forth, would lead to differences in reactivity between high and low hostile individuals, it would not lead a person to expect experimental arrangements that solely involved mental stress (e.g., mental arithmetic, color-word interference tasks, etc.) to induce differences in reactivity between high and low hostile individuals. And in fact, this is what has been found (see Sallis et al., 1988; Smith & Houston, 1988, etc.). Therefore, in the study of anger-related characteristics and reactivity, care needs to be given to the careful selection of theoretically relevant experimental arrangements, rather than routinely administering tasks that frequently have been employed in studies of reactivity (e.g., mental arithmetic, concept formation tasks, cold pressor, etc.).

Another issue in this regard is whether there is evidence from an assessment of subjects' thoughts, feelings, and/or behaviors that the situation engaged the anger-related characteristic in a theoretically meaningful way. For example, congruent with what an investigator might speculate (a priori or even post hoc), did subjects high relative to low on the anger-related characteristic feel more angry or suspicious, behave more aggressively, and so forth, or unlike what the investigator would have wanted, did they dislike more the psychophysiological measuring apparatus, the experimenter, or having to spend their time in an experiment, and so forth? An important implication of this point is that investigators interested in anger/hostility and reactivity should routinely obtain information about the thoughts, feelings, motivations, and/or behaviors of their subjects, without which adequate conclusions about the results cannot be made. Suggestions as to how this can be done may be found in Strube (1989) and Tennenbaum and Jacob (1989).

Interaction Between Personality Characteristics and/or Other Individual Differences

Stemming from the notion that an anger-related characteristic does not influence reactivity separately or directly but in the context of other variables and processes, consideration needs to be given to examining the combined effects of personality characteristics. Besides the prospect of an additive effect, there is the possibility that an interaction of multiple characteristics may affect individuals' reactions to situations. However, interactions between personality characteristics have been studied infrequently in regard to reactivity. A good example of a study in which potential interactions between personality characteristics were investigated was that by Jamner et al. (1991) who found a significant hostility by defensiveness by work setting interaction for HR, which revealed that the greatest HR response was exhibited by subjects who were high in both Ho scale scores and defensiveness when they were in a conflictual work setting.

Consideration also needs to be given to examining the combined effect of an anger-related characteristic and other individual differences besides personality characteristics. An example of a study in which this was done was that by Jorgensen and Houston (1988) in which an interaction was obtained for SBP reactivity between irritability and family history of hypertension, a constitutional variable. SBP reactivity was positively related to irritability for persons without a family history of hypertension, but was negatively related for persons with a family history of hypertension. Thus, a more complete view of the role of anger-related characteristics in reactivity will be obtained not only by considering interactions between personality characteristics, but also by considering interactions between personality and biological characteristics.

Other Issues

An important issue concerning the findings of laboratory studies of psychophysiological reactivity and anger-related variables is their generalizability to natural environments. A few of the studies reviewed above have involved collecting measures of psychophysiological responses in natural environments (e.g., the study of Ho scale scores and daily urinary excretion of cortisol by Pope and Smith, 1990, the study of Ho scale scores, defensiveness, and cardiovascular responses assessed via ambulatory monitoring by Jamner et al., 1991, the study of VSI-derived potential for hostility and psychophysiological responsivity at work by Lundberg et al., 1989, etc.). Generally, the findings of these studies are congruent with those obtained in laboratory settings. Nonetheless, more research needs to be conducted in non-laboratory settings, not only for reasons of generalizability but also to gather information concerning potential differences in daily experiences and psychophysiological responses to these experiences of people who vary in anger-related variables. In regard to the kinds of questions that could be answered by obtaining the latter information, we can consider the study by Jamner et al. (1991). When in the hospital work setting, did high Ho scale subjects exhibit exaggerated DBP and did defensive, high Ho scale subjects exhibit exaggerated HR responses because of their cynically hostile perceptions of the same interpersonally stressful events to which all the paramedics were exposed, because of interpersonal conflict they helped to create, or both? (See Smith, 1992, for a more thorough discussion of the models underlying these alternatives.)

Most of the investigations concerning an association between psychophysiological reactivity and anger-related variables have employed cardiovascular measures only. Considering the role ascribed to sympathetic-adrenal medullary and pituitary-adrenocortical activity in the development of CVD (see Williams, chapter 6), more studies need to be conducted in which changes in measures of other physiological parameters also are obtained (e.g., epinephrine, norepinephrine, cortisol, testosterone, lipids, renin, etc.).

The majority of studies performed to investigate an association between psychophysiological reactivity and anger-related variables have been conducted on men only. Moreover, of the few investigations that have included both men and women as subjects associations between reactivity and anger-related measures were found for men but not women in the majority (Lundberg et al., 1989; Smith & Brown, 1991) though not all (Weidner et al., 1989) of the studies. The issue of sex differences and similarities in associations between anger-related variables and psychophysiological reactivity is of paramount importance in understanding the role of anger-related variables in CVD for both men and women; thus, it deserves much more attention than it has been given heretofore.

Finally, it has been rare that studies have been performed to investigate relations between psychophysiological reactivity and anger-related variables in non-Whites. (See exception by Anderson et al., 1986.) The issue of ethnic/racial similarities and differences in associations between anger-related variables and psychophysiological reactivity is also very important for understanding the role of anger-related variables in CVD for ethnic/racial groups within the United States; thus, it also deserves much more attention than it has received up until now. Research on sex and ethnic/racial differences in relations between psychophysiological reactivity and personality dispositions also may be helpful in shedding light on sex and ethnic/racial differences in the prevalence and incidence of CVD.

REFERENCES

Allred, K. D., & Smith, T. W. (1991). Social cognition in cynical hostility. *Cognitive Therapy and Research, 15*, 399–412.

Anderson, N. B., Williams, R. B., Jr., Lane, J. D., Haney, T., Simpson, S., & Houseworth, S. J. (1986). Type-A behavior, family history of hypertension, and cardiovascular responsivity among Black women. *Health Psychology, 5*, 393–406.

Buss, A. H. (1961). *The psychology of aggression.* New York: John Wiley & Sons.

Chesney, M. A., Ekman, P., Friesen, W. V., Black, G. W., & Hecker, M. H. L. (1990). Type-A behavior pattern: Facial behavior and speech components. *Psychosomatic Medicine, 53*, 307–319.

Christensen, A. J., & Smith, T. W. (1993). *Cynical hostility, self-disclosure, and cardiovascular reactivity. Psychosomatic Medicine, 55*, 193–202.

Cook, W. W., & Medley, D. M. (1954). Proposed hostility and pharisaic-virtue scales for the MMPI. *Journal of Applied Psychology, 38*, 414–418.

Dembroski, T. M. (1978). Reliability and validity of methods to assess coronary-prone behavior. In T. M. Dembroski, S. M. Weiss, J. L. Shields, S. G. Haynes, & M. Feinleib (Eds.), *Coronary-prone behavior* (pp. 95–106). Berlin: Springer-Verlag.

Dembroski, T. M., & Costa, P. T., Jr. (1987). Coronary-prone behavior: Components of the Type-A pattern and hostility. *Journal of Personality, 55*, 211–235.

Dembroski, T. M., MacDougall, J. M., Costa, P. T., Jr., & Grandits, G. A. (1989). Components of hostility as predictors of sudden death and myocardial infarction in the Multiple Risk Factor Intervention Trial. *Psychosomatic Medicine, 51*, 514–522.

Dembroski, T. M., MacDougall, J. M. Shields, J. L., Petitto, J., & Lushene, R. (1978). Components of the Type-A coronary-prone behavior pattern and cardiovascular responses to psychomotor performance challenge. *Journal of Behavioral Medicine, 1*, 159–175.

Diamond, E. L., Schneiderman, N., Schwartz, D., Smith, J. C., Vorp, R., & Pasin, R. D. (1984). Harassment, hostility, and Type-A as determinants of cardiovascular reactivity during competition. *Journal of Behavioral Medicine, 7*, 171–189.

Engebretson, T. O., Matthews, K. A., & Scheier, M. F. (1989). Relations between anger expression and cardiovascular reactivity: Reconciling inconsistent findings through a matching hypothesis. *Journal of Personality and Social Psychology, 57*, 513–521.

Glass, D. C., Lake, C. R., Contrada, R. J., Kehoe, K., & Erlanger, L. R. (1983). Stability of individual differences in physiological responses to stress. *Health Psychology, 2*, 317–341.

Hardy, J. D., & Smith, T. W. (1988). Cynical hostility and vulnerability to disease: Social support, life stress, and physiological response to conflict. *Health Psychology, 7*, 447–459.

Haynes, S. G., Levine, S., Scotch, N., Feinleib, M., & Kannel, W. B. (1978). The relationship of psychosocial factors to coronary heart disease in the Framingham study: I. Methods and risk factors. *American Journal of Epidemiology, 107*, 362–383.

Holroyd, K. A., & Gorkin, L. (1983). Young adults at risk for hypertension: Effects of family history and anger management in determining responses to interpersonal conflict. *Journal of Psychosomatic Research, 27*, 131–138.

Houston, B. K., Smith, M. A., & Cates, D. S. (1989). Hostility patterns and cardiovascular reactivity to stress. *Psychophysiology, 26,* 337–342.

Houston, B. K., & Vavak, C. R. (1991). Hostility: Developmental factors, psychosocial correlates, and health behaviors. *Health Psychology, 10,* 9–17.

Jamner, L. D., Shapiro, D., Goldstein, I. B., & Hug, R. (1991). Ambulatory blood pressure and heart rate in paramedics: Effects of cynical hostility and defensiveness. *Psychosomatic Medicine, 53,* 393–406.

Jorgensen, R. S., & Houston, B. K. (1988). Cardiovascular reactivity, hostility, and family history of hypertension. *Psychotherapy and Psychosomatics, 50,* 216–222.

Kamarck, T. W., Manuck, S. B., & Jennings, J. R. (1990). Social support reduces cardiovascular reactivity to psychological challenge: A laboratory model. *Psychosomatic Medicine, 52,* 42–58.

Kazdin, A. E. (1980). *Research design in clinical psychology.* New York: Harper & Row.

Lundberg, U., Hedman, M., Melin, B., & Frankenhaeuser, M. (1989). Type-A behavior in healthy males and females as related to physiological reactivity and blood lipids. *Psychosomatic Medicine, 51,* 113–122.

MacDougall, J. M., Dembroski, T. M., & Krantz, D. S. (1981). Effects of types of challenge on pressor and heart rate response in Type-A and -B women. *Psychophysiology, 18,* 1–9.

Mills, P. J., Schneider, R. H., & Dimsdale, J. E. (1989). Anger assessment and reactivity to stress. *Journal of Psychosomatic Research, 33,* 379–382.

Pope, M. K., & Smith, T. W. (1991). Cortisol excretion in high and low cynically hostile men. *Psychosomatic Medicine, 53,* 386–392.

Sallis, J. F., Johnson, C. C., Trevorrow, T. R., Kaplan, R. M., & Hovell, M. F. (1987). The relationship between cynical hostility and blood pressure reactivity. *Journal of Psychosomatic Research, 31,* 111–116.

Smith, M. A., & Houston, B. K. (1987). Hostility, anger expression, cardiovascular responsivity, and social support. *Biological Psychology, 24,* 39–48.

Smith, T. W. (1992). Hostility and health: Current status of a psychosomatic hypothesis. *Health Psychology, 11,* 139–150.

Smith, T. W., & Allred, K. D. (1989). Blood pressure responses during social interaction in high- and low-cynically hostile males. *Journal of Behavioral Medicine, 12,* 135–143.

Smith, T. W., & Brown, P. C. (1991). Cynical hostility, attempts to exert control, and cardiovascular reactivity in married couples. *Journal of Behavioral Medicine, 14,* 581–592.

Smith, T. W., & Frohm, K. D. (1985). What's so unhealthy about hostility? Construct validity and psychosocial correlates of the Cook and Medley Ho scale. *Health Psychology, 4,* 503–520.

Spielberger, C. D., Johnson, E. H., Russell, S. F., Crane, R. J., Jacobs, G. A., & Worden, T. J. (1985). The experience and expression of anger: Construction and validation of an anger expression scale. In M. A. Chesney & R. H. Rosenman (Eds.), *Anger and hostility in cardiovascular and behavioral disorders* (pp. 5–30). Washington, DC: Hemisphere.

Strube, M. J. (1989). Assessing subjects' construal of the laboratory situation. In N. Schneiderman, S. M. Weiss, & P. G. Kaufmann (Eds.), *Handbook of research methods in cardiovascular behavioral medicine* (pp. 527–542). New York: Plenum.

Suarez, E. C., & Williams, R. B. (1989). Situational determinants of cardiovascular and emotional reactivity in high and low hostile men. *Psychosomatic Medicine, 51,* 404–418.

Suarez, E. C., & Williams, R. B. (1990). The relationships between dimensions of hostility and cardiovascular reactivity as a function of task characteristics. *Psychosomatic Medicine, 52,* 558–570.

Suarez, E. C., Williams, R. B., Kuhn, C. M., Zimmerman, E. H., & Schanberg, S. M. (1991). Biobehavioral basis of coronary-prone behavior in middle-aged men. Part 2: Serum cholesterol, the Type-A behavior pattern, and hostility as interactive modulators of physiological reactivity. *Psychosomatic Medicine, 53,* 528–537.

Tennenbaum, D. L., & Jacob, T. (1989). Observational methods for assessing psychological state. In N. Schneiderman, S. M. Weiss, & P. G. Kaufmann (Eds.), *Handbook of research methods in cardiovascular behavioral medicine* (pp. 543–569). New York: Plenum Press.

Weidner, G., Friend, R., Ficarrotto, T. J., & Mendell, N. R. (1989). Hostility and cardiovascular reactivity to stress in women and men. *Psychosomatic Medicine, 51*, 36–45.

Williams, R. B., Suarez, E. C., Kuhn, C. M., Zimmerman, E. A., & Schanberg, S. M. (1991). Biobehavioral basis of coronary-prone behavior in middle-aged men. Part 1: Evidence for chronic SNS activation in Type As. *Psychosomatic Medicine, 53*, 517–527.

6

BASIC BIOLOGICAL MECHANISMS

Redford B. Williams, Jr.
Duke University Medical Center

As documented in the other chapters of this book, the 1980s has witnessed a stunning and accelerating rate of progress in research aimed at elucidating the role of hostility and anger in the etiology and course of coronary heart disease and other serious illnesses. To sustain this momentum it will be necessary to begin the process of integrating the research on hostility and disease with the growing corpus of basic research concerned with the neurochemistry of behavior (i.e., hostility/anger) and with the molecular biology underlying pathogenesis of the diseases associated with hostility and anger.

My purpose in this chapter is to stimulate this integrative research by suggesting potential avenues for its pursuit. I begin by engaging in some informed speculation regarding how the impact of one of hostility's biobehavioral correlates—the combination of high cholesterol with enhanced catecholamine reactivity in hostile persons—on the molecular biology of macrophage activation could accelerate atherogenesis. Next I review evidence leading to the hypothesis that the complete array of biobehavioral characteristics found in hostile persons is the result of a single neurochemical factor: diminished brain serotonin function. I conclude by considering the implications of both these concepts—hostility biobehavioral influences on macrophage function and serotonin influences on the biobehavior of hostility—for the biological plausibility of hostility/anger as a pathogenic factor and for the prevention and treatment of diseases associated with increased hostility/anger.

HOSTILITY AND THE MACROPHAGE

Suarez, Williams, Kuhn, Zimmerman, and Schanberg (1991) recently reported a positive association between plasma catecholamine reactivity to a mental stressor and fasting blood cholesterol levels among men with high scores
on the Cook and Medley Ho scale. In contrast, among men with low Ho scores
there was an *inverse* association between cholesterol levels and catecholamine reactivity.

Based on their known pathophysiologic effects, this combination of high
cholesterol and high catecholamine reactivity in hostile men should be an
especially potent stimulant to atherogenesis. We were able to confirm this
synergistic effect on atherogenesis in the Egyptian sand rat model (Mikat et
al., 1991). When fed a high cholesterol diet, sand rats develop characteristic
lipid-filled atherosclerotic lesions with foam cells and intimal hyperplasia, but
only after 6–8 months on the diet. When maintained with high norepinephrine levels (using implanted osmotic minipumps), it only takes 2 months on
the high cholesterol diet for sand rats to develop lesions as severe as those
seen only after 6–8 months on the diet alone.

Mononuclear phagocytes, or macrophages, are known to participate in
the development of atherosclerotic lesions (e.g., as the source of foam cells
in atherosclerotic plaques [Ross, 1986]). It now appears likely that the contribution of macrophages to atherogenesis is determined by changes in their
state of activation, which itself is complexly determined by a variety of
molecular signals (Adams & Hamilton, 1991).

Among the molecules that affect macrophage activation is oxidized-LDL.
Among its effects on macrophage activation are decreased motility and increased release of several growth factors, both of which could contribute to
atherosclerotic plaque formation (Adams & Hamilton, 1991). In contrast to
most cells where cyclic AMP (the second messenger of the beta adrenergic
receptor, BAR) stimulates cellular functions, increasing levels of intracellular cyclic AMP appear to potentiate the *suppressive* effects of oxidized-LDL
on many aspects of macrophage activation (Adams & Hamilton, 1991). Thus,
increased BAR activation could be a significant contributor to alterations in
the molecular biology of macrophage activation that are key elements in
atherogenesis.

Let us now return to the pattern of increased cholesterol associated with
enhanced catecholamine reactivity to stress that is found in hostile men. How
would this combination affect the molecular biology of macrophage activation so that atherogenesis is stimulated?

As noted previously, increased cyclic AMP generation within the macrophage is known to potentiate effects of oxidized-LDL on macrophage activation that are believed to be involved in atherogenesis. Whereas increasing cholesterol concentrations are known to increase the number of BARs

(Tsutsumi, Tsuji, Ogawa, Ito, & Satake, 1988), the effects of increased cate-cholamine levels on macrophage activation would be expected to be poten-tiated in the setting of high cholesterol. Preliminary studies in our laborato-ries (Suarez, Bartolome, Kuhn, Mikat, Schanberg, & Williams, unpublished observations) showed that the high cholesterol diet produces an increased number of liver BARs and increased isoproterenol-stimulated cyclic AMP in both liver and heart in the sand rat.

Let me summarize the proposed sequence of pathogenic events described previously:

1. In hostile people, when cholesterol is elevated, there is also enhanced catecholamine reactivity to stress.
2. The effect of increased cholesterol to upregulate BAR functions com-bines with the increased catecholamine levels to potentiate cyclic AMP levels within the macrophage.
3. The increased intracellular cyclic AMP levels, in turn, potentiate effects of oxidized-LDL (itself increased secondary to the cholesterol elevations) on macrophage activation.
4 The altered pattern of macrophage activation that has been potentiat-ed by the cholesterol-catecholamine effects causes an acceleration of the processes involved in atherosclerotic plaque formation.

I hasten to remind the reader that much research remains to be done be-fore the above scenario can be considered an accurate portrayal of how atherosclerosis is potentiated in any model, whether sand rats given cholester-ol and catecholamines or hostile humans with naturally occurring elevations of these substances. We still do not have a complete final understanding, for example, of "the processes involved in atherosclerotic plaque formation."

But that should not deter us at all from pursuing the studies necessary to document the scenario. For example, my colleague at Duke, Dr. Dolph Adams, has already conducted studies showing that isoproterenol stimulates cyclic AMP formation within macrophages (unpublished results). The next step will be to incubate the macrophages in varying cholesterol concentrations, the goal being to show the isoproterenol-stimulated cyclic AMP dose response curve is shifted to the left by increasing cholesterol concentrations. Success-ful completion of that step will lead to further studies, at first identifying in vitro the specific effects of increased cyclic AMP on the molecular biology of macrophage activation; and ultimately documenting the same effects in lesion-associated macrophages.

Parallel studies can be envisioned using monocytes (the macrophage precursor that circulates in the blood) obtained from hostile humans with high versus low cholesterol levels to document the same effects on macrophage activation that are found important in lesion formation in the sand rat model.

The ultimate goal, of course, will be to use the increased understanding of the molecular basis of cholesterol–catecholamine effects on macrophage activation to identify molecular targets for interventions that can prevent and/or reverse the accelerated atherogenesis responsible for increased coronary heart disease risk in hostile persons.

Let me conclude this foray into macrophage molecular biology with two observations. First, it is possible to use what we have learned about biobehavioral correlates of hostility to formulate innovative, testable hypotheses for our molecular biology colleagues. And second, by expanding our horizons to include knowledge of the molecular biology of the diseases we study, behavioral medicine researchers can advance our field by documenting the biological plausibility of our paradigms, thereby enhancing our ability to contribute to the development of effective prevention and treatment approaches to diseases of major public health significance.

HOSTILITY AND SEROTONIN

Other chapters in this volume provide detailed descriptions of the biobehavioral characteristics that could be responsible for the increased cardiovascular disease risk found among hostile persons in epidemiologic research. Based on a consideration of these characteristics and knowledge of recent research on the role of serotonin in physiology and behavior, I proposed (Williams, 1991) that diminished brain serotonin function is a major determinant of the biobehavioral profile of hostile persons.

I develop this hypothesis by first describing the biobehavioral characteristics that have now been found in hostile persons, described hereafter as the "hostility syndrome." I then present evidence from diverse sources that suggests a role for diminished brain serotonin function in mediating each of these characteristics.

The Hostility Syndrome: Biobehavioral Characteristics

Behavioral. Hostile people are, well, hostile. More specifically, persons who score high on various measures of hostility report (and have been observed to have) more negative interactions with others, increased anger, and irritation during interpersonal conflict, and more overt aggressive expression of their angry feelings (see Smith & Siegman, this volume; Suarez & Williams, 1989).

Autonomic. Hostile persons exhibit increased sympathetic nervous system (SNS)-mediated physiologic reactivity under stress, particularly that arising during interpersonal conflicts that arouse anger and irritation (see Houston, this volume; Suarez & Williams, 1989). In contrast to their enhanced SNS reactivity, hostile persons show decreased parasympathetic responses (Fukudo et al., 1992).

Risk Factors.   As described in Siegler's chapter in this volume, hostile people are more likely to be cigarette smokers, to consume a higher calorie diet (leading to increased body mass index and lipid levels), and to consume more alcohol.

The Hostility Syndrome:
Role of Decreased Serotonin Function

All of the characteristics described previously as part of the hostility syndrome have been shown in diverse areas of research to be potential consequences of decreased brain serotonin function. Here is a brief summary of that evidence.

Hostile Behavior.   It has been known for some time that decreased levels of the serotonin metabolite 5-HIAA are found in the cerebrospinal fluid (CSF) of men with a history of aggressive acting out (Brown, Goodwin, Ballenger, Goyer, & Major, 1979). Even in normal volunteers, low CSF 5-HIAA levels were found in those with high scores on the "urge to act out hostility" subscale of the Hostility and Direction of Hostility Questionnaire (Roy, Adinoff, & Linnoila, 1988). Another index of brain serotonin function—the plasma prolactin response to fenfluramine, a drug known to cause release of serotonin in the brain—was found inversely correlated with scores on the assault and irritability scales of the Buss–Durkee Hostility Inventory (Coccaro et al., 1989).

The most direct evidence for the involvement of brain serotonin in affiliative versus aggressive behaviors comes from a study in which male vervet monkeys were placed on a drug regimen that either raised or lowered brain serotonin levels (Raleigh, McGuire, Brammer, Pollack, & Yuwiler, 1991). Monkeys on the serotonin-lowering regimen displayed more aggressive behaviors toward the females, which led to their becoming subordinate to the other males in the group. Monkeys in whom brain serotonin was increased displayed more affilative behaviors toward the females, leading to their becoming dominant.

These findings make a strong case that reduced brain serotonin function could be responsible for the aggressive, irritable behaviors observed in hostile persons.

Autonomic Balance.   Maneuvers that increase brain serotonin levels (e.g., tryptophan loading with peripheral decarboxylase inhibition) were shown to reduce sympathetic nerve firing and to protect cats with ligated coronary arteries from stress-induced ventricular fibrillation (Verrier, 1986). The effect of increased brain serotonin to decrease SNS outflow appears to be mediated by stimulation of the 5-HT$_{1A}$ class of serotonin receptors. These same receptors when stimulated by serotonin produce an increase in parasympathetic outflow (Saxena & Villalon, 1990).

Thus, stimulation of brain 5-HT$_{1A}$ receptors by serotonin produces the same pattern of autonomic balance—decreased sympathetic outflow and increased parasympathetic outflow—that is observed in nonhostile humans. The opposite pattern, observed in hostile humans, could be a consequence, therefore, of decreased serotonergic stimulation of these same receptors.

Risk Factors. It has long been known that depletion of brain serotonin produces increased food intake, body weight, and adiposity in animal models (Waldbillig, Bortness, & Stanley, 1981). Conversely, maneuvers to increase brain serotonin function decrease food intake, and the serotonin uptake blocker fluoxetine (Prozac), which acts to increase brain serotonin function, was found to decrease appetite and facilitate weight loss in humans (Levine et al., 1989).

Repeatedly confirmed observations of reduced CSF 5-HIAA in alcoholics has led to the conclusion that alcoholics, as a group, have a brain serotonin deficiency and that alcohol is used as a self-medication that remedies the deficit by releasing serotonin (Ballenger, Goodwin, Major, & Brown, 1979). Along with studies showing reduced alcohol consumption after serotonin-enhancing drugs in animals, the human observations led to the suggestion that serotonin-enhancing drugs should be evaluated as potential therapeutic agents in alcoholism (Sellers & Naranjo, 1986).

The rewarding properties of nicotine were found to be mediated in part by serotonergic stimulation of the 5HT$_3$ receptor (Carboni, Acquas, Leone, & Dichiava, 1989). There is also evidence that increasing brain serotonin function by either tryptophan loading (Bowen, Spring, & Fox, 1991) or use of a 5HT$_{1A}$ agonist (buspirone) reduces the negative affects and craving that accompany nicotine withdrawal.

These findings relating reduced brain serotonin function to increased eating, drinking, and smoking indicate that increased expression of these behaviors in hostile persons could result from a functional deficiency of brain serotonin.

Although the evidence I cited earlier relating the biobehavioral features of the hostility syndrome is all circumstantial in nature, it is, in my view, a rather compelling array of circumstantial evidence. Moreover, it suggests specific tests that would confirm the serotonergic basis of the hostility syndrome. For example, during the coming year, we will use the prolactin response to fenfluramine to index brain serotonin function in subjects scoring high and low on the Cook and Medley Ho-scale. If high Ho subjects show a smaller prolactin response to fenfluramine, it will be direct evidence of diminished brain serotonin function in hostile persons. And that, as I consider later, could lead to pharmacologic interventions to prevent and treat the health damaging consequences of the hostility syndrome.

SUMMARY AND IMPLICATIONS

I have presented evidence showing how the combination of elevated cholesterol with enhanced catecholamine reactivity in hostile persons could affect the molecular biology of macrophage activation in ways that would speed the development of atherosclerotic lesions. Although I focused on coronary heart disease in this chapter, it is worth noting that the same alterations of macrophage function could also play a role in tumorogenesis. I also presented evidence suggesting that all the harmful biobehavioral characteristics found in hostile persons—the hostility syndrome consisting of increased aggression/irritability, increased sympathetic function, decreased parasympathetic function, increased eating, drinking, and smoking—are the result of a single "lesion," diminished brain serotonin function.

Although much research will be required to confirm these speculations, the specific studies are easy to conceive and preliminary results are already encouraging. That the studies to advance these hypotheses are worth doing is hard to dispute when we consider the implications of their successful prosecution.

For one thing, being able to apply the tools of molecular biology to demonstrate a specific effect of lipids and catecholamines on macrophage functions that is more pronounced in hostile persons will enhance the scientific credibility of behavioral medicine in general, and the hostility hypothesis in particular, among the biomedical community.

Of more practical import, the demonstration of such effects on macrophage functions would increase our basic understanding of the role of the macrophage in pathogenesis of coronary artery disease, and possibly cancer as well. Armed with such knowledge, we might be able to make significant progress toward more effective prevention and treatment of these major killers.

The demonstration of a serotonergic basis for hostility and its associated health-damaging biobehavioral features would be of enormous theoretical importance. Documenting a neurochemical basis for a coronary-prone personality constellation would greatly strengthen the scientific base for both theorizing and research in behavioral medicine.

Here are some examples of potential future developments that could flow from research that documents a serotonergic basis for the hostility syndrome.

Improved assessment tools could be an early dividend. Rather than the continuing agonizing search for "gold standard" measures of hostility and anger (see Barefoot, this volume), it may be possible one day to simply obtain a blood sample 4 hours after a 60 mg dose of fenfluramine, send it off to the lab for prolactin assay, and let the patient know the next day—with more precision than any behavioral test will ever achieve—whether his "hostility syndrome" test is in the dangerous range.

And if it is, then it would be very likely that effective preventive measures also will have been developed by that time. First of all, by having a more sensitive and specific biological marker for the hostility syndrome, we would be able to make a stronger case to the patient (client) for the need to take preventive measures, even if they may be "only" behavioral to start. As we learn more about the neurochemical basis of the hostility syndrome, it may be possible to retest the patient to see if the serotonin system has been "normalized" by the intervention.

Ultimately, it should be possible to prescribe a pharmacologic approach that would enhance our ability to control the hostility syndrome and ameliorate its health-damaging effects. Drugs are already available that may be useful in this regard—fluoxetine (Prozac) and buspione (Buspar) are good examples.

Does this sound radical? Why not, you may be asking me, focus on behavioral modification, biofeedback, relaxation, stress management training, support groups, and other time-honored and tested tools of behavioral medicine?

I answer this concern by noting that we already use the approach—a combination of behavioral and pharmacologic interventions—I have suggested for the hostility syndrome in controlling other risk factors. If blood pressure or blood cholesterol are too high, the first steps toward their reduction are behavioral—exercise, diet, even relaxation exercises. If these do not achieve the goal, then we move on to pharmacologic approaches—beta blockers, calcium channel blockers, lipid lowering drugs, and so forth.

But we would probably not start with primary prevention in healthy people. Consider the goals so often set for the patient with coronary disease: avoid emotional upsets, stop smoking, cut down on fatty foods (and calories), drink alcohol only in moderation, if at all. Every one of these goals, particularly in the hostile person with his or her shorter temper, strong sympathetic and weak parasympathetic systems, would be served by an intervention that enhanced brain serotonin function. Therefore, controlled clinical trials of serotonergic agents in post-MI patient groups could be the first step toward rational pharmacologic treatment of the hostility syndrome.

Now that would be true behavioral "medicine."

REFERENCES

Adams, D. O., & Hamilton, T. A. (1987). Molecular mechanisms of signal transduction in macrophage activation. *Immunology Today, 8,* 151–158.

Ballenger, J., Goodwin, F. K., Major, L. F., & Brown, G. L. (1979). Alcohol and centeral serotonin metabolism in man. *Archives of General Psychiatry, 36,* 224–227.

Bowen, D. J., Spring, B., & Fox, E. (1991). Tryptophan and high-carbohydrate diets as adjuncts to smoking cessation therapy. *Journal of Behavioral Medicine, 14*, 97–110.

Brown, G. L., Goodwin, F. K., Ballenger, J. C., Goyer, P. F., & Major, L. F. (1979). Aggression in humans correlates with cerebrospinal fluid amine metabolites. *Psychiatry Research, 1*, 131–139.

Carboni, E., Acquas, E., Leone, P., Dichiara, G. (1989). 5HT$_3$ receptor antagonists block morphine- and nicotine- but not amphetamine-induced reward. *Psychopharmacology, 97*, 175–178.

Coccaro, E. F., Siever, L. F., Klar, H. M., Maurer, G., Cochrane, K., Cooper, T. B., Mohs, R. C., & Davis, K. L. (1989). Serotonergic studies in patients with affective and personality disorders. *Archives of General Psychiatry, 46*, 587–599.

Fukudo, S., Lane, J. D., Anderson, N. B., Kuhn, C. M., Schanberg, S. M., McCown, N., Muranaka, M., Suzuki, J., & Williams, R. B. (1992). Accentuated vagal antagonism of beta-adrenergic effects on ventricular repolarization is weaker in hostile Type-A men. *Circulation, 85*, 2045–2053.

Levine, L. R., Enas, G. G., Thompson, W. L., & Byyny, K. L., Daver, A. D., Kirby, R. W., Kreindler, T. C., Levy, B., Lucas, C. P., & McIlwain, H. H. (1989). Fluoxetine as an aid in weight loss programs. *International Journal of Obesity, 13*, 365–369.

Mikat, E. M., Bartolome, J. V., Weiss, J. M., Schanberg, S. M., Kuhn, C. M., & Williams, R. B. (1991). Chronic norepinephrine infusion accelerates atherosclerotic lesion development in sand rats maintained on a high cholesterol diet. *Psychosomatic Medicine, 53*, 212–213. (Abstract)

Raleigh, M. J., McGuire, M. T., Brammer, G. L., Pollack, D. B., & Yuwiler, A. (1991). Serotonergic mechanisms promote dominance acquisition in adult male vervet monkeys. *Brain Research, 559*, 181–190.

Ross, R. (1986). The pathogenesis of atherosclerosis: An update. *New England Journal of Medicine, 314*, 488–500.

Roy, A., Adinoff, B., & Linnoila, M. (1988). Acting out hostility in normal volunteers: Negative correlation with levels of 5-HIAA in cerebrospinal fluid. *Psychiatry Research, 24*, 187–194.

Saxena, P. R., & Villalon, C. M. (1990). Cardiovascular effects of serotonin agonists and antagonists. *Journal of Cardiovascular Pharmacology, 7*, 517–534.

Sellers, E. M., & Naranjo, C. A. (1986). Therapeutic use of serotonergic drugs in alcohol abuse. *Clinical Neuropharmacology, 9*(Suppl. 4), 60–62.

Suarez, E. C., Williams, R. B., Kuhn, C. M., Zimmerman, E. H., & Schanberg, S. M. (1991). Biobehavioral basis of coronary-prone behavior in middle-aged men: Part 2. Serum cholesterol, the Type-A behavior pattern, and hostility as interactive modulators of physiological reactivity. *Psychosomatic Medicine, 53*, 528–537.

Suarez, E. C., & Williams, R. B. (1989). Situational determinants of cardiovascular and emotional reactivity in high- and low-hostile men. *Psychosomatic Medicine, 51*, 404–418.

Tsutsumi, S., Tsuji, K., Ogawa, K., Ito, T., & Satake, T. (1988). Effect of dietary salt and cholesterol loading on vascular adrenergic receptors. *Blood Vessels, 25*, 209–216.

Verrier, R. L. (1986). Neurochemical approaches to the prevention of ventricular fibrillation. *Federation Proceedings, 45*, 2191–2196.

Waldbillig, R. J., Bortness, T. J., & Stanley, B. G. (1981). Increased food intake, body weight, and adiposity following regional depletion of serotonin. *Journal of Comparative Physiology, 95*, 391–398.

Williams, R. B., Jr. (1991). A relook at personality types and coronary heart disease. *Progress in Cardiology, 4*, 91–97.

7

Animal Models of Aggression and Cardiovascular Disease

Jay R. Kaplan
M. Babette Botchin
The Bowman Gray School of Medicine,
Winston-Salem, North Carolina

Stephen B. Manuck
University of Pittsburgh

Behavioral factors have long been implicated in the etiology and expression of coronary heart disease (CHD) and in the development of its underlying condition, coronary artery atherosclerosis. The Type A behavior pattern, defined as a style of coping with challenge and characterized by hostility, time urgency, and competitiveness, is perhaps the best-known psychosocial construct to be associated with increased risk of CHD and atherosclerosis. Recent research suggests that the hostility component of the Type A pattern and, more generally, a high "potential for anger–hostility," are particularly toxic with respect to CHD and atherosclerosis (Siegman, Anderson, Herbst, Boyle, & Wilkinson, 1993; Siegman, Dembrowski, & Ringel, 1987; Costa, McCrae, & Dembrowski, 1989; Dembrowski & Costa, 1988). Further, within the anger–hostility domain, it appears that the expression rather than the experience of these states contributes to the development of disease (Siegman et al., 1993).

Epidemiologic and clinical studies have done much to increase understanding regarding the influence of behavioral factors on CHD and atherosclerosis. However, several characteristics of CHD complicate attempts to define with more certainty the relationships among predisposing behavioral characteristics (e.g., a high potential for anger–hostility), intervening physiological mechanisms (e.g., autonomic arousal), and the disease process. First, the lesions of atherosclerosis develop over a period of decades prior to any appearance of disease. Moreover, there is a low incidence of clinical events, such as heart attacks, within any limited experimental population, even among individuals at high risk for developing CHD. And, although coronary artery atherosclerosis is present to some degree in virtually all adults, it can be assessed only with the use of invasive procedures not ethically applied to asymptomatic individuals (Kaplan, Manuck, Clarkson, & Prichard, 1985). Thus, although numerous studies revealed that psychosocial influences affect CHD and atherosclerosis, many questions, especially those relating to pathogenic mechanisms, remain unanswered.

An obvious alternative research strategy involves the use of appropriate animal models. The choice of such models, however, is not a trivial matter related to convenience and economy. Rather, it depends on the presence of an adequate resemblance to human beings both in the pathological processes underlying the development of CHD and in those behavioral characteristics believed to potentiate such development. In this chapter, we explore first the specific requirements associated with the choice of an animal model for investigating the influence of anger–hostility on atherosclerosis, and then review data and findings from our own laboratory based on the use of one model, the cynomolgus macaque (*Macaca fascicularis*). We conclude the chapter with a review of evidence concerning the mechanisms that mediate the association between behavioral factors and atherosclerosis, and those which may underlie the behavioral factors themselves.

ANIMAL MODELS OF ATHEROSCLEROSIS AND CHD

Atherosclerosis in human beings is a process in which the intimal layer of the large muscular and elastic arteries is thickened as a result of intra- and extracellular accumulation of plasma lipids, cellular proliferation, and macrophage migration (McGill, 1972). The resulting lesions generally progress through several stages of severity from fatty streaks to complicated, fibrous plaques. The presence of severe lesions in the coronary arteries often culminates in a disease spectrum that includes angina pectoris, myocardial infarction, and disturbances of performance, rhythm, and electrical activity of the heart.

The perfect species for modeling atherosclerosis would be one, which, in its normal environment, develops the kind of lesions observed in human beings. Such lesions would progress gradually over an animal's lifetime, with clinical manifestations occurring in middle to old age. At death, atherosclerosis in this model would vary from fatty streaks to raised plaques, the latter characterized by complications such as thrombosis, ulceration, necrosis, and calcification. Further, complicated lesions would occur in about one-fifth of the population, with males affected twice as frequently as females. End-organ complications of myocardial and cerebral infarction would be seen, and occasionally aneurysms in the aorta would develop. Finally, all of this would occur in an animal sufficiently large to allow application of diagnostic and therapeutic measures similar to those found useful in humans. Unfortunately, no animal species has all of the foregoing traits; therefore, the development of close approximations to some of the major characteristics of the atherosclerotic process in people is the most that can be expected (Kaplan et al., 1985).

Many animal species develop atherosclerosis relatively rapidly when fed a diet appropriately high in saturated fat and cholesterol. These species, however, vary considerably in the pathology and location of the lesions, making some more valuable than others for modeling human atherosclerosis. Rats and mice, for example, are widely available, economical, and convenient. Unfortunately, these animals have a cardiovascular morphology that differs significantly from that of people, and the lesions produced in these rodents as a result of dietary or other challenges generally involve the medial rather than intimal arterial layer (Kaplan et al., 1985). Thus, although mice and rats have been used to demonstrate the injurious effects of psychosocial stress on arterial endothelium, the resulting lesions usually do not resemble human atherosclerosis in location or appearance (Henry et al., 1971). Rabbits, which have been used extensively in atherosclerosis research, typically develop lesions affecting the small intramyocardial branches of the coronary vasculature and not the large, proximal coronary arteries, as occurs in people. As a result, these animals are useful for identifying factors (including psychosocial phenomena, Nerem, Levesque, & Cornhill, 1980) that modulate atherogenesis systemically, but not specifically with respect to the coronary arteries. Pigs and some nonhuman primates (e.g., the macaque monkeys), however, develop lesions comparable in severity and distribution to those observed in the coronary arteries of human beings. Further, these animals readily accept diets that approximate the type eaten by people (Kaplan et al., 1985).

Among the aforementioned models, we have emphasized cynomolgus macaques in our research. When fed diets similar to those consumed by people in industrialized countries (i.e., diets high in saturated fat and cholesterol), these animals develop atherosclerosis relatively rapidly. Further, the pathologic characteristics of their coronary lesions, the resultant vasomotor abnormalities, and the relatively high incidence of myocardial infarction resemble the outcomes observed in human beings. Notably, premenopausal females of this species, like their human counterparts, are relatively protected from atherosclerosis in comparison to similarly treated males (Kaplan, Adams, Clarkson, Manuck, & Shively, 1991). For reasons explored later, this species is also suitable for investigating those behavioral features (including anger–hostility) believed to potentiate atherosclerosis and CHD in people.

MODELING ANGER–HOSTILITY

Many investigators believe that the expression, rather than the experience, of anger–hostility is relevant to the development of CHD and atherosclerosis. It is, therefore, reasonable to ask how such expression might be investigated in animal models, which are themselves limited to nonverbal forms of communication. Among human beings, emotions (e.g., anger) and intentions (e.g., hostility) are signaled nonverbally by facial expression, posture, and voice stylistics (Ekman, 1965; Tomkins, 1962). Darwin recognized that a similar signaling of "mood" (i.e., a combination of emotion and intent) occurs in animals that use expressive behaviors emphasizing contrasting characteristics to signal contrasting moods (Darwin, 1872; Sade, 1973).

Intuitively, the expression of anger–hostility in people seems best represented in animals by intraspecific "aggression," a type of behavior commonly observed in most species.[1] Aggression, in turn, is usefully defined as an "overt behavior involving intent to inflict noxious stimulation or to behave destructively toward another organism" (Moyer, 1968). Many investigators consider it helpful to divide intraspecific aggression into offensive (anger-based, attack) and defensive (fear-based, flight) components, as these are thought to be distinct in terms of motor patterns, physiologic concomitants, and neural mechanisms. Anger–hostility, as described for human beings, most plausibly approximates offensive, rather than defensive, aggression in animal models.

Notably, the aggressive behavior of animals is usually indicated by easily recognized, nonverbal signals that distinguish this behavioral state from others. One might, for example, consider the contrast between a dog that is snarling, with face inclined forward and downward, and one that has its head up, a relaxed posture, and a wagging tail. The former animal is signaling its intention to attack whereas the latter is displaying evidence of an affiliative mood. Furthermore, the expressive behaviors used to convey the emotions and intentions associated with aggression or other dimensions of behavior are often inherent, with the signaling gestures of closely related species more similar to each other than to those used by more distantly related animals (Eibl-Eibesfeldt, 1975). It is, therefore, not surprising, perhaps, that the facial expressions, postures, and other outward expressions of agonistic (i.e., combative)[2] behavior in apes and some Old World monkeys are demonstrably homologous with those of people (Sade, 1973; Van Hooff, 1969; Wickler, 1969). Conversely, rodents, cats, and other animals frequently used

---

[1]For purposes of this presentation, aggression refers to behavior directed at conspecifics and does not, therefore, include predation.

[2]Agonism refers to all combative behavior used by animals in fights, whether aggressive, submissive, or a mixture.

in the study of aggression, display agonistic gestures, which, although easily recognizable as indicating an aggressive mood, are, nonetheless, dissimilar to those exhibited by people.

The similarities between human beings and some nonhuman primates in the signals used to communicate a combative mood suggest that the latter animals might be particularly useful for modeling the human expression of anger–hostility. Among macaques, for example, movement of the head and thorax from a high to a low position in the midsagittal plane signals aggressive intent (Sade, 1973). Such movement might be combined with an open mouth, a stare, and a gruntlike vocalization directed toward the target. These gestures, termed *threats*, signal aggressive intent, and thus may represent hostility. The intent becomes more overt when the threatening animal roars and thrusts its shoulders forward in a lunge, which may then grade into a physical charge and chase terminating when the attacking animal grabs and bites the target. The intensity of the attack (which may reflect "anger") is signaled by the degree to which the foregoing gestures are exaggerated and combined with strident vocalizations. It might be noted that macaques signal flight with a series of antithetical gestures emphasizing flexion in the frontal plane (i.e., cowering). Although macaque monkeys occasionally display mixed signals (i.e., an open-mouth threat combined with a grimace and a scream— usually interpreted as defensive aggression), they commonly signal attack or flight unambiguously (Kaplan, 1976; Sade, 1973).

BEHAVIORAL CHARACTERISTICS OF CYNOMOLGUS MACAQUES

Our choice of the cynomolgus macaque as a model for evaluating behavioral influences on atherosclerosis is not based solely on this species' use of aggressive gestures that are homologous to those employed by people. It also is grounded in the observation that these group-living animals are characterized, in the wild, by complex patterns of social interaction and generation-spanning networks of affiliation, alliance, and mutual support (Kaplan et al., 1985; Sade, 1967; Sade, 1972; Seyfarth, 1977). Such features are reminiscent of human society and are present only in rudimentary form in most nonprimate species.

Of particular interest to us, the characteristic natural behavior of macaques readily accommodates to experimental manipulation. Within their social groups, for example, cynomolgus macaques form hierarchies of social status in which some animals (*dominants*) reliably defeat others (*subordinates*) in competitive interactions. Once such hierarchies are formed, fights among individuals are generally unambiguous in outcome, with dominant monkeys using only attack gestures whereas subordinates use only those gestures associated with flight (Bernstein, 1981). The predilection of monkeys to form predictable status hierarchies allows the investigator to categorize animals within groups as customarily either winners (dominants) or losers (subordinates) in response to conspecific challenge and stimulation. Usually, dominant monkeys' behavior is more aggressive (in frequency and intensity) than subordinates. Some subordinates, however, engage in considerable aggressive behavior, targeting animals that are lower ranking than themselves (Kaplan et al., 1985).

Before proceeding, it is worth emphasizing that social status (dominant, subordinate) is an outcome specific to a given social situation and does not necessarily represent an individual behavioral trait. Investigators are sometimes seduced into treating social status as an inherent, individual characteristic because it is easily measured and is predictive of many physiologic and pathophysiologic phenomena. However, social status is more accurately regarded as an outcome dependent on an interaction between the immediate social environment and underlying traits of personality; the latter traits may well be the true correlates or causes of many phenomena usually associated with dominance status. In our own studies, we found the tendency for dominant and subordinate animals to retain their relative rankings in changed social circumstances (see following) as initial evidence that the traits comprising dominance status are stable. One such trait may be aggressivity, as it is clear that dominant animals initiate most fights. Other investigators identified the ready acceptance of subordination by some animals as another individual characteristic that contributes to social status (Rowell, 1974).

In addition to their propensity to establish well-delineated dominance relationships and hierarchies, male cynomolgus macaques are predisposed to respond agonistically to new animals attempting to join their social groupings; such newcomers, in the wild and in captivity, are treated as intruders and a threat to the prevailing social structure (Bernstein, 1981; Kaplan et al., 1985). The disruptive influence of strangers on social relationships within groups provides the basis for an ecologically valid behavioral challenge, and one that was used in many of our studies, namely, the periodic reorganization of social group memberships.

In the following sections, we describe three investigations involving adult male cynomolgus monkeys, and their relevance to the hypothesis that aggressive behavior influences atherosclerosis. In the first experiment, we examined the effects of environmental stress (periodic reorganization of social group membership) and social status (dominant or subordinate) on coronary artery atherosclerosis. The resulting data demonstrated that disruption of the social environment potentiates atherogenesis, but only in habitually aggressive and competitive (i.e., dominant) monkeys. In our second study, we exposed all animals to periodic reorganization of social group memberships while simultaneously giving a beta-adrenergic blocking agent to half of the monkeys. In intact groups, we again observed exacerbated atherosclerosis among dominant individuals; atherosclerosis, however, was inhibited among dominant animals receiving the beta-adrenergic blocking agent. Finally, we described a psychophysiologic finding related to the first two studies; namely, that monkeys exhibiting the largest heart rate responsivity to a common laboratory challenge also had significantly increased atherosclerosis when compared to animals showing a less pronounced cardiac response to stress. The results of these experiments suggested three conclusions for this animal model (a) atherosclerosis is potentiated among individuals that are habitually successful in their aggressive encounters with social strangers, thereby retaining dominant social status in an unstable environment; (b) the increased risk of atherosclerosis experienced by such animals is related, in part, to the autonomic (sympathetic) adjustments they make while responding to the demands of retaining dominant status; and (c) some monkeys may be susceptible to development of atherosclerosis because of a generalized cardiac hyperresponsivity, irrespective of their social environment or status.

Study I. Exacerbation of Atherosclerosis Related to Social Status and Social Disruption

This first study contained 30 animals; of these, 15 monkeys were each assigned to one of three, five-member social groups (Kaplan, Manuck, Clarkson, Lusso, & Taub, 1982). These animals were designated *unstable* (i.e., the stress condition) and were regularly redistributed among the three groups at one- to three-month intervals, on a schedule ensuring that each monkey would be housed with three or four new animals on every reorganization. An additional 15 animals were designated *stable* (i.e., the no-stress condition), and assigned to five-member social groups of unchanging composition. Animals in the unstable and stable groups were treated identically in all other ways. Hence, all animals consumed an atherogenic diet (containing 40% of calories derived from fat and a human equivalent of 700 mg cholesterol per day), designed to mimic that often eaten by North Americans. The monkeys were also evaluated routinely for those clinical characteristics usually associated with atherosclerosis and coronary heart disease (total plasma cholesterol [TPC], high density lipoprotein cholesterol [HDLC], blood pressure, and body size). Finally, routine behavioral observations were made of all animals, allowing us to evaluate the rate and pattern of affiliative and agonistic interaction as well as the social status of each monkey.

The experiment lasted 22 months, during which time dominant animals, in both stressed and not-stressed groups, tended to retain their high rankings; similarly, subordinate animals tended to remain subordinate irrespective of their social condition (stressed or not-stressed). Whereas social condition did not influence the stability of dominance ranks, we did observe that dominant monkeys living in stressed social groups initiated more episodes of contact aggression (grabbing, biting) than did their counterparts living in the not-stressed condition. Fights involving physical contact are relatively atypical of macaques, which generally signal attack and flight at a distance, using ritualized gestures.

At the end of the experiment, the coronary arteries were removed and the extent of coronary artery atherosclerosis measured in each animal (square millimeters), as the average lesion size in 15 sections taken perpendicularly to the long axis of the arteries. Coronary artery atherosclerosis was analyzed according to the social status (dominant or subordinate) and social condition (stable or unstable) of each animal (Fig. 7.1). This analysis revealed that dominant monkeys in unstable social groupings had more extensive atherosclerosis than monkeys in the three other groupings ($p < 0.05$). Thus, dominant monkeys were predisposed to develop exacerbated coronary atherosclerosis, but only under conditions of social instability. More important, the results of this experiment were independent of concomitant variability in TPC, HDLC, and blood pressure. Behavioral influences on CHD are similarly unexplained in epidemiologic investigations involving human beings.

The outcome of this study demonstrated that a behavioral characteristic, dominant social status, can interact with a stressful social environment to exacerbate coronary artery atherosclerosis in monkeys. The outcome of this first study is thus consistent with current hypotheses concerning the role of

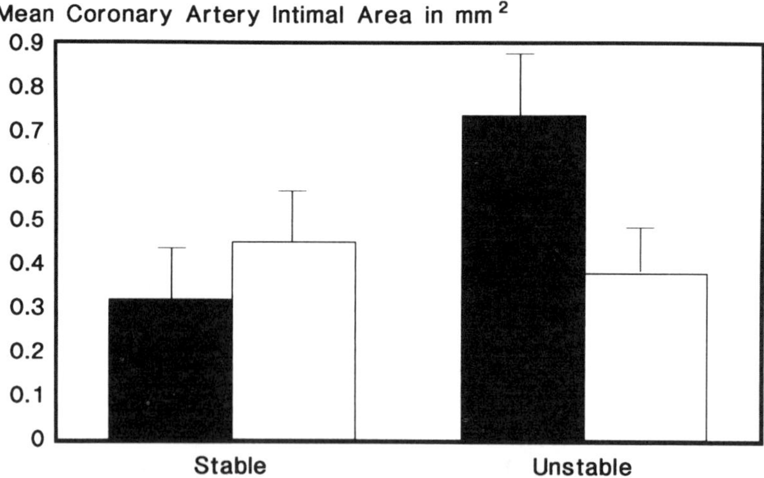

FIG. 7.1. Mean coronary artery intimal area measurements ($\pm$ SEM) among dominant and subordinate monkeys in stable and unstable social conditions. Solid bar = dominant animals, open bar = subordinate animals.

individual behavioral characteristics (such as Type A traits or a high index of hostility–anger) in the development of CHD in human beings. Our data, however, not only suggest that a high degree of antagonism and competitiveness (as observed among dominant monkeys) predisposes individuals to atherogenesis, but also that the pathogenicity of these characteristics may require an appropriately challenging or stressful environment to be fully expressed.

Study 2. The Inhibition of Behaviorally Induced Atherosclerosis in Male Cynomolgus Monkeys by Beta-adrenergic Blockade

The exacerbated coronary artery atherosclerosis of stressed, dominant monkeys in the previous experiment could not be attributed to corresponding group differences in other physiological measurements collected during the experiment—most notably serum lipid concentrations and blood pressure (the so-called traditional risk factors). Based on several lines of evidence, we instead speculated that, as dominant monkeys coped with repeated challenges to their social status, they experienced recurrent sympathetic activation with accompanying increases in heart rate, blood pressure, and catecholamine release; these physiologic responses, in turn, damaged the coronary arteries and resulted in a worsening of atherosclerosis.

If frequent exposure to psychosocial challenge can promote atherogenesis through associated sympathetic mediation, it follows that administration of a beta-adrenergic blocking agent in such circumstances should inhibit the development of atherosclerosis, particularly in behaviorally predisposed (i.e., socially dominant) individuals. We tested this hypothesis in an experiment involving 30 male cynomolgus monkeys fed an atherogenic diet (noted earlier) and housed for two years in repeatedly reorganized social groupings (Kaplan, Manuck, Adams, Weingand, & Clarkson, 1987). Half of the monkeys were administered propranolol HCl in the diet (at a human equivalent of 400 mg/day) throughout the study, and behavior and social status of each monkey were assessed on a recurrent basis. Measurements of blood pressure, heart rate, serum lipid concentrations, and social behavior were made repeatedly over the course of the investigation. At the end of the experiment, atherosclerosis extent (in mm^2) was again evaluated as an average of 15 cross sections of coronary artery from each monkey.

Chronic administration of propranolol was associated with a significant (20%) reduction in heart rate, along with a comparable lowering of blood pressure, relative to untreated controls. Interestingly, propranolol had no effect on the social behavior of the treated monkeys, nor did the drug affect dominance relationships (Kaplan & Manuck, 1989). Thus, the behavioral attributes associated with a predisposition to atherosclerosis in the previous experiment (i.e., the aggressiveness and competitiveness of dominant individuals) were fully expressed in the treated as well as untreated monkeys.

Evaluation of the coronary arteries revealed that, among untreated monkeys, the more aggressive, or dominant, animals had (as in the parallel condition of our first experiment) significantly more atherosclerosis than their subordinate counterparts. In contrast, the atherosclerosis of dominant monkeys treated with propranolol did not differ from that of either treated or untreated subordinate monkeys. These results are summarized in Fig. 7.2, and indicate that the exacerbated atherosclerosis typically observed among dominant monkeys living in disrupted social groups (Figs. 7.1 and 7.2) is inhibited by treatment with a beta-adrenergic blocking agent.

Again, the psychosocial and pharmacological effects on coronary atherogenesis shown in Fig. 7.2 were not associated with concomitant variability in serum lipid concentrations, which were equivalent across experimental groupings. Nor, as noted earlier, was there any evidence that propranolol selectively affected the behavior, and thereby the atherosclerosis, of dominant monkeys. We have demonstrated elsewhere, however, that radiotelemetered heart rate changed substantially, though transiently, in these same monkeys during periods of social reorganization; further, the observed excursions in heart rate were more pronounced in dominant than in subordinate animals (Kaplan et al., 1987; Manuck, Kaplan, Muldoon, Adams, & Clarkson, 1991). To the degree that such substantial alterations in heart rate are indicative of sympathetic arousal, propranolol may have exerted an

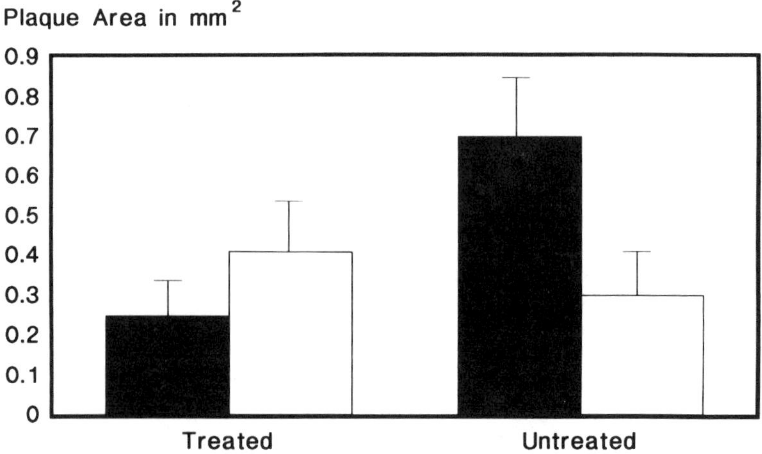

FIG. 7.2.   Coronary artery atherosclerosis ($\pm$ SEM) across all three arteries (n = 15 sections per animal) among monkeys living in unstable groups. Solid bar = dominant animals, open bar = subordinate animals. From Kaplan, Pettersson, Manuck, and Olsson (1991). Reprinted by permission of the American Heart Association.

antiatherogenic influence in this study by attenuating sympathetic activation in those monkeys that were behaviorally challenged most appreciably by exposure to periodic social reorganization, that is, the dominant monkeys.

Study 3. Initial Data Regarding Individual Differences in Cardiac Responsivity and Behavior Associated with Atherogenesis

The first two studies demonstrated that monkeys that successfully retain dominant social status despite repeated challenges, also develop exacerbated coronary atherosclerosis, and possibly do so as a result of frequent activation of the sympathetic nervous system. Additional data from a subset of 26 male monkeys in the study (i.e., no propranolol) support the speculation that a heightened sympathetic responsivity to behavioral stimuli increases the risk for coronary disease (Manuck, Kaplan, & Clarkson, 1983). Specifically, we evaluated individual differences in cardiac reactivity to stress in these monkeys on a single occasion just prior to necropsy. We based our "reactivity" assessments on radiotelemetered heart rate recorded at baseline (i.e., while the animals were in their social groups with no humans in sight) and again during a standardized challenge, in which an experimenter displayed a large monkey catch-glove in a prominent and threatening manner to the target animals. This maneuver was conducted in a stylized manner, mimicking encounters typically preceding capture and physical handling of animals.

The standardized stimulus provoked a relatively large heart rate acceleration across all monkeys (mean = 91 beats per minute [BPM]). There was, nonetheless, considerable interindividual variability in baseline-adjusted responsivity. For example, monkeys comprising the upper and lower thirds of the overall distribution of heart rate reactions differed by more than 35 BPM in their stress period heart rates (mean: "high" reactors = 236 BPM; "low" reactors = 199 BPM, $p < 0.001$); the high and low reactors did not differ in their corresponding baseline values ($M = 126$ and 123 BPM, N.S.). Interestingly, the heart rates of high and low reactors differed significantly, not only in response to deliberate challenge, but also on exposure to a more benign manipulation involving the experimenter's mere appearance in the area where monkeys were housed (M: high reactors = 170; low reactors = 118 BPM, $p < 0.001$). Most important, the high heart rate reactors had intimal lesions twice as extensive as those seen among their low reactive counterparts ($p < 0.04$; Fig. 7.3). High heart rate reactors also had heavier, thicker hearts than did low reactors, suggesting a possible association between the propensity to exhibit heightened heart rate responses to behavioral stimuli and alterations in cardiac morphology (Kaplan et al., 1991).

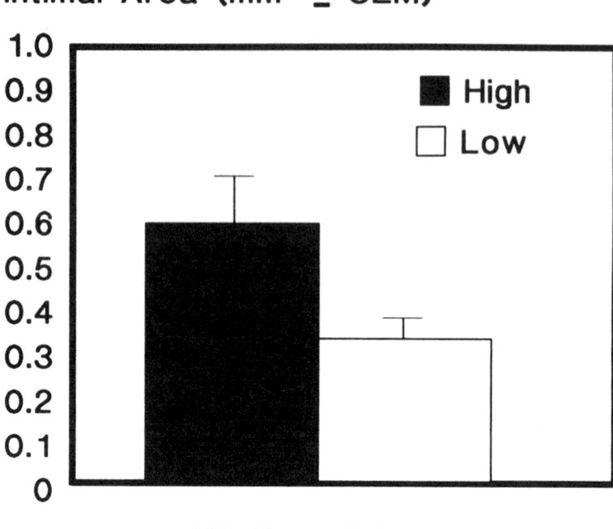

FIG. 7.3. Mean coronary artery atherosclerosis (measured as intimal area) across three coronary arteries among high (dark bar) and low (open bar) heart rate reactors. From Manuck, Kaplan, & Clarkson (1983). Adapted by permission.

In the current context it is notable that high heart rate reactive monkeys engaged in significantly more contact aggression (biting, grabbing, slapping) than did their low heart rate reactive counterparts (Fig. 7.4). By contrast, milder forms of aggression did not vary significantly between groups. Nor did high and low heart rate reactors differ reliably regarding rates of submission or grooming behaviors. Moreover, only contact aggression correlated significantly with individual differences in heart rate reactivity across all 26 experimental animals.

These heart rate findings provide initial support for the hypothesis that an exaggerated cardiac responsivity to behavioral challenge is atherogenic (Kaplan et al., 1987). The data do not, however, offer an explanation for the principal psychosocial finding in Studies 1 and 2 (i.e., that atherosclerosis is exacerbated in dominant monkeys living in unstable social groups). This is because these dominant animals were not disproportionately represented among the high heart rate reactors.

In attempting to reconcile these sets of observations, we have proposed elsewhere that some individuals (e.g., high heart rate reactors) may be sus-

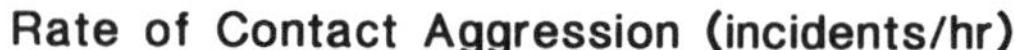

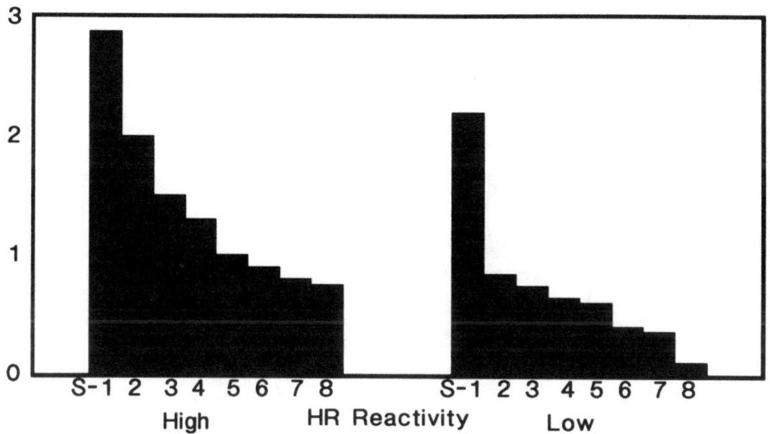

FIG. 7.4. Rate of contact aggression among high and low heart rate (HR) reactive animals. Monkeys ranked S-1 to S-8 by order of aggression within group. From Manuck, Kaplan, & Clarkson (1983). Reprinted by permission.

ceptible to the development of CHD because of an intrinsic sympathoadrenal hyperresponsivity to behavioral stimuli; others (e.g., aggressive/dominant individuals in unstable social environments) may be at increased risk because of frequent elicitation of such responses in stressful environments (Kaplan et al., 1991; Manuck, Kaplan, Adams, & Clarkson, 1988). In both instances, we propose sympathoadrenal activation as the common pathway by which pathogenesis is mediated. Also, in both instances, the two subsets of monkeys at highest risk for developing exacerbated atherosclerosis (dominant males in unstable groupings, cardiac hyperreactors) also exhibit in common an increased tendency to engage in the more extreme forms of aggression.

The foregoing sections have identified dominant social status and heart rate hyperresponsivity to stress as characteristics that potentiate atherosclerosis in cynomolgus monkeys. Although relatively well described in terms of behavioral expression and cardiovascular concomitants and sequelae, little is known regarding the possible role played by the central nervous system (CNS) in the modulation of individual differences in these characteristics. In the following sections, we speculate on the possible influence on aggressivity and sympathetic arousal of a specific CNS neurotransmitter complex that may have links to both phenomena, the serotonergic (5-hydroxytryptamine [5-HT]) system.

HYPOTHESIS CONCERNING CNS CONTROL OF AGGRESSION AND AUTONOMIC AROUSAL

Aggressive Behavior

In the studies reviewed earlier, intense aggressivity was exhibited by dominant animals in unstable social groups and by cardiac hyperresponders, as both subsets of monkeys initiated nonritualized, contact aggression to a greater extent than did their subordinate or hyporesponsive counterparts. The 5-HT synaptic transmitter system is, in turn, prominent among systems identified as potentially regulating intense aggression or violence directed at self or others. A consistent relationship has been observed, for example, between low concentrations of the serotonin metabolite 5-hydroxyindoleacetic acid (5-HIAA) in cerebrospinal fluid (CSF), and the propensity for impulsive aggression in violent criminal offenders (Lidberg, Tuck, Asberg, Scalia-Tomba, & Bertilsson, 1985; Linnoila et al., 1983; Roy, Virkkunen, Guthrie, Poland, & Linnoila, 1986), and suicide attempts in psychiatric populations (Brown et al., 1982; López-Ibor, Saiz-Ruiz, & Pérez de los Cobos, 1985). These results were interpreted as reflective of reduced, presynaptic 5-HT function. Postmortem studies revealed decreases in tritiated-imipramine binding (which is thought to bind to a presynaptic receptor site), in various regions of the brain that support the alterations in presynaptic 5-HT function (Crow et al., 1984; Gross-Isserhoff, Israeli, & Biegon, 1989; Stanley, Virgilio, & Gershon, 1982). Postmortem studies of suicide victims also demonstrated increases in 5-HT$_2$ receptors in prefrontal cortex (Arango et al., 1990). Such up-regulation of 5-HT$_2$ receptors may be secondary to reduced serotonergic activity.

In addition to the results of neuroanatomical investigations, indirect measures of 5-HT function have also shown that reduced activity is associated with aggressivity or suicidal behavior. For instance, serum prolactin concentrations following an infusion of fenfluramine are thought to reflect neurohormonal response to net pre- and postsynaptic activation of the 5-HT system. Not surprisingly, then, fenfluramine infusion is followed by relatively reduced prolactin responses among patients with personality disorders or major affective disorders, particularly those who have attempted suicide, in comparison to normal controls (Coccaro, 1989). Whole blood serotonin is another peripheral index of serotonergic function that has been correlated with aggressive behavior. Specifically, whole blood serotonin was positively correlated with conduct disorder ratings in male adolescents (see review, Coccaro, 1989).

In addition to studies involving human beings, many of which were done with patients referred for psychiatric care, an inverse relationship between central serotonergic activity and indices of aggression has been observed in various animal models. Studies using socially housed rodents, for example, reported a negative correlation between 5-HIAA concentrations in CSF and aggression. Hence, submissive Swiss mice, which had been housed with an α-mouse (i.e., dominant) for two weeks, were found to have significantly lower 5-HIAA concentrations in the hypothalamus, hippocampus, and brain stem compared to α-mice (Hilakivi et al.,1989). Further, among strains of mice socially intermixed to induce spontaneous interstrain aggression, the most aggressive animals had significantly less 5-HT in the amygdala and hypothalamus when contrasted with the least aggressive strains or control mice (Serri & Ely, 1984). Finally, in rats subjected to a resident–intruder model (involving the introduction of an intruder mouse into the established territory of a resident mouse), parachlorophenylalanine-induced serotonin depletion resulted in increased offensive behaviors in both resident and intruders without any difference produced in defensive behavior (Vergnes, Depaulis, & Boehrer, 1986).

Results consistent with those from the foregoing studies were reported for vervet monkeys. In this species, fenfluramine-induced serotonin depletion produced a dose-related decline in whole blood serotonin and CSF 5-HIAA, changes which are significantly correlated with increased movement, human-directed aggression, and aggression directed toward a conspecific. Similarly, it has been observed that fluoxetine (a serotonin reuptake inhibitor) and tryptophan (the amino acid from which 5-HT is produced)[3] caused decreases in aggressive behavior in socially housed subordinate vervets (Raleigh, 1987). Notably, on removal of dominant males from social groups, the subordinate males treated with tryptophan or fluoxetine exhibited decreased aggression and increased affiliative behaviors in comparison to controls, and were able to achieve dominant social status. Conversely, subordinate males treated with fenfluramine and quipazine (a receptor agonist) were not only more aggressive, they also directed significantly more aggression toward females and were unable to achieve dominant social status (Raleigh et al., 1986).

Finally, the dietary manipulations found to influence the aggressive behavior of monkeys also may exert effects through the 5-HT system. Hence, acute administration of a tryptophan-free diet significantly increases spontaneous and food-competitive aggression in male vervet monkeys, an effect that is inhibited in male and female vervets following administration of a tryptophan-supplemented diet (Chamberlain, Ervin, Pihl, & Young, 1987). In our own work, we observed that cynomolgus macaques consuming a diet low in saturated fat and cholesterol engage in significantly more contact aggression than do animals consuming a high-fat, high-cholesterol diet but otherwise treated identically (Kaplan & Manuck, 1990). Notably, fenfluramine-induced increases in serum prolactin concentrations are blunted (indicating

---

[3]There is evidence that serotonin release from brain neurons is decreased when brain tryptophan levels are lowered (Schaechter & Wurtman, 1990).

reduced 5-HT drive) in monkeys eating a low-fat diet in comparison to their high-fat counterparts.

Autonomic Arousal

We suggested earlier that sympathetic arousal was the common pathway through which dominant social status and heart rate hyperresponsivity exerted pathogenic effects. Although admittedly speculative, one reason we chose to emphasize the association between the 5-HT system and aggressive behavior is that there exists evidence linking specific serotonergic receptors and cardiovascular regulation. It is known, for example, that serotonin exerts a variety of responses by stimulation of multiple receptor subtypes located in the central nervous system, autonomic nerve endings, and on smooth muscle tissues (for review, see Saxena & Villalon, 1990). Specifically, the 5-HT_1a and 5-HT_2 receptors appear to be involved in central regulation of cardiovascular responses. For example, 5-HT_1a agonists cause a decrease in heart rate and blood pressure and a reduction in sympathetic neural activity when administered centrally, via vertebral arteries, intracisternally, or directly to cerebral tissue (Saxena & Villalon, 1990). There is also evidence that somatodendritic 5-HT_1a autoreceptors in the raphe nucleus may be involved in the reduction of blood pressure, heart rate, and sympathetic nerve discharge (Kolassa, Beller, & Sanders, 1989; Mir & Fozard, 1987). In contrast to the effects of 5-HT_1a agonists, 5-HT_2 agonists produce an *increase* in blood pressure by stimulation of central sympathetic outflow (McCall & Harris, 1988). This pressor effect is thought to be mediated via pontomedullary serotonergic pathways or spinal 5-HT_2 receptors (Saxena & Villalon, 1990). These observations suggest that the net effect of the serotonergic system on central sympathetic response is dependent on the site of stimulation and the receptor subtype involved (Saxena & Villalon, 1990).

Behaviorally, the 5-HT_1a agonists, such as buspirone and ipsapirone, are reported to have an anxiolytic effect. For example, intraperitoneal administration of buspirone significantly reduces the occurrence of threat and attack behaviors of feral rats in response to threatening stimuli, even including attempted handling by an experimenter (Blanchard, Rodgers, Hendrie, & Hori, 1988). Studies of the role of 5-HT in modulating physiological responses to stress in rats, however, have yielded conflicting results. Intraperitoneal administration of ipsapirone reduced foot-shock bradycardia and immobility in one study (Korte, Koolhas, Schuurman, Traber, & Bohus, 1990), and intraperitoneal administration of buspirone antagonized immobilization-induced increases in heart rate and blood pressure in another (Taylor, Harris, Krieman, & Vogel, 1989). In the latter investigation, however, plasma norepinephrine and epinephrine were significantly increased in stressed and nonstressed rats. The increase in plasma catecholamine levels may be due to the ability of buspirone to stimulate adrenergic cell activity in addition to its central effects on sympathetic outflow. In summary, there is evidence that 5-HT$_1$a agonists, by stimulation of central serotonergic 5-HT$_1$a receptors, alter behavioral and physiological responses to stress. However, further investigation of the effects of 5-HT$_1$a agonists and like compounds on aggressive behavior is necessary to clarify the association between serotonergic activity, aggressivity, and sympathetic arousal.

Conceptual Models Associating Aggressivity, Sympathetic Arousal, and the 5-HT System

As reviewed earlier, dominant animals exposed to psychosocial stress and cardiac hyperresponders share a propensity to exhibit intense aggression. Stressed, dominant animals and cardiac hyperresponders are also characterized by exacerbated coronary artery atherosclerosis. These observations imply that aggressivity may represent, for monkeys as for people, an independent risk factor for the development of CHD and atherosclerosis. We have proposed elsewhere that aggressivity contributes to the development of atherosclerotic lesions via accompanying activation of the sympathetic nervous system and subsequent increases in heart rate, blood pressure, and circulating plasma catecholamines. The foregoing review suggests that both aggressivity and sympathetic responsivity to stress may be influenced by the degree of 5-HT drive expressed in the CNS. More important, it is believed that there exists stable, interindividual differences in central serotonergic drive (Higley, Suomi, & Linnoila, 1991; Raleigh, Brammer, McGuire, Pollack, & Yuwiler, 1991). Hence, it could be hypothesized that some aspect of central serotonergic activity is responsible for those characteristics habitually exhibited by some individuals (i.e., excessive aggressivity and cardiovascular hyperresponsivity) that place them at increased risk for developing exacerbated atherosclerosis and CHD.

To the extent that the 5-HT system influences aggressivity and cardiac responsivity to stress (and thus risk for CHD and atherosclerosis), the relevant interactions within the CNS could conform to any of at least three models:

1. *The 5-HT system potentiates aggressive behavior and the accompanying emotion of anger; the latter change then drives activation of the sympathetic nervous system and subsequent increases in heart rate, blood pressure, and circulating catecholamines (Fig. 7.5A).* In this model, dominant animals and cardiac hyperresponders are both characterized by relatively low serotonergic tone, compared to subordinates and cardiac hyporesponders. When exposed to social challenge (dominant animals) or threatening stimuli (cardiac hyperresponders), these animals would have an increased propensity to behave aggressively. Such aggressive behavior would be accompanied

Conceptual Models

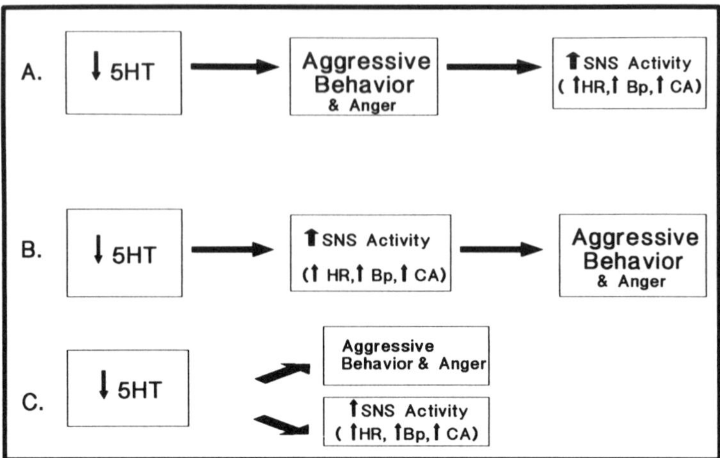

FIG. 7.5.   Conceptual models of how decreased concentrations of the serotonin metabolite 5-hydroxytryptamine (5HT) may act to increase sympathetic nervous system (SNS) activity with accompanying increases in heart rate (HR), blood pressure (Bp), and circulating catecholamines (CA): either directly (Schema A), indirectly through sympathetic activity (Schema B), or through independent actions on the SNS and the system controlling display of aggressive behaviors (Schema C).

by subsequent activation of the SNS and resulting increases in heart rate, blood pressure, and circulating catecholamines. As depicted in this model, the 5-HT system only indirectly influences SNS activity.

   2. *The 5-HT system directly potentiates central sympathetic activity, which is accompanied by peripheral increases in heart rate, blood pressure, and circulating catecholamines. Such central activation then triggers the release of aggressive behavior (Fig. 7.5B).* In this second model, overall low serotonergic tone increases the sensitivity of the neural substrates located in the ventral medulla mediating activity of the SNS such that an appropriate stimulus is likely to increase central sympathetic arousal. Increases in central sympathetic arousal lead to activation of appropriate behavioral responses as well as activation of peripheral sympathetic responses. For dominant animals and cardiac hyperresponders, increases in central sympathetic arousal would most often lead to activation of the centers controlling the release of aggressive behavior.

   3. *The 5-HT system independently increases both the sensitivity of the central sympathetic nervous system to external stimuli and the sensitivity of the system controlling the display of aggressive behaviors (Fig. 7.5C).* In this model, aggression and sympathetic arousal are related to low serotonergic tone, however, the relationships are mediated by independent mechanisms.

The foregoing models are presented as heuristic constructs designed to identify potentially fruitful avenues of investigation. Admittedly, other monoaminergic and peptidergic neurotransmitters may be involved in the activation of the SNS and aggressive behavior; however, current evidence supports a major role for the serotonergic system in these responses.

Future Directions

The preceding evidence and models suggest three hypotheses that might be addressed in future studies. These can be stated as follows:

1. In cynomolgus monkeys, there exist stable, interindividual differences in serotonergic drive that are responsible for differences in the expression of aggressive behavior among individuals. This hypothesis can be tested by analysis of repeated measurements of serotonin metabolites in cerebrospinal fluid and serial assessments of prolactin response to serotonin reuptake inhibitors from animals exposed to a variety of social challenges. We predict that animals with low serotonergic drive will exhibit extreme levels of aggressive behaviors and be at higher risk for the development of atherosclerosis and CHD than their less aggressive counterparts. Essentially, assessment of serotonergic drive may serve as a biological marker of the behavioral risk factor, "potential for anger–hostility."

2. In cynomolgus monkeys, 5-HT_1a receptors modulate central sympathetic outflow. We predict that 5-HT_1a agonists will decrease central sympathetic drive, resulting in lower heart rate and blood pressure responses to either stressful or threatening stimuli in susceptible individuals (i.e., dominant animals and cardiac hyperresponders) and, thereby, reducing atherogenesis and subsequent CHD. Although we have shown that propranolol reduces atherosclerosis in unstable dominant animals, it is not clear whether altering sympathetic response at the level of the central nervous system will have similar effects on atherogenesis.

3. 5-HT_1a agonists reduce the levels of aggressive behavior in dominant animals and cardiac hyperresponders. Although serotonergic involvement in modulation of aggression cannot be ruled out, if aggression is not affected in these groups, it may be determined whether the same serotonergic receptors are activated in both the expression of aggressivity and in the modulation of sympathetic arousal.

Studies such as these, although specific to the 5-HT system, also test the more general hypothesis that stable, inherent characteristics contribute to the risk for atherosclerosis and CHD. To the extent that such characteristics exist and can be identified, investigators may have the opportunity to more readily distinguish those individuals at the greatest risk for developing behaviorally influenced cardiovascular disease.

REFERENCES

Arango, V., Ernsberger, P., Marzuk, P. M., Chen, J., Tierney, H., Stanley, M., Reis, D. J., & Mann, J. J. (1990). Autoradiographic demonstration of increased 5-HT$_2$ and β-adrenergic receptor binding sites in the brain of suicide victims. *Archives of General Psychiatry, 47*, 1038–1047.

Bernstein, I. S. (1981). Dominance: The baby and the bathwater. *Behavioral Brain Sciences, 4*, 419–457.

Blanchard, D. C., Rodgers, R. J., Hendrie, C. A., & Hori, K. (1988). "Taming" of wild rats (*Rattus rattus*) by 5HT$_{1A}$ agonists buspirone and gepirone. *Pharmacology, Biochemistry and Behavior, 31*, 269–278.

Brown, G. L., Ebert, M. E., Goyer, P. F., Jimerson, D. C., Klein, W. J., Bunney, W. E., & Goodwin, F. K. (1982). Aggression, suicide, and serotonin: Relationship to CSF amine metabolites. *American Journal of Psychiatry, 139*, 741–746.

Chamberlain, B., Ervin, F. R., Pihl, R. O., & Young, S. N. (1987). The effect of raising or lowering tryptophan levels on aggression in vervet monkeys. *Pharmacology, Biochemistry and Behavior, 28*, 503–510.

Coccaro, E. F. (1989). Central serotonin and impulsive aggression. *British Journal of Psychiatry, 155*(Suppl. 8), 52–62.

Costa, P. T., McCrae, R. R., & Dembrowski, T. M. (1989). Agreeableness versus antagonism: Explication of a potential risk factor for CHD. In A. W. Siegman & T. M. Dembrowski (Eds.), *In search of coronary prone behavior: Beyond Type A* (pp. 41–63). Hillsdale, NJ: Lawrence Erlbaum Associates.

Crow, T. J., Cross, A. J., Cooper, S. J., Deakin, J. F. W., Ferrier, I. N., Johnson, J. A., Joseph, M. H., Owen, F., Poulter, M., Lofthouse, R., Corselis, J. A. N., Blessed, G., Perry, E. K., Perry, R. H., & Tomlinson, B. E. (1984). Neurotransmitter receptors and monoamine metabolites in brains of patients with Alzheimer-type dementia and depression, and suicides. *Neuropharmacology, 23*, 1561–1569.

Darwin, C. (1872). *The expression of the emotions in man and animals.* Chicago: University of Chicago Press.

Dembrowski, T. M., & Costa, P. T. (1988). Assessment of coronary-prone behavior: A current overview. *Annals of Behavioral Medicine, 10*, 60–63.

Eibl-Eibesfeldt, I. (1975). *Ethology, the biology of behavior* (2nd ed.). New York: Holt, Rinehart & Winston.

Ekman, P. (1965). Differential communication of affect by head and body cues. *Journal of Personality and Social Psychology, 2*(5), 726–735.

Gross-Isseroff, R., Israeli, M., & Biegon, A. (1989). Autoradiographic analysis of tritiated imipramine binding in the human brain postmortem: Effects of suicide. *Archives of General Psychiatry, 46*, 237–241.

Henry, J. P., Ely, D. L., Stephens, P. M., Ratcliffe, H. L., Santisteban, G. A., & Shapiro, A. P. (1971). The role of psychosocial factors in the development of arteriosclerosis in CBA mice. *Atherosclerosis, 14*, 203–218.

Higley, J. D., Suomi, S. J., & Linnoila, M. (1991). CSF monoamine metabolite concentrations vary according to age, rearing, and sex, and are influenced by the stressor of social separation in rhesus monkeys. *Psychopharmacology, 103*, 551–556.

Hilakivi, L. A., Lister, R. G., Durcan, M. J., Ota, M., Eskay, R. L., Mefford, I., & Linnoila, M. (1989). Behavioral, hormonal and neurochemical characteristics of aggressive α-mice. *Brain Research, 502*, 158–166.

Kaplan, J. R., Pettersson, K., Manuck, S. B., & Olsson, G. (1991). Role of sympathoadrenal medullary activation in the initiation and progression of atherosclerosis. *Circulation, 84*(Suppl. 6), 123–132.

Kaplan, J. R., Manuck, S. B., Clarkson, T. B., & Prichard, R. W. (1985). Animal models of behavioral influences on atherosclerosis. In E. S. Katkin & S. B. Manuck (Eds.), *Advances in behavioral medicine* (Vol. 1, 115–163). Greenwich: JAI Press.

Kaplan, J. R., & Manuck, S. B. (1989). The effect of propranolol on social interactions among adult male cynomolgus monkeys (*Macaca fascicularis*) housed in disrupted social groupings. *Psychosomatic Medicine, 51*, 449–462.

Kaplan, J. R., Manuck, S. B., Adams, M. R., Williams, J. K., Selwyn, A. P., & Clarkson, T. B. (1991). Nonhuman primates as a model for evaluating behavioral influences on atherosclerosis, and cardiac structure and function. In A. P. Shapiro & A. Baum (Eds.), *Perspectives in behavioral medicine: Behavioral aspects of cardiovascular disease* (pp. 105–129). Hillsdale, NJ: Lawrence Erlbaum Associates.

Kaplan, J. R., Adams, M. R., Clarkson, T. B., Manuck, S. B., & Shively, C. A. (1991). Social behavior and gender in biomedical investigations using monkeys: Studies in atherogenesis. *Laboratory Animal Science, 41*(4), 334–342.

Kaplan, J. R., & Manuck, S. B. (1990). The effects of fat and cholesterol on aggressive behavior in monkeys. *Psychosomatic Medicine, 52*, 246–247.

Kaplan, J. R., Manuck, S. B., Clarkson, T. B., Lusso, F. M., & Taub, D. M. (1982). Social status, environment, and atherosclerosis in cynomolgus monkeys. *Arteriosclerosis, 2*(5), 359–368.

Kaplan, J. R., Manuck, S. B., Adams, M. R., Weingand, K. W., & Clarkson, T. B. (1987). Inhibition of coronary atherosclerosis by propranolol in behaviorally predisposed monkeys fed an atherogenic diet. *Circulation, 76*, 1364–1372.

Kaplan, J. R. (1977). Patterns of fight interference in free-ranging rhesus monkeys. *American Journal of Physical Anthropology, 47*, 279–288.

Kolassa, N., Beller, K. D., & Sanders, K. H. (1989). Evidence for the interaction of urapidil with 5-HT$_1$a receptors in the brain leading to a decrease in blood pressure. *American Journal of Cardiology, 63*(Suppl. C), 36–39.

Korte, S. M., Koolhas, J. M., Schuurman, T., Traber, J., & Bohus, B. (1990). Anxiolytics and stress-induced behavioral and cardiac responses: A study of diazepam and ipsapirone (TVX Q 7821). *European Journal of Pharmacology, 179*, 393–401.

Lidberg, L., Tuck, J. R., Asberg, M., Scalia-Tomba, G. P., & Bertilsson, L. (1985). Homicide, suicide and CSF 5-HIAA. *Acta Psychiatrica Scandinavia, 71*, 230–236.

Linnoila, M., Virkkunen, M., Scheinen, M., Nuutila, A., Rimon, R., & Goodwin, F. K. (1983). Low cerebrospinal fluid 5-hydroxyindoleacetic acid concentration differentiates impulsive from nonimpulsive violent behavior. *Life Sciences, 33*, 2609–2614.

López-Ibor, J. J., Jr., Saiz-Ruiz, J., & Pérez de los Cobos, J. C. (1985). Biological correlations of suicide and aggressivity in major depression (with melancholia): 5-hydroxyindoleacetic acid and cortisol in cerebrospinal fluid, dexamethasone suppression test and therapeutic response to 5-hydroxytryptophan. *Neuropsychobiology, 14*, 67–74.

Manuck, S. B., Kaplan, J. R., & Clarkson, T. B. (1983). Behaviorally-induced heart rate reactivity and atherosclerosis in cynomolgus monkeys. *Psychosomatic Medicine, 45*, 95–108.

Manuck, S. B., Kaplan, J. R., Muldoon, M. F., Adams, M. R., & Clarkson, T. B. (1991). The behavioral exacerbation of atherosclerosis and its inhibition by propranolol. In P. M. McCabe, N. Schneiderman, T. M. Field, & J. S. Skylar (Eds.), *Stress, coping and disease* (pp. 51–72). Hillsdale, NJ: Lawrence Erlbaum Associates.

Manuck, S. B., Kaplan, J. R., Adams, M. R., & Clarkson, T. B. (1988). Effects of stress and the sympathetic nervous system on coronary artery atherosclerosis in the cynomolgus macaque. *American Heart Journal, 116*, 328–333.

McCall, R. B., & Harris, L. T. (1988). 5-HT2 receptor agonists increase spontaneous sympathetic nerve discharge. *European Journal of Pharmacology, 151*, 113–116.

McGill, H. C., Jr. (1972). Atherosclerosis: Problems in pathogenesis. *Atherosclerosis Reviews, 2*, 27–66.

Mir, A. K., & Fozard, J. R. (1987). Cardiovascular effects of 8-hydroxy-2-(di-n-propylamino) tetralin (8-OH-DPAT). In C. T. Dourish, S. Ahlenius, & P. H. Hutson (Eds.), *Series in biomedicine: Brain 5-HT1a receptors. Behavioral and neurochemical pharmacology* (pp. 120–134). Chichester: Elis Horwood.

Moyer, K. E. (1968). Kinds of aggression and their physiological basis. *Communications on Behavioral Biology, 2*(A), 65–87.

Nerem, R. M., Levesque, M. J., & Cornhill, J. F. (1980). Social environment as a factor in diet-induced atherosclerosis. *Science, 208,* 1475–1476.

Raleigh, M. J., Brammer, G. L., McGuire, M. T., Pollack, D. B., & Yuwiler, A. (1992). Individual differences in basal cisternal cerebrospinal fluid 5-HIAA and HVA in monkeys: The effects of gender, age, physical characteristics, and matrilineal influences. *Neuropsychopharmacology, 7,* 295–304.

Raleigh, M. J., Brammer, G. L., Ritvo, E. R., Geller, E., McGuire, M. T., & Yuwiler, A. (1986). Effects of chronic fenfluramine on blood serotonin, cerebrospinal fluid metabolites, and behavior in monkeys. *Psychopharmacology, 90,* 503–508.

Raleigh, M. J. (1987). Differential behavioral effects of tryptophan and 5-hydroxytryptophan in vervet monkeys: Influence of catecholaminergic systems. *Psychopharmacology, 93,* 44–50.

Rowell, T. (1974). The concept of social dominance. *Behavioral Biology, 11*(2), 131–159.

Roy, A., Virkkunen, M. B. M., Guthrie, S., Poland, R.,& Linnoila, M. (1986). Monoamines, glucose metabolism, suicide and aggressive behaviors. *Psychopharmacology Bulletin, 22*(3), 661–665.

Sade, D. S. (1967). Determinants of dominance in a group of free-ranging rhesus monkeys. In S. Altmann (Ed.), *Social communication among primates* (pp. 99–114). Chicago: The University of Chicago Press.

Sade, D. S. (1973). An ethogram for rhesus monkeys: I. Antithetical contrasts in posture and movement. *American Journal of Physical Anthropology, 38,* 537–542.

Sade, D. S. (1972). Sociometrics of *Macaca mulatta.* I. Linkages and cliques in grooming matrices. *Folia Primatologica, 18,* 196–223.

Saxena, P. R., & Villalon, C. M. (1990). Cardiovascular effects of serotonin agonists and antagonists. *Journal of Cardiovascular Pharmacology, 15*(Suppl. S), (7) 17–34.

Schaechter, J. D., & Wurtman, R. J. (1990). Serotonin release varies with brain tryptophan levels. *Brain Research, 532,* 203–210.

Serri, G. A., & Ely, D. L. (1984). A comparative study of aggression related changes in brain serotonin in cba, c57bl, and dba mice. *Behavioral Brain Research, 12,* 283–289.

Seyfarth, R. M. (1977). A model of social grooming among adult female monkeys. *Journal of Theoretical Biology, 65,* 671–698.

Siegman, A. W., Dembrowski, T. M., & Ringel, N. (1987). Components of hostility and the severity of coronary heart disease. *Psychosomatic Medicine, 45,* 539–549.

Siegman, A. W., Anderson, R., Herbst, J., Boyle, S., & Wilkinson, J. (1992). Dimensions of anger-hostility and cardiovascular reactivity in provoked and angered men. *Journal of Behavioral Medicine, 15,* 257–272.

Stanley, M., Virgilio, J., & Gershon, S. (1982). Tritiated imipramine binding sites are decreased in the brain of suicide victims. *Science, 216,* 1337–1339.

Taylor, J., Harris, N., Krieman, M., & Vogel, W. H. (1989). Effects of buspirone on plasma catecholamines, heart rate, and blood pressure in stressed and nonstressed rats. *Pharmacology, Biochemistry and Behavior, 34,* 349–353.

Tompkins, S. S. (1962). *Affect, imagery, and consciousness.* New York: Springer-Verlag.

Van Hooff, J. (1969). The facial displays of the catarrhine monkeys and apes. In D. Morris (Ed.), *Primate ethology* (pp. 9–88). Garden City, NY: Anchor Books.

Vergnes, M., Depaulis, A., & Boehrer, A. (1986). Parachlorophenylalanine-induced serotonin depletion increases offensive but not defensive aggression in male rats. *Physiology and Behavior, 36,* 653–658.

Wickler, W. (1969). Sociosexual signals and their intraspecific imitation among primates. In D. Morris (Ed.), *Primate ethology* (pp. 89–189). Garden City, NY: Anchor Books.

8

PERSONALITY AND ANGER IN CARDIOVASCULAR DISEASE: TOWARD A PSYCHOLOGICAL MODEL

Richard J. Contrada
Rutgers University

The purpose of this chapter is to present a framework for conceptualizing anger-related personality characteristics that have been implicated in the etiology and the course of cardiovascular disorders. This task is approached by first presenting an overview of essential concepts, and then by attempting to organize those concepts within a single model. Relevant research findings are presented where they serve to illustrate key points. The main goals are to describe the elements of a unified theoretical perspective where that is possible, to highlight issues that appear in particular need of conceptual and empirical analysis, and to discuss implications for research methodology.

MAJOR CONCEPTUAL DOMAINS

The focus of the present analysis lies at the intersection of the two major conceptual domains implied by the constructs of personality and psychological stress. Each of these domains entails specific conceptual elements that are essential to the explanation of linkages between anger and cardiovascular disease. An additional prerequisite is an analysis of mechanisms whereby psychological factors may promote physical disorders.

From the study of personality can be drawn two sets of principles whose apparent incompatibility has often been a source of confusion and controversy: Principles of personality *process* provide a means of conceptualizing the organization of person systems whose operation generates activity and change; principles of personality *structure* are required to account for stability and invariance in human functioning (Allport, 1937, 1961). Thus, a process view is necessary for understanding how environmental events may provoke anger, whereas structural concepts are needed to account for observations indicating that individuals show temporal and cross-situational consistency in the frequency or intensity with which they experience anger.

From the study of psychological stress has emerged a means of conceptualizing the processes whereby major life events, minor hassles, and chronic environmental conditions give rise to anger and other negative emotions (Lazarus & Folkman, 1984). These processes include *primary appraisal*, the evaluation of events as threatening to physical and/or psychological well-being; *secondary appraisal*, the evaluation of available means of managing threatening events; and *coping*, the effort to manage threatening circumstances and their effects on the person. As elaborated later, appraisal and coping may be viewed as a distinct subset of the larger domain of regulatory activities carried out by the personality system.

There are at least three distinct pathways whereby the interplay between personality and psychological stress might contribute to the development of cardiovascular disease (Krantz, Glass, Contrada, & Miller, 1981). First, the *direct, psychophysiologic concomitants* of anger and of other negative emotional states include cardiovascular and neuroendocrine responses that appear related to mechanisms involved in the etiology of essential hypertension and coronary disease. Second, *overt, health-damaging behaviors*, such as cigarette smoking and poor diet, may reflect personality-based styles of coping with anger and other negative emotions. Third, *reactions to disease* already in progress may reflect the effects of personality and negative emotions on processes that play a role in determining the course of an illness episode, such as the detection and interpretation of cardiac symptoms and the decision to seek health care.

The following sections discuss separately the domains of personality and psychological stress. Each discussion begins with a brief theoretical rationale for drawing from the domain in question in developing the more general framework. Essential concepts are then defined. After considering issues unique to each domain, attention is turned to issues of between-domain interaction.

Personality

Pervasiveness and Persistence of Influence. Personality is relevant to the development of cardiovascular disease to the degree that it provides a basis for understanding the operation of one or more of the three disease-producing mechanisms outlined earlier. Such a basis can be developed, and rests in part on the *pervasiveness* and *persistence* of personality influences. By pervasiveness of influence I refer first to the fact that, traditionally, personality has been viewed as having effects on multiple domains of human functioning, including cognitive, affective, behavioral, and biological activity. To the degree that personality processes actually have such pervasive effects on the person system, it becomes more probable that personality influences the development and course of cardiovascular disease through all three pathways to disease. By contrast, if the scope of personality in general, or that of a particular personality construct such as hostility, is relatively narrow, this, by itself, might reduce its relevance to cardiovascular disease, perhaps by limiting its effects to just one of the three disease-promoting mechanisms, or even to a single, highly circumscribed role within one mechanism category.

Pervasiveness of influence also refers to the emphasis that personality theory places on cross-situational consistency in human functioning. Cross-situational consistency refers to the stability of individual differences in human functioning from one environmental condition to another. To the degree that a given personality variable is activated in a wide variety of circumstances, the individual with a high level of the trait experiences an increased frequency of exposures to its pathogenic effects. Increased exposure strengthens the relationship between personality and disease. It enhances the probability that processes representing one or more disease-generating mechanism will compromise health. For example, if the hostile person's cynical, distrusting attitudes extend to interactions involving health care providers, he or she may be slower to act on cardiac symptoms, or to comply with medical prescriptions, than if those attitudes are confined to closer personal relationships.

The persistence of personality influences derives from the temporal stability of personality characteristics. Temporal stability refers to the consistency of individual differences in human functioning across significant time periods. Like cross-situational consistency, temporal stability enhances risk of disease by increasing exposure to pathogenic events (e.g., more episodes of sympathetic–adrenomedullary activity will be associated with anger that is recurrent). In addition, temporal consistency may permit personality to play a special role in exerting pathogenic effects through health-damaging mechanisms that unfold gradually. For example, the catecholamine theory of coronary disease involves slowly operating mechanisms, such as the gradual accumulation of atheromatous plaque, as well as more rapidly developing mechanisms, such as the precipitation of myocardial infarction (MI) through the production of thrombosis (Schneiderman, 1983). Although individual differences in response to a single event may represent a pathway linking personality to disease (the hostile person experiences an MI during an angry discussion), personality influences may be particularly important for outcomes that reflect responses accumulated over multiple occasions (repeated angry exchanges gradually promote the development of atherosclerosis in the hostile person).[1]

Personality Structure.   The preceding paragraph referred to the "influences" or "effects" of personality. Many readers may have objected to the apparently glib implication that personality can be viewed as a causal antecedent to parameters of human functioning. If personality is a pattern of consistencies in cognition, affect, overt action, and biological activity, how then can personality also cause the production of such patterns?

One way to approach this apparent circularity is to distinguish explicitly the notions of *statistical* structure and *personality* structure. Statistical structure refers to the two forms of behavioral consistency discussed earlier, that is, individual differences in overt behavior that are consistent over time and across situations. These forms of consistency can be thought of as statistical structures because they refer to response-patterns that are organized, that manifest regularity, and that have an enduring quality. But the structure is in the numbers, and in the behavioral observations that the numbers represent. The patterns of consistency do not correspond to unobservable personality characteristics; they reflect the causal effects of those characteristics.

Personality structures exist beneath the person's skin. Like patterns of temporal and cross-situational consistency, personality structures have organization, but here, the organization is real, rather than statistical (Loevinger, 1957). Structures in the person are conceptually distinct from the observable behavior patterns they produce. Like those patterns, the personality structures have organization, manifest regularity, and endure. But these qualities do not describe a set of numbers, or a set of observed behaviors; they describe biological entities such as neural circuits, or psychological entities such as internal representations of the self and of the world.

Personality Process.   Personality process refers to those aspects of human functioning that involve the operation of personality structures. Implicit in the preceding discussion are processes whereby personality structures produce overt responses comprised by the two forms of statistical structure. In addition, because personality does not operate in a situational vacuum, processes must be specified to account for interactions between personality structures and environmental conditions that are relevant to those structures. Conceptual and empirical analysis of process is essential if we are to escape circular

---

[1]Personality attributes are not unique in their potential for contributing to coronary disease through slowly operating mechanisms. For example, chronic conditions, such as repeated exposure to a demanding work environment, also may promote disease through gradually accumulating effects. Moreover, a personality attribute may exert a pathogenic effect by promoting chronic exposure to stressful environments, a point that is discussed later.

arguments in which both cause (personality structure) and effect (statistical structure) are inferred from the same set of observations. Such an analysis depends on further development of concepts drawn from the study of psychological stress, to which we now turn.

Psychological Stress

Earlier it was stated that the study of psychological stress has generated three process concepts that are critical to the present discussion: primary appraisal, secondary appraisal, and coping. These processes define a sequence of events initiated when the individual is confronted by conditions in the environment that may be referred to as stressors. Introduction of the concepts of appraisal and coping made it possible to reconcile findings indicating a probabilistic, rather than invariant relationship between the occurrence of stressful events and negative adaptive outcomes (e.g., Rabkin & Struening, 1976). Individual differences in outcome could now be attributed to variability in appraisal and coping among individuals experiencing objectively equivalent exposure to stressful events. The absence of strong, stress main effects, and the considerable between-person variability in the effects of stressors also stimulated interest in the characteristics of the person and of the social context that may moderate the stress-outcome association by influencing the processes of appraisal and coping (e.g., Cassel, 1976; Kobasa, 1979). Thus, appraisal and coping, the main conceptual elements of psychological stress theory, may be thought of as personality concepts in that they provide a means of explaining individual differences in thought, feeling, behavior, and biological activity elicited by a certain class of situations.

Psychological Stress and Regulation.   For purposes of the present analysis it is useful to distinguish two phases of the processes mediating responses to stressors.[2] *Problem representation* subsumes primary and secondary appraisal and refers to processes whereby the individual constructs an internal representation of the stressful transaction. In addition to the evaluation of potential harm to physical and/or psychological well-being (something is at stake in this encounter), this representation includes features of the stressor, subjective and somatic reactions to the stressor, and alternative courses of action (this is what is at stake, this is how I feel about it, and there are several ways to respond with varying probabilities of success).

---

[2]The distinctions between primary and secondary appraisal, and between problem representation and response generation, are presented for purposes of analysis and exposition, and should not be taken as sharply demarcated, time-ordered events. For discussions of this issue, see Lazarus (1991, pp. 149–152), Lazarus and Folkman (1984, pp. 31–38), and Leventhal and Everhart (1979).

Response generation includes, but is not limited to, coping. It involves the initiation of regulatory responses aimed at countering elements of the problem as represented by the individual. Coping refers to cognitive and behavioral responses to the stressor that are effortful and deliberate (nonautomatic regulation), whereas other regulatory responses are relatively effortless and require no deliberation (automatic regulation). Either type of regulatory response may focus primarily on the environment or on the self, a distinction that subsumes that between problem-focused and emotion-focused coping (Lazarus & Folkman, 1984). Once initiated, the outcome of initial coping efforts is appraised, which permits an updating of the problem representation, possibly leading to modification of coping strategy (Leventhal, Suls, & Leventhal, in press).

The processes of problem representation and response generation cannot be observed directly but can be inferred from indicators reflecting the activity of affective, expressive-behavioral, and physiological systems. Among the physiologic effects of stress are cardiovascular and neuroendocrine responses that may represent the direct psychophysiologic pathway to disease discussed earlier (Krantz & Manuck, 1984; Schneiderman, 1983). It has long been suspected that, among the negative emotions, anger and associated coping activity may be linked to a specific pattern of physiologic adjustments that is particularly damaging to cardiovascular health (Glass & Contrada, 1984). This response pattern, characterized by pronounced sympathetic–adrenomedullary (SAM) activity and consequent effects on target organs possessing adrenergic receptors, has also been associated with circumstances that are not specifically anger-inducing, but that share with anger the generation of a readiness to perform effortful muscle activity (Obrist, 1981). Thus, the preparation for active, environment-focused, self-regulatory behavior may be the basis for the direct, health-damaging, physiologic correlates of anger-related personality attributes.

The "physiologic reactivity" mechanism appears biologically plausible, and has received considerable attention in empirical research. However, the role of personality and anger in cardiovascular disease may not be confined to this mechanism. As noted earlier, it is conceivable that anger-related attributes influence affective- and expressive-behavioral processes involved in the development and maintenance of overt, health-damaging lifestyle variables such as cigarette smoking, alcohol abuse, and poor diet. Moreover, the signs and symptoms of existing disease may be conceptualized as health threats in response to which the individual may evidence stress-reducing, self-regulatory activity that may further the course of the disorder. For example, anger-related personality attributes may disturb the relationship between patient and health-care provider and undermine compliance with medical regimens.

CONCEPTUALIZING THE PERSONALITY–STRESS INTERFACE

As noted earlier, between-person variability in the stress response indicates that the environmental stressor is not the sole determinant of that response. If two individuals walking together are confronted by the same menacing mugger, and one prepares to attack whereas the other prepares to flee, it may be assumed that each constructed a different representation of the problem, or that similar problem representations generated different regulatory responses. Some factor or factors that distinguish the two individuals interacted with the presence of a menacing mugger to produce different behavioral reactions.

By themselves, individual differences in response on a single occasion do not necessarily reflect personality. More transient, contextual factors, such as differences in environmental exposures immediately prior to the occasion in question, may suffice to explain the between-person variability. For example, to the more aggressive of the two potential victims, the mugger's imminent attack may have been a last straw, the latest in a series of anger instigations that occurred, by chance, on a particular, bad day. The person–situation interaction represented by the mugging scenario becomes relevant to the personality–stress interface only if we add cross-situational and temporal consistency to the picture. Let us assume, then, that these two individuals differ in the degree to which they respond aggressively to a range of different stressful situations, and that this is a rather long-standing pattern. This deceptively simple example implies an array of constructs that provide a model for conceptualizing interactions between personality and anger.

Statistical Structure

The term *respond aggressively* might refer to individual differences in affect (intensity of anger), expressive–motor behavior (facial display of anger; threatening posture; verbal/physical assault), and physiological activity (SAM activation). In the simplest case, these response parameters would form a single (i.e., unidimensional) pattern of response with both temporal and cross-situational consistency. This form of response covariation would support the inference that a single, enduring personality structure underlies differences in the degree to which the two potential mugging victims exhibit a coordinated, defensive reaction involving the affective, behavioral, and physiological elements described earlier.

However, research concerned with the role of anger-related personality traits in cardiovascular disease has relied heavily on assessment tools that were not constructed with a broad, aggressiveness construct in mind. For example, the Structured Interview (SI) (Rosenman, 1978) was first used to derive global ratings of Type A behavior, which included hostility as but one of several descriptive elements. The remaining elements—achievement-striving, competitiveness, and time-urgency—have conceptual linkages to anger, but an explicit formulation of those linkages and their relation to structured interview assessments has not been developed. The SI subsequently was used to derive a single, "potential for hostility" rating (Matthews, Glass, Rosenman, & Bortner, 1977), and then to assess separately a number of specific, anger-related dimensions. The latter involve distinctions between hostile style (antagonistic vocal tone), hostile content (self-report of intense/frequent anger experience), and anger expression (stated reluctance to communicate anger).

There is growing interest in another measure of anger-related personality attributes, the Cook and Medley (1954) Hostility scale (Ho). The Ho was constructed for the purpose of distinguishing teachers with good versus bad rapport with students, and later came to be used to measure individual differences in hostility. As in the case of the SI, the Ho has been subjected to empirical and conceptual analyses aimed at determining the number of distinct personality attributes they measure and the nature of those attributes (Contrada & Jussim, 1992). Among several proposed facets of Ho-measured hostility are cynicism, mistrust, and paranoid alienation. Internal analyses of the Ho, like those involving the SI, are necessarily constrained by features of a measurement tool that was not constructed with explicit reference to a conceptual definition of hostility.

Although a clear picture of the internal statistical structure of SI and Ho responses has yet to emerge, there is a basis for suggesting some preliminary hypotheses concerning the types of personality structures that may be responsible for anger-related behaviors measured by these instruments. As discussed next, these include both what may be thought of as psychological personality structures, and what might be referred to as biological personality structures.

Psychological Versus Biological Structures

What "real" personality structures might account for individual differences in anger-related behavior? Social and personality psychologists have proposed numerous types of *cognitive-affective* structures that might qualify, including possible selves, schemas, scripts, goal hierarchies, implicit personality theories, and worldviews. Although specific conceptualizations vary, all of these constructs have been ascribed three properties that fit the present definition of psychological structure: They exist within the individual, they are enduring, and they are representational. By representational it is meant that these structures have the property of being stored knowledge, or records of information. They "stand for" features of the self or of the world (Markus & Zajonc, 1985).

To be relevant to anger-related behavior, a cognitive–affective structure must have additional features that promote the frequent, intense, and/or prolonged experience of anger. Recently, Lazarus (1991) suggested that a *"demeaning offense against me and mine* is the best shorthand description of the provocation to adult human anger" (p. 222). It follows that a cognitive–affective structure that favors the occurrence of stress appraisals characterized by this theme may constitute the personality structure underlying individual differences in anger-related behavior. Conceptual and empirical analyses of the hostility component of Type A behavior suggest such a construct. It consists of a *hostile world-view*, or an internal representation of life "as a competitive struggle for survival and advancement, in which other people use unfair, deceptive, and manipulative means in the pursuit of selfish goals" (Contrada, Leventhal, & O'Leary, 1990, p. 653).

There is also a theoretical rationale for positing that one or more *biological structures* contribute to individual differences in anger and related behavioral and physiologic activity. By biological personality structures I refer to characteristics of lower brain centers and the somatic and autonomic nervous system. Like their psychological counterparts, biological personality structures exist within the individual and are enduring over time. The difference is that whereas biological personality structures may interact with cognitive and affective structures, the biological structures themselves are not representational. Although peripheral physiologic systems have some of the properties of information-processing systems (Rushmer, 1989), their primary function is not to serve as internal records where information about the self or about the outside world is encoded. Rather, the primary function of biological personality structures, as defined here, is to support the muscular activity whereby the person acts on the environment.

Krantz and Durel (1983) described a somatopsychic feedback model of Type A behavior involving a constitutional predisposition to SAM hyperreactivity. In this model, SAM responses reflect, in part, the operation of a biological substrate. That substrate may be a characteristic of central nervous system structures responsible for sympathetic outflow, of adrenergic receptors that mediate cardiovascular and other somatic effects of SAM activation, and/or of target organs themselves. In the somatopsychic feedback model, this biological structure interacts with cognitive structures to produce the outward manifestation of hostility and other emotional Type A behaviors.

To return to our mugging scenario, the personality of the more aggressive of the two potential victims may differ from that of his counterpart in two ways. One possibility is that his aggressive stance reflects his view of the world, and the other posits an underlying biological predisposition. These alternatives are neither exhaustive, nor mutually exclusive. However, they do suffice to illustrate two major types of anger-related personality structure, and lend themselves to an analysis of processes of person–situation interaction that may account for anger-related behavior.

Processes of Person–Situation Interaction

The stage is now set to discuss the processes whereby a hostile worldview and a constitutionally based tendency toward SAM hyperreactivity might influence psychological stress parameters. Although a number of specific processes are implied by this analysis, a useful way to proceed is to distinguish between three general types of processes. This distinction is based on three points at which personality structures may come in contact with the stress process, namely, the points of *exposure, problem representation*, and *response generation*.

The exposure notion refers to the possibility that personality structures influence the frequency and duration of contact with potentially stressful conditions. The idea that personality traits influence exposure to trait-relevant situations was essential to Eysenck's (1965) conceptualization of introversion–extraversion, and is reflected in Bandura's (1978) principle of reciprocal determination. According to an analysis described by Buss (1987), exposure may involve *self-selection* into situations (e.g., through choice of marital partner or career), the unintentional *evocation* of responses from the environment (e.g., the attractive person receives more attention), or active *manipulation* (e.g., the dependent individual deliberately elicits social support from others). In the present context, exposure would involve the effects of these processes on the frequency, intensity, and/or duration of objectively real, anger-provoking events. For example, the office worker with a hostile worldview might have an interpersonal style that creates a more hostile work environment than existed when he/she was originally hired (through a combination of evocation and manipulation effects). In the mugging scenario, it may be that the more aggressive of the two potential victims was responsible for their entering a high-crime part of town (an example of selection).

Objectively real differences in exposure aside, hostile individuals may differ from their less hostile counterparts at the problem representation stage of the stress process. A hostile worldview might be expected to favor anger-provoking appraisals, particularly in situations involving a degree of ambiguity. For example, Dodge (1980) reported that children characterized by an aggressive, antisocial behavior pattern are more likely than less aggressive children to perceive hostile intent in a videotaped depiction in which one child causes another to spill a drink. Thus, preemptive action on the part of the aggressive member of our duo might actually be a miscalculation based on an erroneous interpretation of the "mugger's" intentions. However, the hostile construal of the situation need not be inaccurate. It is equally plausible to posit that anger-related personality structures influence problem representation by enhancing the individual's ability to detect threats that actually have a basis in reality.

Finally, personality-based variability in anger responses may emerge at the response-generation stage of the stress process. Here, following identical appraisals of the same, objectively real provocation, anger-related personality structures influence response tendencies. For example, individual differences in SAM reactivity may be associated with a tendency to emit vigorous behavioral responses (Krantz & Durel, 1983; Matthews, 1982). To the degree that behavioral and physiologic elements of this response pattern are integrated subcortically, they may not be accompanied by between-person variability in cognitive or affective responses to provocation. Instead, individual differences may not emerge until the stage at which lower-level systems rather proximal to overt responding are activated. In this case, the more aggressive response to the potential mugging might reflect a response tendency produced by feedback from heightened SAM and cardiovascular activity. Individual differences in problem-representation need not be posited, but might occur as a byproduct of somatopsychic feedback.

EXTENDING THE MODEL

Previous sections sketch the bare elements of a framework for conceptualizing the relationship between personality and anger. Although there are many lines along which the model might be elaborated, there are three general issues in particular need of conceptual work. First, further analysis of personality structure must be conducted to determine the number of distinct, anger-related personality attributes and to characterize both their individual operating characteristics and their interrelationships. This issue is particularly important for its implications for personality assessment. A second point discussed shortly concerns the need for further consideration of the processes whereby personality structures influence problem representation and regulation. Much of the laboratory work in the area of anger and cardiovascular disease has involved the study of stressors that are judged to be relevant to the personality attribute in question without reference to explicit theory. A fine-grained analysis of personality structure in relation to the stress process may facilitate the development of research protocols with the potential for improving our understanding of the person–situation interactions that have health-damaging consequences. The third issue addressed in the following section concerns the interaction between psychological and biological personality structures. Although much of the work in this area has been driven by the notion of SAM hyperreactivity as a biological substrate, there is a theoretical basis for an alternative view in which the mental representation of physiologic responses plays a key role.

Conceptualizing Anger-Related Personality Structures

At present, the question is open as to what personality structures might contribute to anger. In addition to the notion of a predisposition to SAM hyperreactivity (Krantz & Durel, 1983), biological characteristics that have been studied in relation to anger-related personality attributes include the density and sensitivity of beta-adrenergic receptors (Kahn, Perumal, & Gully, 1987), and degree of parasympathetic tone (Muranaka et al., 1988). This work may be expected to expand as new techniques continue to be developed and refined for the study of neurophysiological structure and function in humans, such as magnetic resonance imaging (Coffey, Figiel, Djang, & Weiner, 1990), receptor binding techniques (Mills & Dimsdale, 1988), and positron emission tomography (PET) scanning (Reiman, Fusselman, Fox, & Raichle, 1989).

Regarding the *form* of cognitive–affective structures relevant to the domains of anger and hostility, several possibilities were listed earlier, including schemas, implicit theories, and goal hierarchies. The reader is referred elsewhere for discussions of alternative conceptualizations of the formal properties of mental representations (Markus & Zajonc, 1985). As to the *content* of these mental representations, it may be of heuristic value to turn to two principles that emerged from the study of psychological stress and emotion. The first is the notion that stress inheres in the appraisal of a disturbed relationship between the person and the environment. The second is the idea that regulation consists of both self-focused and environment-focused activity. These principles suggest that the psychological structure of hostile individuals may be characterized in terms of representational structures with both self- and environment-related features, and that those representations include descriptive, evaluative, and procedural elements.

The self-environment dichotomy is relatively straightforward and refers to the distinction between beliefs, attitudes, and other psychological structures that are *self*-referent and those that are *nonself*-referent (see, for example, Carver & Scheier, 1981; Higgins & Bargh, 1987; Markus & Zajonc, 1985). A concrete example would be the distinction between features of one's self-concept (I am hostile) and one's beliefs about people in general (people are unfair, deceitful, and manipulative). Both beliefs are internal representations, but one refers to an attribute of self and the other to an attribute of "the nonself," in the example given, of people in general.

The descriptive–evaluative–procedural trichotomy refers to the distinction between representations of the self or nonself as they *actually are*, representations of *desired states* of self and nonself, and representations of *strategies* for acting on perceived reality so as to bring about desired states (see Cantor, 1990, for a discussion of this distinction). Statements such as "I am aggressive," and "People are unfair, deceitful, and manipulative" are descriptive representations; whether veridical or not, they refer to what to the person is a representation of an actual state of affairs. Other statements, such as "One should be free of external constraints," or "It is best not to express one's anger" are evaluative standards. They refer to states that are more or less desired or acceptable, but do not necessarily describe the person's view of reality. Still other statements, such as "One must lie to get ahead," or "It is useful to ask probing questions to uncover people's true motives" describe strategies or procedures for reducing the discrepancy between what is perceived as actual and what is perceived as desirable.

Personality Structure, Problem Representation, and Regulation

The distinction between descriptive, evaluative, and procedural facets of anger-related personality structure leads to several specific suggestions regarding the nature of relevant, stressful, person–situation interactions. For example, the process of primary appraisal may be construed in terms of the detection of a *match* between perceived events and a *descriptive* mental representation. Thus, an anger-producing appraisal may reflect a perceived correspondence between ongoing events and a "hostile worldview." As noted earlier, it has yet to be determined whether the effects of a hostile worldview on appraisal involve a cognitive *bias*, leading to the nonveridical perception of threat in objectively benign social situations, or a cognitive *skill*, allowing the hostile person to detect actual interpersonal threats that others might not notice. Primary appraisals culminating in anger also may reflect a *mis*match between perceived events and an *evaluative* mental representation. For example, the desire to be free of external constraints and intrusions might be threatened by an inquisitive interviewer, leading to antagonistic verbal responses reflecting anger and an effort to reassert control (Dembroski, MacDougall, & Musante, 1983).

Regulatory responses generated by hostile threat are likely to be constrained by the situation, but they also may be influenced by *procedural* cognitive–affective structures favoring one strategy or another. In addition to retaliatory aggression (*aggressive responding*), environmentally focused regulation might involve efforts aimed at further characterizing the threat (*detection procedures*), or at escaping from the situation (*social avoidance*). Alternatively, it may be at this point that a biological predisposition produces a tendency to act in a particular manner. In other words, individual differences in the aggressiveness of behavioral responses to social threats need not reflect the top-down effects of an internal representation ("hostile worldview→hostile appraisal→aggressive response"). They may instead reflect a process initiated by individual differences in fist-clenching or cardiac acceleration, attributable, in turn, to individual differences in biological structure.

Self-focused regulatory activity may be influenced by appraisal of the ongoing stressful encounter in relation to self-referent, *evaluative standards* (Carver & Scheier, 1981). For example, once anger has been provoked, self-referent evaluative standards pertaining to the expression of anger may be activated ("Don't let them know you are angry"). Instead of influencing environment-focused regulatory responses (e.g., detection procedures, aggressive responding, social avoidance), perceived discrepancies involving self-referent, evaluative structures may influence self-focused regulatory activity, such as the masking or suppression of emotional expression (Newton & Contrada, 1992) or use of palliatives such as alcohol and tranquilizers.[3]

Personality Structure and the Internal Representation of Biological Responses

As noted earlier, Krantz and Durel (1983) proposed that hostility, and other emotional components of Type A behavior reflect the outcome of an interaction between cognitive and biological structures. This view was based, in part, on Schachter and Singer's (1962) two-factor theory, in which emotion is generated when peripheral autonomic activity is labeled by a cognitive process involving emotion-related cues available in the environment. In effect, Krantz and Durel added a personality component to the Schachter–Singer model by positing that the frequency and intensity with which anger is generated is a function of two individual difference factors, a cognitive-attitudinal structure favoring Type A relevant appraisals, and a constitutionally based predisposition to SAM hyperreactivity. In this model, the cognitive-affective and biological parameters are distinct from one another, and their interaction involves a somatopsychic feedback loop that allows peripheral autonomic activity to influence the experience and behavioral expression of emotion.

More recent theorizing in the area of human emotion provides a basis for an alternative view. For example, in his bioinformational model of emotional imagery, Lang (1979) suggested that emotion reflects the operation of a cognitive–affective structure that includes components representing the situational provocation to emotion (descriptive elements), as well as behavioral impulses and bodily responses such as cardiac symptoms (response elements).

---

[3]Extended discussions of the relationship between cognitive structures and the process of appraisal may be found in Lazarus (1991) and Mandler (1982).

A similar view forms the basis of Leventhal's (1984) perceptual–motor theory of emotion. Although the response elements posited by these models resemble the procedural facets of anger-related personality structures described earlier, their somatic and visceral character allows them to play a special role in organizing actual efferent activity. The activation of behavioral and bodily elements of the internal representation is therefore critical to the generation of a full-blown emotional response that includes experiential, behavioral, and physiologic activity. That is, the *mental representation* of physiologic activity may be involved in the generation of observable emotional responses, including *actual* physiological activity.

Perceptual–motor theories of emotion suggest that it may be worth considering a modification of the Krantz–Durel (1983) somatopsychic hypothesis. Rather than an *interaction* between psychological and biological structures, personality-based emotional responding may reflect a *representational integration* of those structures. Individuals prone to the intense experience of anger and concomitant SAM responses may differ from their less anger-prone counterparts in the degree to which they possess cognitive–affective structures in which response elements such as cardiac symptoms and aggressive action are well represented. These representations may be the developmental consequence of repeated episodes in which anger provocations were followed by actual SAM reactivity. Thus, the Krantz–Durel model may describe an early stage in the development of anger-related personality attributes. Over time, this stage may be superseded by one in which anger provocations come to elicit pronounced, multichannel, emotional responses as a consequence of a strong associative connection between descriptive and response-encoding cognitive structures.

METHODOLOGICAL IMPLICATIONS

There has been a marked methodological bifurcation in research concerned with the health-damaging effects of anger-related personality attributes. Research on the psychological underpinnings of these traits has largely been limited to correlational analysis. The primary goal of this work has been to characterize distinct facets of anger-related traits such as hostility on the basis of their differential patterns of association with other personality constructs. Experimental research in this area has focused almost exclusively on the association between personality and physiologic reactivity to psychological stressors. The primary goal of this work has been to demonstrate the viability of hypotheses positing a direct psychophysiologic link between hostility and disease-promoting mechanisms. In some, although not all cases, selection of psychological stressors was based on their conceptual relevance to anger-related personality attributes (e.g., Glass et al., 1980; Suarez & Williams, 1989).

However, there have been few experimental analyses of psychological aspects of the person–situation interactions that link personality to physiologic reactivity. A clear conception of the points of contact between an explicit model of personality structure and an explicit model of the stress process provides a means of guiding efforts to integrate correlational and experimental approaches in the study of personality and anger.

Measuring Psychological Structure

One way to investigate a more elaborated model of anger-related, cognitive–affective structures would be through the development of new psychometric instruments. For example, following a traditional trait-measurement approach (e.g., Jackson, 1970; Messick, 1981), the self-nonself and description–evaluation–strategy distinctions described earlier could be used to generate a pool of anger-related personality items. This would involve systematically pairing each value of the two distinctions with each other, as in a multifactorial analysis of variance. The resulting framework would accommodate constructs that have emerged from content analyses of the Ho (e.g., Barefoot, Dodge, Peterson, Dahlstrom, & Williams, 1989). For example, most "Cynicism" and "Hostile Attribution" items reflect descriptions of people in general, whereas "Aggressive Responding" and "Social Avoidance" items would be categorized as strategies. Following a series of iterations between item-writing and statistical analysis of inter-item and item-scale correlations, it should be possible to generate a new measure based on a comprehensive framework describing the cognitive–affective structure of hostility, with subscales for facets of that structure that are not well represented in the Ho as it now exists.

The foregoing suggestion is intended only as an illustration. The underlying psychometric model is but one of several plausible alternatives. It is possible that techniques of subject-clustering, item-clustering, or multidimensional scaling provide a better model for investigating the psychological structure of anger-related personality attributes. However, any approach based entirely on correlational methods possesses a critical disadvantage. Causal analysis of personality structure requires experimentation. Psychometric instruments provide a means of distinguishing individuals with respect to differences in personality structure. To demonstrate the causal impact of anger-related personality structure on responses that reflect disease-promoting mechanisms, an experimental analysis of the effects of anger provocation is required. In addition, many aspects of cognitive–affective structure, such as the representation of somatic and visceral responses emphasized in perceptual–motor theories of emotion, may not be readily accessible through conventional, self-report measurement approaches.

Transaction Versus Interaction

The study of personality influences on environmental exposure reflects a dynamic view of the person–situation relationship. This view has sometimes been referred to as a *transactional* perspective, to distinguish it from a less dynamic, person–situation *interactionism*. In the more traditional, interactionist approach, analysis focuses on individual differences in response to equivalent exposure, which, in the present context, could involve effects located either at the stage of problem representation or response generation. It will require research reflecting both transactional and interactional paradigms to explicate fully the interface between anger-related personality attributes and the stress process.

There are many ways anger-related personality attributes might increase the frequency and duration of exposures to objectively real anger provocations. Among them are several processes that may have long-lasting effects on the person, such as mate selection, vocational choice, and interpersonal dynamics in the family and work environments. Through effects in these two major life domains, hostility and other anger-related traits may seriously limit the availability of supportive social relationships, and set in motion health-damaging patterns of social interaction (Smith & Frohm, 1985; Smith, Pope, Sanders, Allred, & O'Keeffe, 1988). Only by investigating personality from an ecological perspective will it be possible to gauge the degree to which hostile individuals actually create a more hostile world for themselves and for the people in their lives.

This is not to say that laboratory experimentation is without its place in research concerning the effects of personality on exposure to anger provocation. Smith (1989) reviewed a number of laboratory studies that reflect a transactional approach to the study of the global Type A pattern. For example, in a test of Glass's (1977) controllability hypothesis, Miller, Lack, and Astroff (1985) demonstrated that Type A individuals prolong exposure to a difficult task situation rather than relinquishing control to a more capable partner. With minor variations, the experimental procedures they employed could be adapted for the study of personality and the prolongation of hostile interpersonal situations. Another example is a study reported by Strube, Boland, Manfredo, and Al-Falaij (1987). The results suggest that the Type A individual's motivation to generate information diagnostic about his or her abilities may result in greater contact with demanding environments. Similar methodology could provide a means of evaluating the hypothesis that the hostile individual causes interpersonal conflict through his or her efforts to detect hostile motives for the behavior of others. Still another experimental approach to the study of hostility and exposure to anger provocation may be adapted from research on interpersonal communication (e.g., Levenson

& Gottman, 1985). For example, in a behavioral analysis of married couples, Smith, Sanders, and Alexander (1990) found evidence linking hostility to an interaction style likely to promote and maintain marital conflict.

Experimental Activation of Anger-Related Personality Structures

The study of anger-related personality attributes in relation to the problem representation and response generation phases of the stress process would be facilitated by several modifications of the "physiologic reactivity" paradigm. One modification would involve designing experimental manipulations that allow comparisons of anger provocations that vary in degree of subtlety. It would be expected that individual differences in reactivity reflecting effects on problem representation would be maximized under conditions in which threat is ambiguous. An analogous finding has been reported in the area of gender differences in aggression, where the tendency for males to be more aggressive than females appears stronger under conditions of low compared to high provocation (Frodi, Macauley, & Thome, 1977). By contrast, in order to isolate effects occurring at the stage of response generation, it would be necessary to present subjects with clear provocations in response to which individual differences in problem representation are minimized. Under these conditions, personality-related, between-person differences in stress response might be attributable to effects reflecting the generation of different regulatory responses to a similarly perceived threat.

In addition to designing experimental manipulations with a process model of stress in mind, there is a need for multivariate measurement of responses to the stressor. A focus on the direct, psychophysiologic correlates of anger-related personality attributes may be responsible for the relative neglect of dependent measures that may reflect the appraisal of anger provocations and nonphysiological regulatory responses. All too frequently, investigators have failed to obtain or to report data on self-reported affect and other psychological concomitants of heightened SAM activity. A more comprehensive assessment of affect, cognitive appraisal, and regulation might be obtained through the use of techniques such as thought sampling (Brunson & Matthews, 1981), videotape reconstruction (Cacioppo, Martzke, Petty, & Tassinary, 1988), and the analysis of facial expression (Chesney, Ekman, Friesen, Black, & Hecker, 1990) and other channels of nonverbal communication (Aiello, 1987). Although multivariate assessment of emotion complicates research protocols and statistical analysis, it has, in some cases, confirmed hypotheses linking personality to specific patterns of verbal, physiologic, and/or behavioral response (e.g., Newton & Contrada, 1992).

The present framework also argues for a more multivariate approach on the predictor side of the equation. To the degree that further examination of personality structure confirms the existence of multiple, distinct, anger-promoting structures, it will be necessary to investigate these constructs in relation to the stress process. Consider, by way of illustration, the simple case involving a single cognitive–affective structure and a single biologic structure. For the sake of argument, let us make the not all together unreasonable assumption that the Ho turns out to be primarily a marker for the cognitive–affective structure, and stylistic ratings based on the SI, primarily a marker for the biologic structure.

One direction for experimental analysis would be to include both measures as independent predictors of responses to an anger provocation. The Krantz–Durel (1983) somatopsychic model would suggest that the interaction of Ho and SI-derived personality assessments would be an important predictor of anger-related responses, with subjects with high scores on both measures showing greatest reactivity (see Carver, 1989, for a discussion of analytic issues in research involving multifaceted personality attributes). Specific hypotheses also might be tested regarding differential associations between these two predictors and measures reflecting effects of problem representation as opposed to response generation. The "hostile worldview" reflected in Ho scores might be expected to produce stronger associations with individual differences in problem representation; by contrast, SAM hyperreactivity and vigorous behavioral responses tendencies reflected in SI assessments might be more strongly associated measures reflecting response generation.

As a final methodological note in this section, it may be useful to return to the problem of demonstrating causal associations between personality structure and the stress response. Measures that show validity as markers for individual differences in personality structure (e.g., the SI and Ho) have fruitfully been used as predictors in experimental research examining the effects of anger provocation. The manipulation of a situational parameter (presence versus absence of interpersonal threat) may indicate that the social context plays the role of a causal moderator variable. That is, it elicits an association between personality marker and response measure. However, that association is correlational. The prospective design of such a study (personality is measured prior to the laboratory session) may make it reasonable to rule out the possibility that the experimental manipulation caused the dependent measure to influence the personality marker. Nonetheless, the data remain open to alternative explanations in terms of third variables, correlated with the hypothesized personality structure, that may have been activated by the experimental manipulation and produced the obtained effect on the dependent measure.

The problem of causal analysis has no easy solution, but can best be approached by an integration of experimental and correlational methods. One example of such an integration combines path analysis with experimentation. Although frequently used as means of probing causal hypotheses in correlational data sets, path analysis can be a powerful adjunct to randomized experiments. With the use of path analysis it is possible to test hypotheses concerning the role of psychological states in mediating the effects of experimental manipulations on dependent measures (Strube, 1989). By extending this approach, it would be possible to evaluate hypotheses concerning the pathways (e.g., problem representation, response generation) whereby the situational activation of anger-related personality structures influences the stress response.

Another strategy for evaluating causal hypotheses involving the effects of personality structure involves the use of pharmacological manipulations. For example, in a test of the Krantz–Durel (1983) somatopsychic feedback model, Krantz et al. (1988) found that a drug that blocks SAM influences on the cardiovascular system reduces the intensity of global Type A behavior. Similarly, research involving other pharmacological agents has provided evidence suggesting that Type B individuals may be less reactive to psychological stress than their Type A counterparts by virtue of having greater parasympathetic tone (Muranaka et al., 1988). Although methods of pharmacological stimulation and blockade entail numerous logistical and interpretative problems, their integration with more traditional research methods has the potential for adding considerable analytic power to the study of biological structures responsible for individual differences in anger.

CONCLUDING COMMENT

It is difficult to call attention to the need for more psychological theory without appearing at least a bit strident. This situation is only made worse by the fact that, at the early stages of theorizing, the ratio of constructs to operations is often alarmingly high, and any practical payoff seems remote, at best. Still, readers familiar with the history of health psychology are aware that many of the pioneers in this field were psychologists who were just as committed to developing basic theory as they were to solving problems, and who saw the inherent interdependence of these two goals. We would do well to emulate those pioneers in investigating the role of hostility and anger in cardiovascular disease, lest the signal fade again.

REFERENCES

Aiello, J. R. (1987). Human spatial behavior. In D. Stokols & I. Altman (Eds.), *Handbook of environmental psychology* (pp. 389–504). New York: Wiley.

Allport, G. W. (1937). *Personality: A psychological interpretation.* New York: Holt, Rinehart & Winston.

Allport, G. W. (1961). *Pattern and growth in personality.* New York: Holt, Rinehart, & Winston.

Bandura, A. (1978). The self system in reciprocal determinism. *American Psychologist, 33,* 344–358.

Barefoot, J. C., Dodge, K. A., Peterson, B. L., Dahlstrom, W. G., & Williams, R. B. (1989). The Cook–Medley Hostility Scale: Item content and ability to predict survival. *Psychosomatic Medicine, 51,* 46–57.

Brunson, B. I., & Matthews, K. A. (1981). The Type-A coronary-prone behavior pattern and reactions to uncontrollable events: An analysis of learned helplessness. *Journal of Personality and Social Psychology, 40,* 906–918.

Buss, D. M. (1987). Selection, evocation, and manipulation. *Journal of Personality and Social Psychology, 53,* 1214–1221.

Cacioppo, J. T., Martzke, J. S., Petty, R. E., & Tassinary, L. G. (1988). Specific forms of facial EMG response index emotions during an interview: From Darwin to the continuous flow hypothesis of affect-laden information processing. *Journal of Personality and Social Psychology, 54,* 592–604.

Cantor, N. (1990). From thought to behavior: "Having" and "doing" in the study of personality and cognition. *American Psychologist, 45,* 735–750.

Carver, C. S. (1989). How should multifaceted personality constructs be tested? Issues illustrated by self-monitoring, attributional style, and hardiness. *Journal of Personality and Social Psychology, 56,* 577–585.

Carver, C. S., & Scheier, M. F. (1981). *Attention and self-regulation: A control-theory approach to human behavior.* New York: Springer-Verlag.

Cassel, J. (1976). The contribution of the social environment to host resistance. *American Journal of Epidemiology, 104,* 107–123.

Chesney, M. A., Ekman, P., Friesen, W. V., Black, G. W., & Hecker, M. H. L. (1990). Type A behavior pattern: Facial behavior and speech components. *Psychosomatic Medicine, 52,* 307–319.

Coffey, C. E., Figiel, G. S., Djang, W. T., & Weiner, R. D. (1990). Subcortical hyperintensity on magnetic resonance imaging: A comparison of normal and depressed elderly patients. *American Journal of Psychiatry, 147,* 187–189.

Contrada, R. J., & Jussim, L. (1992). What *does* the Cook–Medley hostility scale measure? In search of an adequate measurement model. *Journal of Applied Social Psychology, 22,* 615–627.

Contrada, R. J., Leventhal, H., & O'Leary, A. (1990). Personality and health. In L. A. Pervin (Ed.), *Handbook of personality: Theory and research* (pp. 638–669). New York: Guilford.

Cook, W. W., & Medley, D. M. (1954). Proposed hostility and pharisaic-virtue scales for the MMPI. *The Journal of Applied Psychology, 38,* 414–418.

Dembroski, T. M., MacDougall, J. M., & Musante, J. L. (1983). Desirability of control versus locus of control. *Health Psychology, 3,* 15–36.

Dodge, K. A. (1980). Social cognition and children's aggressive behavior. *Child Development, 51,* 162–170.

Eysenck, H. J. (1965). *Fact and fiction in psychology.* Baltimore: Penguin Books.

Frodi, A., Macauley, J., & Thome, P. R. (1977). Are women always less aggressive than men? A review of the experimental literature. *Psychological Bulletin, 84,* 634–660.

Glass, D. C. (1977). *Behavior patterns, stress, and coronary disease.* Hillsdale, NJ: Lawrence Erlbaum Associates.

Glass, D. C., & Contrada, R. J. (1984). Type A behavior and catecholamines: A critical review. In C. R. Lake & M. Ziegler (Eds.), *Frontiers of Clinical Neuroscience: Vol. 2, Norepinephrine: Clinical aspects* (pp. 346–367). Baltimore: Williams & Wilkins.

Glass, D. C., Krakoff, L. R., Contrada, R. J., Hilton, W. F., Kehoe, K., Mannucci, E., Collins, C., Snow, B., & Elting, E. (1980). Effect of harassment and competition upon cardiovascular and plasma catecholamine responses in Type A and B individuals. *Psychophysiology, 17,* 453–463.

Higgins, E. T., & Bargh, J. A. (1987). Social cognition and social perception. *Annual Review of Psychology, 38,* 369–425.

Jackson, D. N. (1970). A sequential system for personality scale development. In C. D. Spielberger (Ed.), *Current topics in clinical and community psychology* (Vol. 2, pp. 61–96). New York: Academic Press.

Kahn, J. P., Perumal, A. S., & Gully, R. J. (1987). Correlation of Type A behavior with adrenergic receptor density: Implications for coronary artery disease. *Lancet, 1,* 937–939.

Kobasa, S. C. (1979). Stressful life events, personality, and health: An inquiry into hardiness. *Journal of Personality and Social Psychology, 37,* 1–11.

Krantz, D. S., Contrada, R. J., Durel, L. A., Hill, D. R., Friedler, E., & Lazar, J. D. (1988). Comparative effects of different beta-blockers on cardiovascular reactivity and Type A behavior in hypertensives. *Psychosomatic Medicine, 50,* 615–626.

Krantz, D. S., & Durel, L. A. (1983). Psychobiological substrates of the Type A behavior pattern. *Health Psychology, 2,* 393–411.

Krantz, D. S., Glass, D. C., Contrada, R. J., & Miller, N. E. (1981). Behavior and health. In the National Science Foundation's *Five year outlook on science and technology: 1981 Source Materials* (Vol. 2, pp. 561–588). Washington, DC: U.S. Government Printing Office.

Krantz, D. S., & Manuck, S. B. (1984). Acute psychophysiologic reactivity and risk of cardiovascular disease: A review and methodological critique. *Psychological Bulletin, 96,* 435–464.

Lang, P. J. (1979). A bio-informational theory of emotional imagery. *Psychophysiology, 16,* 495–512.

Lazarus, R. S. (1991). *Emotion and adaptation.* New York: Oxford University Press.

Lazarus, R. S., & Folkman, S. (1984). *Stress, appraisal, and coping.* New York: Springer-Verlag.

Levenson, R. W., & Gottman, J. M. (1985). Physiological and affective predictors of change in relationship satisfaction. *Journal of Personality and Social Psychology, 49,* 85–94.

Leventhal, E., Suls, J., & Leventhal, H. (in press). Hierarchical analysis of coping: Evidence from life-span studies. In H. Krohne (Ed.), *Attention and avoidance: Strategies and coping with aversiveness.* Toronto, Canada: Hogrese & Huber.

Leventhal, H. (1984). A perceptual–motor theory of emotion. In L. Berkowitz (Ed.), *Advances in experimental social psychology* (Vol. 17, pp. 117–182). San Diego, CA: Academic Press.

Leventhal, H., & Everhart, D. (1979). Emotion, pain, and physical illness. In C. E. Izard (Ed.), *Emotions in personality and psychopathology* (pp. 261–299). New York: Plenum Press.

Loevinger, J. (1957). Objective tests as instruments of psychological theory. *Psychological Reports, 3*(Monograph Suppl. 9), 635–694.

Mandler, G. (1982). The structure of value: Accounting for taste. In M. S. Clark & S. T. Fiske (Eds.), *Affect and cognition: The 17th Annual Carnegie Symposium on Cognition* (pp. 3–36). Hillsdale, NJ: Lawrence Erlbaum Associates.

Markus, H., & Zajonc, R. B. (1985). The cognitive perspective in social psychology. In G. Lindzey & E. Aronson (Eds.), *Handbook of social psychology* (pp. 137–230). New York: Random House.

Matthews, K. A. (1982). Psychological perspectives on the Type A behavior pattern. *Psychological Bulletin, 91,* 293–323.

Matthews, K. A., Glass, D. C., Rosenman, R. H., & Bortner, R. W. (1977). Competitive drive, Pattern A, and coronary heart disease: A further analysis of some data from the Western Collaborative Group Study. *Journal of Chronic Diseases, 30,* 489–498.

Messick, S. (1981). Constructs and their vicissitudes in educational and psychological measurement. *Psychological Bulletin, 89,* 575–588.

Miller, S. M., Lack, E. R., & Astroff, S. (1985). Preference for control and the coronary-prone behavior pattern: "I'd rather do it myself." *Journal of Personality and Social Psychology, 49,* 492–499.

Mills, P. J., & Dimsdale, J. E. (1988). The promise of receptor studies in psychophysiologic research. *Psychosomatic Medicine, 50,* 555–566.

Muranaka, M., Monou, H., Suzuki, J., Lane, J. D., Anderson, N. B., Kuhn, C. M., Schanberg, S. M., McCown, N., & Williams, R. B. (1988). Physiological responses to catecholamine infusions in Type A and Type B men. *Health Psychology, 7*(Suppl.), 145–163.

Newton, T. L., & Contrada, R. J. (1992). Verbal–autonomic response dissociation in repressive coping: The influence of social context. *Journal of Personality and Social Psychology, 62*, 159–167.

Obrist, P. A. (1981). *Cardiovascular psychophysiology: A perspective.* New York: Plenum Press.

Rabkin, J. G., & Struening, E. L. (1976). Life events, stress, and illness. *Science, 194*, 1013–1020.

Reiman, E. M., Fusselman, M. J., Fox, P. T., & Raichle, M. E. (1989). Neuroanatomical correlates of anticipatory anxiety. *Science, 243*, 1071–1074.

Rosenman, R. H. (1978). The interview method of assessment of the coronary-prone behavior pattern. In T. M. Dembroski, S. M. Weiss, J. L. Shields, S. G. Haynes, & M. Feinleib (Eds.), *Coronary-prone behavior* (pp. 55–69). New York: Springer-Verlag.

Rushmer, R. F. (1989). Structure and function of the cardiovascular system. In N. Schneiderman, S. M. Weiss, & P. G. Kaufman (Eds.), *Handbook of research methods in cardiovascular behavioral medicine* (pp. 5–22). New York: Plenum Press.

Schachter, S., & Singer, J. E. (1962). Cognitive, social, and physiological determinants of emotional state. *Psychological Review, 69*, 379–399.

Schneiderman, N. (1983). Animal models of coronary disease. In D. S. Krantz, A. Baum, & J. E. Singer (Eds.), *Handbook of psychology and health: Vol. 3. Cardiovascular disorders* (pp. 19–56). Hillsdale, NJ: Lawrence Erlbaum Associates.

Smith, T. W. (1989). Interactions, transactions, and the Type-A pattern: Additional avenues in the search for coronary-prone behavior. In A. W. Siegman & T. M. Dembroski (Eds.), *In search of coronary-prone behavior* (pp. 91–116). Hillsdale, NJ: Lawrence Erlbaum Associates.

Smith, T. W., & Frohm, K. D. (1985). What's so unhealthy about hostility? Construct validity and psychological correlates of the Cook and Medley Ho scale. *Health Psychology, 4*, 503–520.

Smith, T. W., Pope, M. K., Sanders, J. D., Allred, K. D., & O'Keefe, J. L. (1988). Cynical hostility at home and work: Psychosocial vulnerability across domains. *Journal of Research in Personality, 22*, 525–548.

Smith, T. W., Sanders, J. D., & Alexander, J. F. (1990). What does the Cook and Medley Hostility Scale measure? Affect, behavior, and attributions. *Journal of Personality and Social Psychology, 58*, 699–708.

Strube, M. J. (1989). Assessing subjects' construal of the laboratory situation. In N. Schneiderman, S. M. Weiss, & P. G. Kaufman (Eds.), *Handbook of research methods in cardiovascular behavioral medicine* (pp. 527–542). New York: Plenum Press.

Strube, M. J., Boland, S. M., Manfredo, P. A., & Al-Falaij, A. (1987). Type A behavior pattern and the self-evaluation of abilities: Empirical tests of the self-appraisal model. *Journal of Personality and Social Psychology, 52*, 956–974.

Suarez, E. C., & Williams, R. B. (1989). Situational determinants of cardiovascular and emotional responses in high and low hostile men. *Psychosomatic Medicine, 51*, 404–418.

9

CARDIOVASCULAR CONSEQUENCES OF EXPRESSING AND REPRESSING ANGER

Aron Wolfe Siegman
University of Maryland Baltimore County

Psychoanalytic theory's pathogenic view of repression gave rise to the belief that the expression of anger is beneficial to mental and physical health. During the 1940s and 1950s this belief gained widespread adherence not only in lay circles but also among mental health professionals. Some went as far as to recommend the periodic full-blown expression of anger for therapeutic purposes (as in the encounter group movement). It was believed that such periodic release of pent-up anger has cathartic effects and helps reduce the occurrence of aggressive behavior. However, a systematic research program by Leonard Berkowitz and associates (1970) demonstrated that far from raising the threshold for subsequent aggressive behavior, the verbal and physical expression of anger has the very opposite effect: it reduces the threshold for subsequent aggression. But even Berkowitz (1970) conceded that such expressions of anger have a beneficial effect on the cardiovascular system, in that they reduce anger induced blood pressure (BP) elevations. However, recent experimental and epidemiological studies show that the expression of anger per se is in fact associated with heightened levels of systolic and diastolic BP reactivity—in some cases with dangerously high elevations. Because there is evidence that heightened CV reactivity is associated with coronary artery disease (CAD) and coronary heart disease (CHD) (Manuck, Muldoon, Kaplan, Adams, & Polefrone, 1989; Manuck, Olson, Hjemdahl, Renq-

173

vist, 1992; Williams, 1989), and also with essential hypertension (EH) (Fredrikson & Matthews, 1990; Light, Dolan, Davis, & Sherwood, 1992; Manuck, Kasprowicz, & Muldoon, 1990; Menkes, Matthews, Krantz et al., 1989), these findings are of more than theoretical interest; they have direct implications for the diagnosis and management of CHD, CAD, and EH. In fact, we now have epidemiological evidence that links the expression of anger to CAD and CHD. On the other hand, there is no convincing evidence that the suppression or repression of anger is related to CVR, CAD, and CHD. The present chapter reviews this literature in greater detail.

THE PARAVERBAL EXPRESSION OF ANGER AND CARDIOVASCULAR REACTIVITY IN MEN AND WOMEN: SOME EXPERIMENTAL FINDINGS

The major objective of two recent experiments (Siegman, Anderson, & Berger, 1990; Siegman & Boyle, 1992) was to test the hypothesis that the expression of anger is associated with heightened levels of cardiovascular (CV) reactivity. Anger is expressed physically (physical aggression)[1] and verbally, but given the social inhibitions against physical aggression, mostly verbally. This takes the form of loud, rapid, and interruptive speech (Scherer, 1979, 1981; Siegman, 1985, 1987a, 1987b, 1993). Loud and rapid speech is to anger what slow and soft speech is to depression: They represent the expressive vocal dimension of these affective experiences. (In this context it should be noted that in natural speech loudness and speech rate are confounded: as loudness goes up, so does speech rate, and vice versa, Bond & Feldstein, 1982). The purpose of our two experimental studies was to ascertain whether it is possible to amplify and/or to attenuate cardiovascular reactivity[2] (CVR) during angry interactions by modifying the participants' expressive vocal behavior. Specifically, we wanted to ascertain whether an increase in speech rate and loudness during an angry exchange, that is, an increase in anger expression, is associated with a corresponding increase in CVR, and, conversely, whether a decrease in speech rate and loudness during angry communications, that is, a decrease in anger expression, is associated with a decrease in CVR. Positive results would provide experimental support for the hypothesized positive relationship between the *expression* of anger and CVR, that is, the more a person expresses his/her anger, the greater his/her CVR level.

---

[1]According to many psychologists, the distinction between anger, hostility, and aggression is that the first refers to an emotion, the second to attitudes, and the last to behavior. These distinctions are accepted as a working hypothesis, although it is recognized that they may require some qualifications.

[2]Reactivity is defined as CV deviations from baseline, as a function of stress, challenge, or some other stimulation.

A second objective of these studies was to ascertain the role of gender in the anger expression–CVR relationship. This objective is of interest because of the demonstrated gender difference in relation to CHD, with men experiencing about twice the age-adjusted mortality and morbidity rates from CHD relative to women (Lerner & Kennel, 1986).[3] One of the rationales that has been offered in explanation of this gender difference is that compared to women, men experience greater CV reactivity to challenge and stress. The empirical evidence relevant to this question is contradictory (Contrada & Krantz, 1988), but it is difficult to evaluate these findings because the standardized challenging and stressful situations that are used in these studies could be perceived differently by females than by males. This problem was minimized in the present series of studies in which we used personalized anger-arousing stimuli: Each participant discussed events that caused him or her to become very angry.

In the first study (Siegman, Anderson, & Berger, 1990) in this series, which was conducted at Ben Gurion University in Israel, we asked 36 undergraduates, 18 males and 18 females, to describe nine neutral and nine anger-arousing events. One-third of these events were described in a loud and rapid voice, that is, in an angry voice, another third in a normal voice, and the remaining third in a soft and slow voice, that is, in a decidedly nonangry or mood incongruent voice. Subjects' systolic BP levels, diastolic BP levels, and HRs were monitored throughout the descriptions. After each set of descriptions, subjects rated themselves on three anger-relevant adjectives. Speech style had a highly significant effect on the participants' systolic, diastolic, and HR reactivity scores when they discussed the anger-arousing experiences [$Fs(2,68)$ = 351.23, 30.79, and 14.15, respectively; ps < .0001; ε^2 = .91, .47, and .29, respectively]. The highest systolic BP, diastolic BP, and HR responses occurred during the loud–fast condition, that is, when the participants expressed their anger (138 mm Hg, 79 mm Hg, and 88 BPM, respectively), the intermediate SBP, DBP, and HR responses occurred during the normal speech style condition (126 mm Hg, 72 mm Hg, and 80 BPM, respectively), and the lowest SBP and DBP responses occurred during the soft–slow condition, that is, when the participants did *not* express their anger (120 mm Hg, 65 mm Hg, and 81 BPM, respectively) (Fig. 9.1). The participants' average increase in CVR from the normal to the loud and fast condition was 18 mm Hg for systolic BP, 12 mm Hg for diastolic BP, and 7 BPM for HR. For some individuals, the average increase was as much as 30 mm Hg for systolic BP and 25 mm Hg for diastolic BP. The average drop in CVR from the normal to the soft–slow condition was less dramatic: 6 mm Hg for systolic BP and 5 mm Hg for diastolic BP. Compared to the descriptions of the neutral events, the descriptions of the anger-arousing events elicited significantly

---

[3]For a comprehensive review of potential mediators of gender differences in CHD, see Stoney and Engebretson (in press).

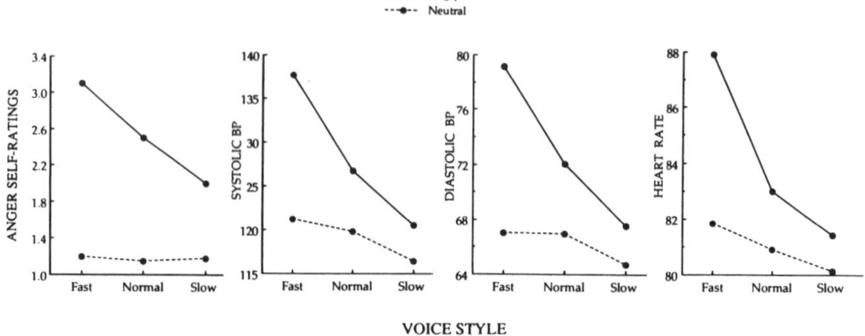

FIG. 9.1.   Anger self-ratings, SBP, DBP, and HR measurements as a function of voice, style, and topic in Study I.

higher levels of BP and HR. However, the differences were of a substantial magnitude, that is, sufficient to be a potential risk factor for CAD and CHD, only when the participants expressed their anger (when they spoke loudly and quickly). The differences were trivial when the participants spoke softly and slowly. In fact, for the female participants, the anger-arousing descriptions were not associated with significantly higher CV reactivity than the neutral descriptions, when they used a mood incongruent speech style (Table 9.1). There was yet another gender difference: Only males showed a significant increase in CVR as a function of loud and rapid speech during the descriptions of neutral events (Table 9.1).

One methodological shortcoming of this study was that each participant discussed both anger-arousing and neutral events. Consequently, at least for some subjects, there may have been a carry over from the anger-arousing topics to the neutral ones. We, therefore, did another study in which the anger-arousing and the neutral events were described by different subjects.

In this replication study (Siegman & Boyle, 1992), 36 participants discussed nine anger-arousing events, three in an angry voice, another three in a normal voice, and yet another three in a soft and slow voice. Another 36 participants discussed nine neutral events, using the same three speech styles. As in the first study, the participants who discussed the anger-arousing events obtained the highest BP and HR scores in the loud–fast speech condition, the intermediate BP and HR scores in the normal speech condition, and the lowest BP and HR scores in the soft–slow condition (Fig. 9.2). Again, these differences were highly significant [$Fs(2,68)$ = 198.91 and 42.68 for systolic BP, and diastolic BP, respectively; ps < .0001]. Speech rate also had a significant effect on the participants' HR levels, but at a lower level of significance than for the BP measures [$F(2,68)$ = 7.92, p < .001]. The mean difference in CVR when speaking about the anger-arousing events loudly and quickly versus speaking about such events softly and slowly was 17 mm Hg for SBP, 10 mm Hg for DBP, and 4 BPM for HR. All comparisons between conditions,

TABLE 9.1

Mean CV Reactivity as a Function of Speech Conditions and Gender in First Anger Study

Speech Conditions	Gender	Systolic BP		Diastolic BP		Heart Rate	
		Mean	t	Mean	t	Mean	t
Angry L–F vs. Angry Norm.	Ma	139 vs. 129	13.70***	78 vs. 72	4.26**	88 vs. 82	2.50*
	Fe	136 vs. 124	12.85**	80 vs. 72	2.91**	88 vs. 83	2.92**
Angry Norm. vs. Angry S–S	Ma	129 vs. 123	7.01***	72 vs. 69	2.42*	82 vs. 80	2.07*
	Fe	124 vs. 117	9.18***	72 vs. 67	2.50*	84 vs. 83	.46
Angry L–F vs. Angry S–S	Ma	139 vs. 123	13.04***	78 vs. 68	5.54***	88 vs. 80	4.44***
	Fe	136 vs. 117	16.63***	80 vs. 67	4.90***	88 vs. 83	1.59
Neut. L–F vs. Neut. Norm.	Ma	124 vs. 120	3.44**	71 vs. 66	3.53**	82 vs. 77	2.04
	Fe	118 vs. 119	−.47	63 vs. 67	−2.23*	82 vs. 84	−1.54
Neut. Norm. vs. Neut. S–S	Ma	120 vs. 117	1.86	66 vs. 65	.79	77 vs. 76	.44
	Fe	119 vs. 116	3.69**	67 vs. 64	1.64	84 vs. 83	.40
Neut. L–F vs. Neut. S–S	Ma	124 vs. 117	6.72***	71 vs. 65	3.00**	82 vs. 77	2.97**
	Fe	118 vs. 116	1.37	63 vs. 64	−.53	82 vs. 83	−.89
Angry L–F vs. Neut. L–F	Ma	139 vs. 124	11.77***	78 vs. 71	3.34**	88 vs. 82	2.37*
	Fe	136 vs. 118	9.94***	80 vs. 63	7.11***	88 vs. 82	2.28*
Angry Norm. vs. Neut. Norm.	Ma	129 vs. 120	6.81***	72 vs. 66	3.98***	82 vs. 77	2.90**
	Fe	124 vs. 119	3.61**	72 vs. 67	2.44*	84 vs. 84	−.39
Angry S–S vs. Neut. S–S	Ma	124 vs. 117	3.92**	68 vs. 65	2.09*	80 vs. 76	2.37*
	Fe	117 vs. 116	1.45	67 vs. 64	1.39	83 vs. 89	−.37

L–F = Loud–Fast, S–S = Soft–Slow
*p < .05. **p < .01. ***p < .001.

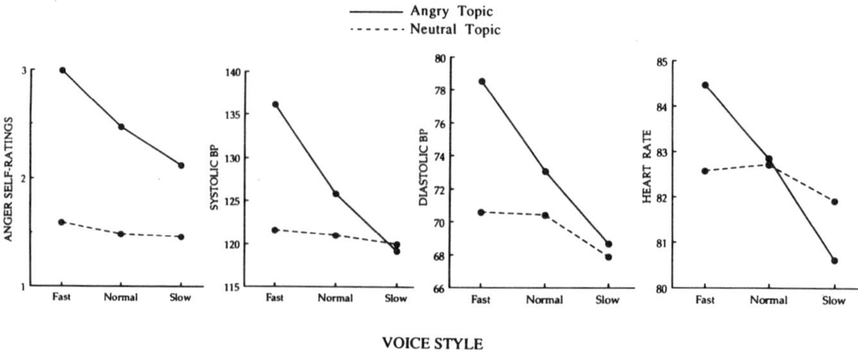

FIG. 9.2.   Anger self-ratings, SBP, DBP, and HR measurements as a function of voice, style, and topic in Study II.

that is, fast–loud versus normal, normal versus slow–soft, and fast–loud versus slow–soft, were significant (Table 9.2). As far as the effects of speech rate and loudness on CVR during anger arousing communications are concerned, the results of this study replicate those of our first study. In fact, the male participants' systolic and diastolic BP scores associated with the description of the anger-arousing events in this replication study were almost identical to those obtained in the original study (Fig. 9.3).

In this replication study, the angry topics were associated with significantly higher levels of systolic reactivity than the neutral topics only when the participants spoke loudly and quickly, that is, when they expressed their anger (the mean difference was 14 mm Hg), or normally (although the mean difference was only 4.9 mm Hg), but not when they spoke slowly and softly (Table 9.2). The angry communications were associated with significantly higher diastolic reactivity scores than the neutral communications, but only when they spoke loudly and quickly (the mean difference was 7.9 mm Hg) (Table 9.2). The angry communications were not associated with significantly heightened HR reactivity levels (Table 9.2). These findings indicate (a) that anger arousal is associated primarily with heightened BP reactivity, not HR reactivity; and

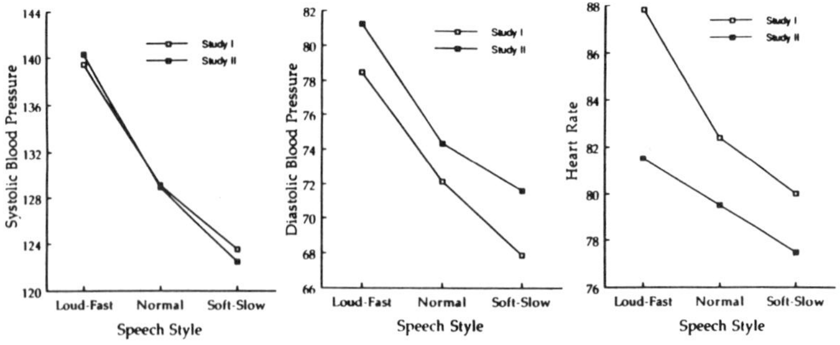

FIG. 9.3.   Cardiovascular responses of male participants in Anger Study I and II.

TABLE 9.2
Mean CV Reactivity as a Function of Speech Conditions in Second Anger Study

Speech Conditions	Systolic BP		Diastolic BP		Heart Rate	
	Mean	t	Mean	t	Mean	t
Angry L–F vs. Angry Norm.	136.1 vs. 125.8	13.15***	78.5 vs. 73	5.15***	84.5 vs. 82.8	1.84
Angry Norm. vs. Angry S–S	125.8 vs. 119.2	9.40***	73 vs. 68.6	4.33***	82.8 vs. 81.6	2.45*
Angry L–F vs. Angry S–S	136.1 vs. 119.2	16.28***	78.5 vs. 68.6	8.60***	84.5 vs. 81.6	3.52**
Neut. L–F vs. Angry S–S	121.6 vs. 121	1.37	70.6 vs. 70.4	.22	82.6 vs. 82.7	−.19
Neut. Norm. vs. Neut. S–S	121 vs. 120	2.43**	70.4 vs. 67.9	2.43	82.7 vs. 81.9	1.24
Neut. L–F vs. Neut S–S	121.6 vs. 120	2.95**	70.6 vs. 67.9	2.25*	82.6 vs. 81.9	.98
Angry L–F vs. Neut. L–F	136.1 vs. 121.6	6.58***	78.5 vs. 70.6	4.38***	84.5 vs. 82.6	.74
Angry Norm. vs. Neut. Norm.	125.8 vs. 121	2.36*	73 vs. 70.4	1.44	82.9 vs. 82.7	.05
Angry S–S vs. Neut. S–S	119.2 vs. 120	−.38**	68.6 vs. 67.9	.44	80.6 vs. 81.9	−.51

L–F = Loud–Fast, S–S = Soft–Slow

*$p < .05$. **$p < .01$. ***$p < .001$.

(b) that only the expression of anger, not its mere experience, is associated with appreciable increases in BP reactivity.

THE EXPRESSION OF ANGER AND CVR: CORRELATIONAL STUDIES

Prior to the aforementioned experimental investigations, we conducted several correlational studies on the relationship between trait measures of the experience of anger, the expression of anger, and CVR. The distinction between the experience versus the expression of anger is based on the results of several factor analytic studies of the Buss–Durkee Hostility Inventory (BDHI) (Buss & Durkee, 1957) conducted in our laboratory and elsewhere (Bendig, 1962a; Buss & Durkee, 1957; Edmunds & Kendrick, 1980; Sarason, 1961; Siegman, Dembroski, & Ringel, 1987). The BDHI consists of several rationally constructed subscales: Physical aggression (Item example: When I really lose my temper, I am capable of slapping someone), Verbal aggression (When I get mad, I say nasty things), Indirect aggression (When I am mad, I sometimes slam things), Irritability (I am irritated a great deal more than people are aware of), Negativism (When someone is bossy, I do the opposite of what he asks), Suspicion, and Resentment. Clearly, the BDHI subscales and items are not only limited to hostility, as one might be led to believe from the name of this test, but also cover anger and aggressive behavior. These factor analyses of the BDHI items or of the BDHI subscales have consistently identified two factors. The first is defined by items or subscales that measure the frequency with which the individual *experiences* feelings of anger and hostility, including feelings of mistrust and suspicion. The first factor, then, is a measure of the experience of anger–hostility. This factor has substantial positive correlations with indices of trait anxiety or neuroticism (Siegman, Dembroski, & Ringel, 1987), and, therefore, can be viewed as a measure of neurotic hostility. The second factor is defined by items and subscales that measure the expression of anger that occurs in response to provocation. Apparently, the extent to which one experiences feelings of anger and hostility and the tendency to express or not to express these feelings represent two orthogonal personality dimensions or traits. It should be noted that the tendency to express anger has significantly lower correlations with indices of neuroticism than does experiential anger–hostility.

Our first study (Siegman, Dohm, & Gjesdal, 1988) investigated the relationship between BDHI-derived experience of anger–hostility scores, expression of anger–hostility scores, and CVR during a serial subtraction task. The participants were 42 male and 33 female undergraduates. There were no significant correlations between the participants' expression of anger and CVR scores. In the male group there was a borderline negative correlation between the experience of anger–hostility and HR. Perhaps the failure to obtain the expected positive relationship between the expression of anger and CVR is due to the fact that the participants were not deliberately angered.[4] Perhaps for the relationship to occur, it is essential that the participants actually be angered. In our next study (Siegman, Anderson, Herbst, Boyle, & Wilkinson, 1992), therefore, 39 male undergraduates were administered the same serial subtraction test, once with and once without harassment and provocation. There were two significant correlations: a positive correlation between the expression of anger–hostility and systolic reactivity, and a positive correlation between the expression of anger–hostility and diastolic reactivity—but only in the provoked condition [partial $rs(34)$ = .41 and .36, respectively, ps < .02 and .05, respectively]. These findings confirm that for the positive relationship between BDHI-derived expression of anger scores and CVR to occur, it is necessary that the participants be harassed or provoked, that is, that they be angered. An experiment (Boyle & Siegman, 1992) recently completed in our laboratory replicated the above findings. Eighty-two male subjects participated in a serial subtraction task. One half of the participants were provoked and angered. They were all administered Spielberger's Anger Expression Scale (Spielberger et al., 1985). Anger-out correlated positively with systolic, diastolic, and HR reactivity (partial r's = .41, .45, and .39 respectively), but only in the angered group. The correlations between Anger-in (the experience of anger) and CVR were either not significant or negative. This much is clear then: The two traits, that is, the expression of anger and the experience of anger, relate differentially to CVR, with only the expression of anger, not its mere experience, correlating positively with CVR, provided that the participants have been angered.

Similar findings were obtained in other laboratories. Suarez and Williams (1990) investigated the relationship between the BDHI-derived expression of anger and experience of anger–hostility scores and CVR in a group of male undergraduates who worked on a series of anagrams. One half of the participants were provoked and harassed, the others were not. Only the expression of anger was positively and significantly associated with systolic reactivity, provided the participants were provoked and harassed. There was no parallel association between the experience of anger–hostility and BP reactivity.

Similar results were also obtained by Engebretson, Matthews, and Scheier (1989). In their study, participants worked on a task either with a pleasant or with a harassing confederate. The authors found a significant positive relationship between the outward expression of anger—as measured by Spielberger's (Spielberger, Johnson, Russel, et al., 1985) Anger Expression Scale—and BP and HR reactivity, but only when the participants were harassed.

---

[4]I am indebted to Professor R. B. Williams, Jr., for bringing this point to my attention.

In four studies, then, conducted in three different laboratories, significant positive correlations obtained between trait measures of the expression of anger and BP reactivity during an anger-arousing task. It would seem, then, that individuals who habitually express their anger, respond to harassment and provocation with heightened BP reactivity even when they have no opportunity to express their anger, as was the case in three of the four studies.

THE EXPRESSION OF ANGER, THE EXPERIENCE OF ANGER, CAD AND CHD

Actually the first study (Siegman, Dembroski, & Ringel, 1987) that suggested that hostility, no less than global Type A, has many components, and that only some of them are toxic involved severity of CAD rather than CVR as an endpoint. Given the factor analytic findings regarding the distinction between the expression of anger versus the experience of anger–hostility, we felt that it was important to ascertain the relationship between these two anger–hostility dimensions, with CAD and CHD. Our first study (Siegman, Dembroski, & Ringel, 1987) in this series involved 79 patients referred for coronary angiography. All patients were administered the BDHI. We found that only the scales measuring the expression of anger correlated significantly and positively with the severity of the patients' stenosis. In fact, the scales measuring the participants' experience of anger–hostility and a measure of neuroticism correlated negatively with the severity of the patients' CAD (Table 9.3). We also performed an item analysis to determine which items in the BDHI correlated significantly with the severity of CAD in this group of angiographic patients. As can be seen in Table 9.4, it is the *expression* of anger, not the mere experience of these feelings, that seems to be the toxic factor in CAD. It should be pointed out that the significant positive relationship between the expression of anger and CAD was independent of traditional risk factors, such as cholesterol level and blood pressure. It should also be noted that the significant correlation between the expression of anger and

TABLE 9.3

Partial Correlations Between Buss–Durkee Factor Scores and Number of Blocked Vessels in Younger (<60) and Older (>60) Patients

Factor Scores	Younger Patients (N = 36)	Older Patients (N = 36)
Expressed anger–hostility	+.40*	+.11
Experienced anger–hostility	−.22	−.08

*p < .05.

Note. Traditional risk factors were partialled out.

TABLE 9.4
Buss–Durkee Hostility Scale Items That Correlate Significantly[a] with
CAD Endpoints in Siegman, Dembroski, and Ringel (1987) Study

Items Affirmed	*Items Denied*
I lose my temper easily but get over it	I don't get what's coming to me
When people yell, I yell back	I feel resentful when I look back
I am capable of slapping someone	If I am made fun of, my blood boils
I have had temper tantrums	Being forgiven for my sins concerns me
I raise my voice when arguing	People have a hidden reason for doing something nice
People push me so far, we come to blows	I feel I get a raw deal out of life
	I would rather concede than argue

[a]$p < .05$.

the severity of CAD was limited to patients up to age 65, a finding previously reported by Williams and associates (Williams, Barefoot, Haney, et al., 1988).

Other findings of this study also are consistent with the conclusion that the expression of anger is the "toxic" agent in the Type-A–CAD relationship. In addition to the BDHI, the patients in this study (Siegman, Feldstein, Tommaso, Ringel, & Lating, 1987) were administered the Structured Interview (SI) developed by Rosenman (1978) for the assessment of the Type-A Behavior Pattern (TABP). There was no significant relationship between the patients' global Type-A scores and the severity of their coronary artery disease. However, the patients' responses to the SI were also scored, by means of an automated scoring system, for a variety of speech and vocal parameters, including response latency, loudness, pause durations, speech rate, and frequency of interruptive, simultaneous speech. Previous research conducted in our laboratory (Siegman, 1985) showed that the BDHI-derived expression of anger scales are associated with loud, rapid, and interruptive speech, whereas the BDHI-derived experience of anger scales and hostility scales tend to be associated with the very opposite speech style (soft and slow speech). In the present study (Siegman, Feldstein et al., 1987), two out of these three markers of expressed anger, namely, loud and interruptive speech, accounted for as much as 38% of the variance in the severity of the younger patients' coronary occlusion scores. These findings, then, are consistent with the conclusion that the expression of anger is a significant risk factor for CHD.

The finding that only the expression of anger factor of the BDHI, but not the experience of anger–hostility factor, is positively and significantly related to CAD was recently replicated in a study by Helmig, Houston, Vavak, and Mullin (1991). A third study (Mendes de Leon, 1992) used the Spielberger et. al (1985) scales to measure these two anger–hostility dimensions, and also found that only the expression of anger–hostility, not their mere experience, are related to the severity of CAD.

There is evidence to suggest that the distinction between the expression versus the experience of anger–hostility may also apply to CHD. In the reanalysis of the MRFIT data by Dembroski, MacDougall, Costa, and Grandits (1989) the authors divided the SI-derived clinical ratings of the potential-for-hostility into three components: content, intensity, and style. References to past experiences and expressions of anger or hostility provide the basis for the *Content* scores. The intensity with which these events are described provide the basis for the *Intensity* scores. Direct expressions of anger–hostility toward the interviewer provide the basis for the *Style* scores. Only hostile style, that is, direct expressions of anger–hostility during the interview, was prospectively related to CHD. In discussing their findings, the authors stated that: Research using well known anger–hostility measures such as the MMPI Cook and Medley HO scale, the Buss-Durkee Hostility Inventory (1957), and SI-derived hostility indicates that each of those measures reflects to varying degrees two basic dimensions of personality. One dimension is *neuroticism*, which refers to the tendency to experience distressing emotions, including anger, irritability, resentment, and suspicion. The other personality dimension tapped by anger/hostility measures is *agreeableness–antagonism*, which refers to the quality of one's attitudes and behaviors toward others, including the tendency to express anger and hostility directly to others. Of the three SI hostility components, the style rating that reflects instances of rude, uncooperative, and disagreeable behavior toward the interviewer, is the purest measure of antagonism. The authors conclude that their finding is consistent with that of Siegman, Dembroski, and Ringel (1987) that only the expression of anger–hostility, not its mere experience, is associated with CHD.

A major objective of a recent study by Siegman, Lating, Johnston, and Boyle (1992) was to ascertain whether the aforementioned findings by Dembroski et al. (1989) can be replicated in female and male patients referred for stress exercise tomographic thallium studies: A computerized imaging technique for determining the severity of coronary perfusion defects. The use of angiographic studies for determining coronary risk has been criticized on the grounds that the patients referred for such examinations typically suffer from severe CHD symptoms or are otherwise seriously at risk for a MI, and that one cannot readily generalize from findings obtained with such patients to more healthy individuals. Pickering (1986) pointed out that even some of the established risk factors for CHD, such as high BP levels, frequently are not associated with severity of CAD in angiographic studies. Such findings moved Pickering to question the appropriateness of using angiographic patients for the study of CHD risk factors. Instead, Pickering (1986) recommended the use of patients referred for thallium testing on the assumption that, as a group, such patients tend to be less severely ill. In this study, therefore, we used thallium stress test results as a measure of CHD. The patients were 57 women and 51 men. All patients were administered the SI, which was scored according to the method developed by Dembroski et al. (1989). This scoring procedure yields the following variables: vocal stylistic variables (response latency, loudness, rapid accelerated speech, and explosive speech), a global Potential for Hostility score and its three component scores referred to earlier (Hostile Content, Intensity of Hostility, and Hostile Style), Anger-In, Verbal Competition, and a global Type A score. The following SI-derived scores correlated positively and significantly with the patients' severity of perfusion scores: PoHo, Hostile Content, Intensity of Hostility, Hostile Style, and Verbal Competition. When separate regression analyses were conducted for the female and the male patients, Hostile Style and Intensity of Hostility emerged as a significant source of variance for the females, although the latter was significant only for younger females. Verbal Compeition and all the hostility components, except Hostile Style, emerged as significant sources of variance for the male patients. However, only Verbal Competition and PoHo remained significant in a multivariate analysis. Competition for control was clearly a significant source of variance for the males [$F(1, 50) = 4.48$, partial $r = .29$, $p < .05$], and marginally significant for the females [$F(1, 48) = 3.57$, partial $r = .26$, $p = .06$]. The results of this study, then, are consistent with the hypothesis that anger–hostility is no less a risk factor for women than it is for men, although somewhat different patterns of anger–hostility expression seemed to be involved in the two genders. Ironically, the conclusion reached by Dembroski et al. (1989) that of the various hostility components only Hostile Style is a risk factor for CHD, was confirmed in females but not in males.

Also of interest is the finding that the SI-derived Verbal Competition Scores correlated significantly with the patients' severity of perfusion defects scores. An earlier reanalysis of the WCGS by Matthews, Glass, Rosenman, and Bortner (1977) found a significant relationship between Verbal Competition and CHD endpoints. Because interruptions of the interviewer are a major constituent of this SI component and because, as pointed out earlier, such interruptions are a manifestation of expressed anger (Siegman, 1985), the findings regarding Verbal Competition and CHD can be viewed as part of the expressed anger–CHD relationship. On the other hand, interrupting one's partner is also an expressive correlate of dominance and assertiveness (Siegman, 1987b, p. 368). Perhaps this personality trait, which is related to the original conceptual definition of the Type-A behavior pattern is yet another risk factor for CHD, independent of anger–hostility. The results of a recent study by Houston, Chesney, Black, Cates, and Hecker (1992) suggest that this is indeed the case. In this context, it should be noted that Kaplan, Botchin, and Manuck (this volume) report that dominant social status in combination with heart rate reactivity potentiate atherosclerosis in cynomolgus monkeys.

The weight of the evidence, then, indicates that it is the expression of anger and hostility, rather than their mere experience, that is related to CVR and the severity of CAD. Perhaps the mere experience of anger–hostility is not a significant risk factor for CAD and CHD because, as we have demonstrated (Siegman, Anderson, & Berger, 1991), such passive experiences are not associated with appreciable increases in BP and HR, but more about this later in this chapter.

Negative Relationships Between Neuroticism and CAD: Real or Artifactual?

In our very first study on the relationship between anger–hostility and CAD (Siegman, Dembroski, & Ringel, 1987), we found a significant negative correlation between our patients' BDHI-derived experience of anger–hostility scores and the severity of their CAD. In this study (Siegman, Dembroski, & Ringel, 1987), we also found a negative correlation between the patients' Bendig (1962b) anxiety (or neuroticism) scores and the severity of their CAD. Because there is a substantial positive correlation (about .70) between the BDHI experience of anger–hostility and the Bendig scales, these two correlations should be viewed as reflecting the same basic finding: a significant negative relationship between neuroticism and CAD. Our original explanation of these findings was that they are artifactual—a function how patients are selected for coronary angiography. Neurotic individuals seem to be prone to hypochondriacal anginalike pains in the absence of any evidence of CHD or CAD (Costa, Zonderman, McCrae, & Williams, 1986). When such individuals persist with their complaints, as they are prone to do, and are selected for coronary angiography, researchers are likely to obtain wholly artifactual negative correlations between neuroticism, or between scales that are highly correlated with neuroticism, such as the experience of anger–hostility scales, and the severity of CAD. However, one cannot rule out the possibility that the negative correlation between neurotic anxiety and CAD is real and not artifactual.

What leads us to suggest that the negative relationship between neuroticism and CAD may be real and nonartifactual are the negative correlations that we found between the experience of anger–hostility, anxiety–neuroticism, and CVR (Siegman, Dohm, & Gjesdal, 1988; Siegman, Anderson, & Boyle, 1991). Significant negative correlations were also obtained between neuroticism and resting measurements BP and HR measurements (Davies, 1970; Siegman, Anderson, Herbst, et al., 1992; Watson & Pennebaker, 1989). Clearly, these negative correlations between neuroticism and CV measurements during baseline and during task performance cannot be so readily dismissed as artifacts of subject selection.

Although these negative relationships appear to be nonartifactual, they are, at first glance, puzzling, because state anxiety is typically associated with heightened rather than reduced BP and HR reactivity. Perhaps we need to distinguish between state and trait anxiety. Perhaps chronically anxious individuals become habituated to relatively low levels of anxiety arousal, or perhaps they acquire methods to cope with such low levels of arousal. The same explanation has been invoked by Eysenck (1983, 1984) to account for the negative association between neuroticism and cancer. If correct, we have a basis for arguing that the significant negative associations between trait anxiety, neurotic hostility, and the severity of CAD that have been obtained by us (Siegman, Dembroski, & Ringel, 1987) and others (Blumenthal, Thompson, Williams, & Kong, 1979; Elias, Robbins, Rice, & Edgecomb, 1982) are also real and not artifactual.

THE EXPRESSION OF ANGER, THE EXPERIENCE OF ANGER-HOSTILITY, AND OTHER CHD RISK FACTORS

Additional support for the position that only the expression of anger, not its mere experience, is a significant behavioral risk factor for CAD and CHD comes from a study undertaken more than 20 years ago by Persky, Smith, and Basu (1971) on the role of trait anger expression in testosterone production. They found a significant positive correlation between the expression of anger–hostility, as measured by the appropriate Buss–Durkee hostility scales, and plasma testosterone levels [$r(16) = .52, p < .05$] and testosterone production rate [$r(16) = .69, p < .001$] in a group of 18 young males. By way of contrast, the experience of hostility, or neurotic hostility, as measured by the appropriate Buss–Durkee scales, barely related to testosterone production rate at the 5% level. Furthermore, in a regression analysis in which these two measures of hostility plus two other indices of overt–reactive hostility were entered as independent variables and testosterone production rate as the dependent variable, both types of hostility contributed significantly to the variance in the participants' testosterone production rates, but in opposite directions: expressive hostility positively, and the experience of hostility negatively. Between them, they accounted for 82% of the variance in the participants' testosterone production rates. More recently, Olweus (1986) also found a significant positive relationship between expressed anger, defined in terms of verbal and physical aggression in response to provocation, and testosterone production. It should be noted that levels of testosterone production have been identified as yet another link, besides CV reactivity, between behavioral risk factors and CHD (Williams, 1989).

Platelet hyperaggregability is yet another variable that can play a role in the pathophysiology of CHD, and it too is differentially affected by the expression versus the experience or the repression of anger–hostility. In a

recent study (Wenneberg, Schneider, McLean et al., 1992), which used Spielberger's (Spielberger et al., 1985) Anger Expression Scale to assess how the
participants coped with anger, only Anger-out, but not Anger-in, correlated
positively and significantly with collagen induced platelet aggregation. Similar results were obtained in another recent study (Markovitz, Matthews, &
Kiss, 1992), which correlated SI-derived clinical ratings of anger–hostility and
stress induced platelet reactivity. Of the three SI-derived hostility components
(content, intensity, style), only intensity and style, the two components that
are conceptually related to the actual expression of anger, showed significant positive associations with platelet reactivity.

The evidence, then, seems to be fairly clear: the two dimensions of anger–
hostility—experience versus expression—relate differentially not only to CHD
outcome variables, but also to the physiological–neurohormonal variables
that mediate the relationship between anger–hostility and CHD, with the expression of anger appearing to be the toxic personality variable.

SOME THEORETICAL AND APPLIED CONSIDERATIONS

Why is it that only the expression of anger, not its mere experience, produces
exceedingly high levels of CVR that ultimately results in CAD and CHD? To
answer this question, we need to understand the role of expressive behavior
in emotions. Contemporary students of emotions (Buck, 1987; Leventhal, 1986;
Plutchik, 1986) believed that the expressive behaviors that are associated with
the different emotions, such as the loud and rapid voice that is associated
with anger, are not mere secondary consequences of emotions, but represent
an integral dimension of emotional experiences, conceptually on par with
their physiological and cognitive dimensions. This point of view has its roots
in the writings of Charles Darwin (1955), who believed that the various expressive behaviors that are associated with emotions have a biological basis,
that they serve communicative functions, and that they have clear-cut survival values. In a somewhat similar vein, Lange and James (1962) argued that
the expressive and physiological changes that occur during emotional behavior trigger the subjective feeling of emotion, not the other way around.
We do not run because we are scared; we are scared because we run. A contemporary version of this theory, articulated by Tomkins (1962) and Ekman
(1972) proposed that emotions start in the face, and that feedback from facial expressions to the brain starts a process that brings about autonomic,
hormonal, and behavioral changes, as well as the subjective emotional experience. Of course, facial expressions are not the sole manifestations of emotions. Studies conducted in our laboratory and elsewhere showed that
emotions also have specific vocal correlates: a loud and rapid voice with anger,

a soft and slow voice with sadness–depression, and a rapid and high-pitched voice with fear–anxiety (Siegman, 1985, 1987a, 1987b, 1993).

Beyond the importance of recognizing the multidimensional nature of emotions, that is, their cognitive, physiological, and expressive nonverbal and paraverbal manifestations, it is also important to realize that there is feedback between these different dimensions, that is, that they interact with each other in a dynamic, reciprocal fashion (Fig. 9.4). Thus, people who are angry experience an increase in BP, HR, cortisol, epinephrine, and so forth. They also raise their voice, accelerate their speech rate, and interrupt their partner. However, the heightened levels of BP, HR, and catecholamines will further intensify the speaker's angry voice and subjective feelings of anger. Similarly, an angry voice will further intensify physiological arousal and subjective feelings of anger. This accounts for the escalating nature of emotions: anger turns into rage, fear into panic, and sadness into despair. But emotions have yet another characteristic: they are contagious. With the best intentions to remain calm, it is very difficult to interact with an angry person without becoming angry oneself. Here, too, nonverbal and paraverbal behavior plays a significant role. There is considerable evidence that participants in dyadic interactions match each other's paraverbal behavior, including each other's loudness level and speech rate, even if these interactions are of a neutral character (Feldstein & Welkowitz, 1987). Thus, when an angry person raises his or her voice and accelerates his or her speech rate, so will that person's partner. This is likely to raise the partner's blood pressure and feelings of anger. This accounts not only for the contagion effect, but also contributes to the spiraling nature of emotions, because the listener's reactions will, in turn, affect the speaker, and so on.

The evidence indicates that anger is uniquely associated with heightened levels of blood pressure reactivity, much more so than fear–anxiety or sadness–

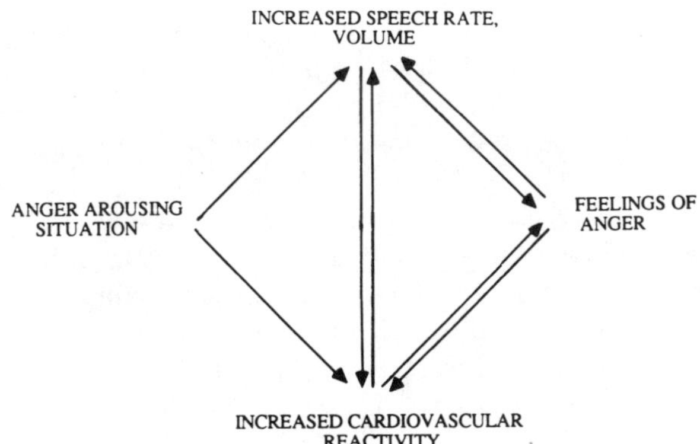

FIG. 9.4.   Schematic representation of the reciprocal interactions of anger, expressive vocal behavior, and CVR.

depression (Siegman, 1992, 1993). Given the escalating and contagious nature of emotions, anger can result in sufficiently high levels of CVR to result in CAD and CHD. However, given the critical role of the expressive dimension in producing escalation and contagion of emotions, it is easy to understand why only the expression of anger, not its mere experience, produces exaggerated levels of CVR that ultimately results in coronary heart disease.

There are, then, good reasons, both of a theoretical–conceptual and an empirical nature, for the position that expression of anger is a serious behavioral risk factor for hyperreactivity, CAD, and CHD.

The point of view that expressive vocal behavior is an integral feature of anger on par with, for example, the physiological manifestations of anger, has important implications for the management of anger, and ultimately of CAD and CHD. It implies that by modifying the expressive manifestation of anger, for example, by training people to speak softly and slowly when they are angry, it should be possible to short-circuit the escalation of anger. In fact, two of our experiments (Siegman, Anderson, & Berger, 1990; Siegman & Boyle, 1992) demonstrated just that. In these two studies, a mood incongruent speech style, that is, soft and slow speech during angry communications significantly reduced our subjects' feelings of anger, and completely canceled all CV elevations normally associated with anger. Furthermore, we have used this procedure with CHD patients and with patients in ICC units and found that it helped reduce their feelings of stress, in general, as well as their levels of CV arousal (Siegman, 1992, 1993).

THE REPRESSION OF ANGER, CVR, AND CHD

We introduced this chapter by suggesting that psychoanalytic theory's pathogenic view of repression is responsible for the still widely held belief that the expression of anger has prophylactic and therapeutic properties. The evidence reviewed so far suggests that far from being beneficial the expression of anger is actually associated with heightened CVR and is a risk factor for CAD and CHD. But what about the CV consequences of anger repression? Is there any evidence for a positive relationship between anger repression, CVR, and CHD, as suggested by psychoanalytic authors?

The empirical evidence in regard to this question is relatively sparse, probably because, at least until recently, we lacked satisfactory instruments for the measurement of the personality trait of repression. Although there are a number of instruments purporting to measure *Anger-in*, such as the Anger-In questions that were used in the Framingham study (Haynes, Levine, Scotch, Feinleib, & Kannel, 1978), the Anger-in subscale of Spielberger's (Spielberger, Johnson, Russel et al., 1985) Anger-expression scale, and SI-derived clinical ratings of Anger-In (Dembroski & McDougall, 1983, 1989), these do not distinguish between suppressing (simply not expressing) anger and repressing anger. At any rate, most studies on the relationship between Anger-in and CVR report null findings (e.g., Mills, Schneider, & Dimsdale, 1989; Smith & Houston, 1987; for a more comprehensive discussion, see Houston, in press). Of course, these negative findings may be due to the fact that in these studies the participants were not specifically angered. It will be recalled that even trait anger expression scales do not correlate significantly with CVR unless the participants are actually angered.

The study of the physiological and health consequences of the repressive coping style received a major impetus from the results of a study by Weinberger, Schwartz, and Davidson (1979). These authors used their participants' Bendig (1962b) Manifest Anxiety Scale (MAS) and Marlowe–Crowne (Crowne & Marlowe, 1964) Social Desirability Scale (SDS) scores to measure trait repression. Participants were classified as *repressors* when reporting low anxiety but scoring high on the SDS, as *low anxious* when reporting low anxiety and scoring low on the SDS, and as *high anxious* when reporting high anxiety and scoring low on the SDS. It should be noted that, based on the results of several studies, Weinberger et al. (1979) took the position that the SDS is not merely a measure of impression management, that is, the attempt to deceive others, but rather more generally, of the defensive, or repressive coping style (Weinberger, 1990). In their study, Weinberger et al. (1979) were concerned, among others, with the ANS correlates of repression. The task was to respond to a sentence completion task, which included aggressive, sexual, and neutral items. ANS reactivity indices, including HR, GSR, and EMG, were obtained throughout. The repressors obtained the highest GSR and EMG scores. Repressors also obtained higher HR scores than the nonanxious participants. This study did not include BP measures, but a subsequent study by Siegman, Anderson, and Boyle (1991) which did, did not find a significant relationship between the repressive coping style and heightened BP reactivity, although it confirmed the findings of Weinberger et al. (1979) in regard to HR.

Pennebaker and associates (Pennebaker, Hughes, & O'Heeron, 1987) assessed trait repression in terms of their participants' failure to self-disclose when asked to describe traumatic experiences. They found that repression was associated with heightened ANS reactivity as measured by indices of skin conductance level (SCL), but not with heightened CV reactivity.

Weinberger et al. (1979) assumed that the repression of anxiety implies a tendency for the repression of negative affectivity in general. This may very well be the case. On the other hand, it is also possible that some individuals tend to repress anxiety but not anger, or vice versa. Therefore, in a recent study (Siegman, Anderson, & Boyle, 1991), we focused specifically on the effects of anger repression on CV reactivity. Anger repression was measured in a manner similar to the method used by Weinberger et al. (1979).

The participants' BDHI-derived experience of anger scale scores and their SDS scores were used to create a group of anger-repressors (low BDHI and high SDS scorers), true nonangry subjects (low BDHI and low SDS scorers), and angry subjects (high BDHI and low SDS scorers). The participants were provoked and harassed while they worked on a serial subtraction task. Systolic BP, diastolic BP, and HR measures were obtained throughout. Although the anger-repressors obtained significantly higher HR reactivity scores than the nonangry subjects, there were no significant group differences in relation to BP reactivity. It is especially worthy to note that in the same group of subjects the BDHI-derived expression of anger scores did correlate positively and significantly with both systolic and diastolic reactivity but not with HR reactivity. Similarly, in our second "angry voice" experiment (Siegman & Boyle, 1992), the expression of anger was associated with heightened levels of BP reactivity but not with heightened levels of HR reactivity. It would seem, then, that the expression of anger is primarily associated with heightened pressor reactivity, the *repression* of anger is primarily associated with accelerated HRs.

Finally, it is of interest to note that although recent reanalyses of both the WCGS and MRFIT studies (Dembroski et al., 1989; Hecker, Chesney, Black, & Frautschi, 1988) indicated that the expression of anger is related to CHD endpoints, there was no evidence in these studies for a significant relationship between Anger-in and CHD endpoints. Similarly, in our thallium study (Siegman, Lating, Johnston, & Boyle, 1992), there was no significant evidence for a relationship between patients' SI-derived Anger-In scores and perfusion positive defects. In fact, for the male patients, there was a near-significant, negative relationship between Anger-In and thallium stress scores. Although in two other studies with angiographic patients, Dembroski and associates (Dembroski et al., 1985; MacDougall et al., 1985) did find significant positive

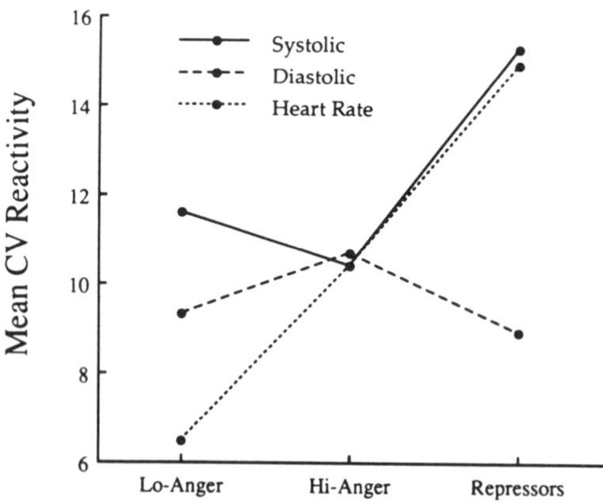

FIG. 9.5. Cardiovascular reactivity scores of low anger, high anger, and anger repressors during an anger-arousing subtraction task.

correlations between SI-derived Anger-In scores and severity of CAD. Dembroski and Costa (1987) made a convincing case that in these patients Anger-In is a consequence of CHD rather than an etiological factor.

Of course, none of the aforementioned should be taken as evidence that repression, including anger-repression, does not come at a price. Although repression apparently is not associated with heightened BP reactivity, it is, as pointed out earlier, associated with heightened ANS reactivity as indexed by EMG and SCL. Furthermore, there is evidence that repression has significant immunological consequences (Esterling, Antoni, Kumar, & Schneiderman, 1990; Pennebaker, Kiecolt-Glaser, & Glaser, 1988) and is related to increased risk or worsened course of some neoplastic diseases (e.g., Dattore, Schonz, & Coyne, 1980; Jensen, 1987; Temoshok, 1987).

It would seem, then, that different autonomic measures selectively tap psychological processes associated with anger-repression and anger-expression, and that they put one at risk for different diseases: anger repression for neoplastic diseases and anger expression for CHD.

COPING WITH ANGER: A THIRD OPTION

If both the repression and the expression of anger have untoward health consequences, how else, then, is one to cope with feelings of anger? Clearly, the repression and expression of anger do not exhaust the available options. A number of years ago, Holt (1970) pointed out that Freud really never advocated the full-blown expression of anger, in all its expressive paraverbal intensity, as a desirable form of catharsis. Rather, he advocated insight into the unconscious determinants of one's emotional behavior and the bringing of such behavior under conscious control. This is also the approach now widely favored by various self-assertion training groups: Not to repress anger, nor to express these feelings in their full paraverbal intensity, but to discuss them coolly and rationally. Our findings that the communication of anger arousing experiences in a normal, or even better, in a soft and slow voice, does not produce CV upheaval, suggest that such purely verbal discussions of anger-arousing events without their accompanying paraverbal and nonverbal expressions are not likely to produce physiological hypertension and coronary heart disease.

ACKNOWLEDGMENT

The preparation for this chapter and some of the research reported therein were supported by a grant from the National Heart, Lung, and Blood Institute (HL-036027).

REFERENCES

Bendig, A. W. (1962a). Factor analytic scales of covert and overt hostility. *Journal of Consulting Psychology, 26*, 200.

Bendig, A. W. (1962b). The development of a short form of the manifest anxiety scale. *Journal of Consulting Psychology, 20*, 384.

Berkowitz, L. (1970). Experimental investigations of hostility catharsis. *Journal of Consulting and Clinical Psychology, 35*, 1–7.

Blumenthal, J. A., Thompson, L. W., Williams, R. S., & Kong, Y. (1979). Anxiety-proneness and coronary heart disease. *Journal of Psychosomatic Research, 23*, 17–21.

Bond, R. N., & Feldstein, S. (1982). Acoustical correlates of perception of speech rate: An experimental investigation. *Journal of Psychological Research, 11*, 539–557.

Boyle, S., & Siegman, A. W. (1992). *Dimensions of anger expression and CVR in angered men.* Unpublished manuscript, University of Maryland, Baltimore County.

Buck, R. (1987). The psychology of emotion. In J. E. Ledoux & W. Hirst (Eds.), *Mind and brain.* Cambridge: Cambridge University Press.

Buss, A. H., & Durkee, A. (1957). An inventory for assessing different kinds of hostility. *Journal of Consulting Psychology, 21*, 343–349.

Contrada, R. J., & Krantz, D. S. (1988). Stress, reactivity, and Type-A behavior: Current status and future directions. *Annals of Behavioral Medicine, 10*(2), 64–71.

Costa, P. T., Jr., Zonderman, A. B., McCrae, R. R., & Williams, R. B., Jr. (1986). Cynicism and paranoid alienation in the Cook & Medley Ho-scale. *Psychosomatic Medicine, 48*, 283–285.

Crowne, D. P., & Marlowe, D. (1964). *The approval motive: Studies in evaluative dependence.* New York: Wiley.

Darwin, C. R. (1955). *The expression of emotions in man and animals.* New York: Philosophical Library. (Original work published 1896)

Dattore, P. J., Shontz, F. C., & Coyne, L. (1980). Premorbid personality differentiation of cancer and noncancer groups: A list of the hypotheses of cancer proneness. *Journal of Consulting and Clinical Psychology, 48*, 388–394.

Davies, M. (1970). Blood pressure and personality. *Journal of Psychosomatic Research, 14*, 89–104.

Dembroski, T. M., & MacDougall, J. M. (1983). Behavioral and psychophysiological perspectives on coronary-prone behavior. In T. M. Dembroski, T. H. Schmidt, & G. Blumchen (Eds.), *Biobehavioral bases of coronary heart disease.* New York: Karger.

Dembroski, T. M., & Costa, P. T., Jr. (1987). Coronary-prone behavior: Components of the Type-A pattern and hostility. *Journal of Personality, 55*, 211–236.

Dembroski, T. M., & MacDougall, J. M. (1985). Beyond global Type A: Relationships of paralinguistic attributes, hostility and anger-in to coronary heart disease. In T. Field, P. McAbe, & N. Schneiderman (Eds.), *Stress and Coping* (pp. 223–242). Hillsdale, NJ: Lawrence Erlbaum Associates.

Dembroski, T. M., MacDougall, J. M., Costa, P. T., & Grandits, G. A. (1989). Components of hostility as predictors of sudden death and myocardial infarction in the Multiple Risk Factor Intervention Trial. *Psychosomatic Medicine, 51*, 514–522.

Edmunds, G., & Kendrick, D. C. (1980). *The measurement of human aggressiveness.* West Sussex, England: Ellis Horwood.

Ekman, P. (1972). Universal and cultural differences in facial expression of emotion. In J. K. Cole (Ed.), *Nebraska Symposium on Motivation* (pp. 207–283). Lincoln: The University of Nebraska Press.

Elias, M. F., Robbins, M. A., Rice, A., & Edgecomb, J. L. (1982). Symptom reporting, anxiety and depression in arteriographically classified middle-aged chest pain patients. *Exploratory Aging Research, 8*, 45–81.

Engebretson, T. D., Matthews, K. A., & Scheier, M. F. (1989). Relations between anger expression and cardiovascular reactivity: Reconciling inconsistent findings through a matching hypothesis. *Journal of Personality and Social Psychology, 57*, 513–521.

Esterling, B. A., Antoni, M. H., Kumar, M., & Schneiderman, N. (1990). Emotional repression, stress disclosure responses, and Epstein-Barr viral capsid antigen titers. *Psychosomatic Medicine, 52,* 397–410.

Eysenck, H. J. (1983). Stress, disease and personality: The "inoculation effect." In C. L. Cooper (Ed.), *Stress research* (pp. 121–146). New York: Wiley.

Eysenck, H. J. (1984). Personality, stress and lung cancer. In S. Rachman (Ed.), *Contributions to medical psychology* (Vol. 3, pp. 151–171). Oxford: Pergamon Press.

Feldstein, S., & Welkowitz, J. (1987). A chronography of conversation: In defense of an objective approach. In A. W. Siegman & S. Feldstein (Eds.), *Nonverbal behavior and communication.* Hillsdale, NJ: Lawrence Erlbaum Associates.

Fredrikson, M., & Matthews, K. A. (1990). Cardiovascular responses to behavioral stress and hypertension: A meta-analytic review. *Annals of Behavioral Medicine, 12*(1), 17–39.

Haynes, S. G., Levine, S., Scotch, N., Feinleib, M., & Kannel, W. B. (1978). The relationship of psychosocial factors to coronary heart disease in the Framingham Study. I. Methods and risk factors. *American Journal of Epidemiology, 107,* 362–383.

Hecker, H. L., Chesney, M. A., Black, G. W., & Frautschi, N. (1988). Coronary-prone behaviors in the Western Collaborative Group Study. *Psychosomatic Medicine, 50,* 153–164.

Helmig, L., Houston, B. K., Vavak, C. R., & Mullin, J. (March 1991). *Hostility related variables, self-schemata and CHD.* Paper presented at the meetings of the Society for Behavioral Medicine, Washington, DC.

Holt, R. (1970). On the interpersonal and intrapersonal consequences of expressing or not expressing anger. *Journal of Consulting and Clinical Psychology, 35,* 8–12.

Houston, B. K. (in press). Anger, hostility, and psychophysiological reactivity. In A. W. Siegman & T. Smith (Eds.), *Anger, hostility, and the heart.* NJ: Lawrence Erlbaum Associates.

Houston, B. K., Chesney, M. A., Black, G. W., Cates, D. S., & Hecker, H. L. (1992). Behavioral clusters and coronary heart disease risk. *Psychosomatic Medicine, 54,* 447–461.

Jensen, M. R. (1987). Psychobiological factors predicting the course of breast cancer. *Journal of Personality, 55,* 317–342.

Lange, C. G., & James, W. (1962). *The emotions.* New York: Hafner. (Original work published 1922)

Lerner, D. J., & Kennel, W. B. (1986). Patterns of coronary heart disease morbidity and mortality in the sexes: A 26-year follow-up of the Framingham population. *American Heart Journal, 111,* 383–390.

Leventhal, H. A. (1986). Perceptual motor theory of emotion. In K. Scherer & P. Ekman (Eds.), *Approaches to emotion.* Hillsdale, NJ: Lawrence Erlbaum Associates.

Light, K. C., Dolan, C. A., Davis, M. R., & Sherwood, A. (1992). Cardiovascular responses to an active coping challenge as predictors of blood pressure patterns 10 to 15 years later. *Psychosomatic Medicine, 54,* 217–230.

MacDougall, J. M., Dembroski, T. M., Dimsdale, J. E., & Hackett, T. (1985). Components of Type A Hostility and Anger-In: Further relationships to angiographic findings. *Health Psychology, 24,* 137–152.

Manuck, S. B., Muldoon, M. F., Kaplan, J. R., Adams, M. R., & Polefrone, J. M. (1989). Coronary artery atherosclerosis and response to stress in cynomolgus monkeys. In A. W. Siegman & T. M. Dembroski (Eds.), *In search of coronary-prone behavior: Beyond Type-A.* Hillsdale, NJ: Lawrence Erlbaum Associates.

Manuck, S. B., Kasprowicz, M. S., & Muldoon, M. F. (1990). Behaviorally evoked cardiovascular reactivity and hypertension: Conceptual issues and potential associations. *Annals of Behavioral Medicine, 12*(1), 17–29.

Manuck, S. B., Olson, G., Hjemdahl, P., & Renqvist, N. (1992). Does cardiovascular reactivity to mental stress have prognostic value in postinfarction patients? A pilot study. *Psychosomatic Medicine, 54,* 102–108.

Markovitz, J. H., Matthews, K. A., & Kiss, J. E. (1992, March 31–April 4). *Platelet reactivity to stress in coronary heart disease.* Paper presented at 50th anniversary international meeting of the *American Psychosomatic Society,* New York.

Matthews, K. A., Glass, D. C., Rosenman, R. H., & Bortner, R. W. (1977). Competitive drive, pattern A, and coronary heart disease: A further analysis of some data from the Western Collaborative Group Study. *Journal of Chronic Disease, 30*, 489–498.

Mendes de Leon, C. F. (1992). Anger and impatience/irritability in patients of low socioeconomic status with acute coronary heart disease. *Journal of Behavioral Medicine, 15*, 273–284.

Menkes, M. S., Matthews, K. A., Krantz, D. S., Lundberg, V., Mead, L. A., Qadish, B., Liang, K. Y., Thomas, C. B., & Pearson, T. A. (1989). Cardiovascular reactivity to the cold pressor test as a predictor of hypertension. *Hypertension, 14*, 524–530.

Mills, P. J., Schneider, R. H., & Dimsdale, J. E. (1989). Anger assessment and reactivity to stress. *Journal of Psychosomatic Research, 33*, 379–382.

Olweus, D. (1986). Aggression and hormones: Behavioral relationship with testosterone and adrenaline. In D. Olweus, J. Block, & Radke-Yarrow (Eds.), *Development and antisocial and prosocial behavior*. New York: Academic Press.

Pennebaker, J. W., Hughes, C., & O'Heeron, R. C. (1987). The psychophysiology of confession: Linking inhibitory and psychosomatic processes. *Journal of Personality and Social Psychology, 52*, 781–793.

Pennebaker, J. W., Kiecolt-Glaser, J., & Glaser, R. (1988). Disclosure of traumas and immune function: Health implications for psychotherapy. *Journal of Consulting and Clinical Psychology, 56*, 239–245.

Persky, H., Smith, K. D., & Basu, G. K. (1971). Relation of psychological measures of aggression and hostility to testosterone production in men. *Psychosomatic Medicine, 33*, 265–277.

Pickering, T. C. (1986). Should studies of patients undergoing coronary angiography be used to evaluate the role of behavioral risk factors for coronary heart disease? *Journal of Behavioral Medicine, 8*, 203–213.

Plutchik, R. (1986). Emotions: A general psychoevolutionary theory. In J. D. Maser (Ed.), *Approaches to emotion*. Hillsdale, NJ: Lawrence Erlbaum Associates.

Rosenman, R. H. (1978). The interview method of assessment of the coronary-prone behavior pattern. In T. M. Dembroski, S. Weiss, J. Shields, S. Haynes, & M. Feinleib (Eds.), *Coronary-prone behavior*. New York: Springer-Verlag.

Sarason, I. (1961). Intercorrelations among measures of hostility. *Journal of Clinical Psychology, 17*, 192–195.

Scherer, K. R. (1979). Personality markers in speech. In K. R. Scherer & H. Giles (Eds.), *Social markers in speech*. New York: Cambridge University Press.

Scherer, K. R. (1981). Vocal indicators of stress. In J. K. Darby (Ed.), *Speech evaluation in psychiatry*. New York: Grune & Stratton.

Siegman, A. W. (1985). Expressive correlates of affective states and traits. In A. W. Siegman & S. Feldstein (Eds.), *Nonverbal behavior: A multichannel perspective*. Hillsdale, NJ: Lawrence Erlbaum Associates.

Siegman, A. W. (1987a). The pacing of speech in depression. In J. D. Maser (Ed.), *Depression and expressive behavior*. Hillsdale, NJ: Lawrence Erlbaum Associates.

Siegman, A. W. (1987b). The telltale voice: Nonverbal messages of verbal communication. In A. W. Siegman & S. Feldstein (Eds.), *Nonverbal behavior and communication* (2nd ed.). Hillsdale, NJ: Lawrence Erlbaum Associates.

Siegman, A. W. (1992, July 19–24). *The role of expressive vocal behavior in negative emotions: Implications for stress management*. Paper presented at XXV International Congress of Psychology, Brussels.

Siegman, A. W. (1993). Paraverbal correlates of stress: Implications for stress identification and stress management. In L. Goldberger & S. Breznitz (Eds.), *Handbook of stress: Theoretical and clinical aspects*. NY: The Free Press.

Siegman, A. W., Anderson, R. W., & Berger, T. (1990). The angry voice: Its effects on the experience of anger and cardiovascular reactivity. *Psychosomatic Medicine, 52*, 631–643.

Siegman, A. W., Anderson, R. W., & Boyle, S. (1991, March). Repression, impression management, trait anxiety, and cardiovascular reactivity in men and women. Paper presented at annual meeting of the Society for Behavioral Medicine, Washington, DC.

Siegman, A. W., Anderson, R. A., Herbst, J., Boyle, S., & Wilkinson, J. (1992). Dimensions of anger–hostility and cardiovascular reactivity in provoked and angered men. *Journal of Behavioral Medicine, 15*, 257–272.

Siegman, A. W., & Boyle, S. (1992, March 31–April 4). *The expression of anger and cardiovascular reactivity in men and women: An experimental investigation.* Paper presented at 50th anniversary international meeting of the *American Psychosomatic Society*, New York.

Siegman, A. W., Dembroski, T. M., & Ringel, N. (1987). Components of hostility and the severity of coronary artery disease. *Psychosomatic Medicine, 49*, 127–135.

Siegman, A. W., Dohm, F. A., & Gjesdal, J. (April, 1988). *The effects of repressive coping style on the relationship between hostility, neuroticism, and cardiovascular reactivity.* Symposium paper presented at the annual meetings of the Society for Behavioral Medicine, Boston.

Siegman, A. W., Feldstein, S., Tommaso, C., Ringel, N., & Lating, J. (1987). Expressive vocal behavior and the severity of coronary artery disease. *Psychosomatic Medicine, 49*, 545–561.

Siegman, A. W., Lating, J., Johnston, G. S., & Boyle, S. (1992, March 31–April 4). *Structured interview derived hostility scores and thallium stress results in men and women.* Paper presented at 50th anniversary international meeting of the *American Psychosomatic Society*, New York.

Smith, M. A., & Houston, B. K. (1987). Hostility, anger expression, cardiovascular responsivity, and social support. *Biological Psychology, 24*, 39–48.

Spielberger, C. D., Johnson, E. H., Russel, S. F., Crane, R. J., Jacobs, G. A., & Worden, T. J. (1985). The experience and expression of anger: Construction and validation of an anger expression scale. In M. Cheney & R. Rosenman (Eds.), *Anger and hostility in cardiovascular and behavioral disorders*. New York: McGraw-Hill.

Stoney, C. M., & Engebretson, T. O. (in press). Anger and hostility: Potential mediators of the gender difference in coronary heart disease. In A. W. Siegman & T. Smith (Eds.), *Anger, hostility, and the heart*. NJ: Lawrence Erlbaum Associates.

Suarez, E. C., & Williams, R. B. (1990). The relationships between dimensions of hostility and cardiovascular reactivity as a function of task characteristics. *Psychosomatic Medicine, 52*, 558–570.

Temoshok, L. (1987). Psychoimmunology and AIDS. *Clinical Immunology Newsletter, 9*, 113–116.

Tomkins, S. S. (1962). *Affect, imagery, consciousness: I. The positive affects*. New York: Springer-Verlag.

Watson, D. A., & Pennebaker, J. W. (1989). Health complaints, stress, and distress. Exploring the central role of negative affectivity. *Psychological Review, 96*, 239–254.

Weinberger, D. A. (1990). The construct validity of the repressive coping style. In J. L. Singer (Ed.), *Repression and dissociation: Implications for personality theory, psychopathology, and health*. Chicago: The University of Chicago Press.

Weinberger, D., Schwartz, G., & Davidson, R. (1979). Low-anxious, high-anxious, and repressive coping styles: Psychometric patterns and behavioral and physiological responses to stress. *Journal of Abnormal Psychology, 88*, 4.

Wenneberg, S. R., Schneider, R. H., McLean, C. R., Levitsky, D. K., Walton, K. G., Mendarino, J. P., & Wallace, R. K. (1992, March 31–April 4). *Anger/hostility correlates with platelet aggregation during mental stress.* Paper presented at 50th anniversary international meeting of the American Psychosomatic Society, New York.

Williams, R. B. (1989). Biological mechanisms mediating the relationship between behavior and coronary heart disease. In A. W. Siegman & T. M. Dembroski (Eds.), *In search of coronary-prone behavior: Beyond Type A*. Hillsdale, NJ: Lawrence Erlbaum Associates.

Williams, R. B., Barefoot, J. C., Haney, T. L., Harrell, F. E., Blumenthal, J. A., Pryor, D. B., & Peterson, B. (1988). Type-A behavior and angiographically documented coronary atherosclerosis in a sample of 2,289 patients. *Psychosomatic Medicine, 50*, 139–152.

10

HOSTILITY AND RISK: DEMOGRAPHIC AND LIFESTYLE VARIABLES

Ilene C. Siegler
Duke University Medical Center
and
University of North Carolina

OVERVIEW AND METHODS

Demographic and lifestyle variables have played an important role in understanding the pathogenesis of coronary heart disease. The major CHD risk factors include both demographic (e.g., age, gender) and "lifestyle" variables (lipids, smoking and hypertension) (e.g., Dawber, 1980; Feinleib, Brand, Remington, & Zyanski, 1978; Leaverton et al., 1987; MRFIT, 1982). The literature on coronary-prone behavior—originally Type A and now hostility—was reviewed in volumes by Chesney and Rosenman (1985), Houston and Snyder (1988), Williams (1989), and Friedman (1992). There is a current consensus that hostility is the component of the Type A behavior pattern with the strongest relationship to coronary heart disease. This chapter focuses on the relationship of hostility to factors with known CHD associations. Whereas the typical approach to this problem has been to control for known demographic and lifestyle risk factors to rule out any "covariable bias" (Brand, 1978), confirmation of the status of hostility as an independent risk factor for coronary heart disease (CHD) awaits further data.

Definitions of Hostility. Measures of hostility come from three large classes: personality tests, anger and hostility inventories, and interviews.

1. Measures derived from personality tests include the Minnesota Multiphasic Personality Inventory (MMPI; Hathaway & McKinley, 1943; Butcher,

Dahlstrom, Graham, Tellegen, & Kaemmer, 1989) based measures of hostility such as the Cook–Medley hostility scale and the series of measures derived from it (Cook & Medley, 1954; Barefoot, Dodge, Peterson, Dahlstrom, & Williams, 1989) and the content dimension of cynicism (Costa, Zonderman, McCrae, & Williams, 1985). The Cattell 16 PF has a measure of suspiciousness—Factor L (Cattell, Eber, & Tatsuoka, 1970); and the NEO Personality Inventory has a measure of Agreeableness versus Antagonism (Costa & McCrae, 1985; Costa, Stone, McCrae, Dembroski, & Williams, 1987).

2. The second class of measures includes findings from the Buss–Durkee Hostility scale (Buss & Durkee, 1957), Multidimensional Anger Inventory (Siegel, 1992), Spielberger Anger scales (Spielberger, Jacobs, Russel, & Crane, 1983), the Anger-in scale of the Framingham Type A (Haynes, Levine, Scotch, Feinleib, & Kannel, 1978), and trust subscale of the Philosophies of Human Nature (Wrightsman, 1974).

3. The third class of measures are ratings of hostile behavior from interviews such as the original Type A Structured Interview (see Friedman & Rosenman, 1974). For a detailed discussion of the construct validity of hostility, see the chapters by Barefoot (1992; infra) and Smith and Christensen (1992).

Risk Factors as a Mechanism for CHD.   Risk factors are variables that have been associated with an increased probability of disease (Fletcher, Fletcher, & Wagner, 1982). The health behavior model postulates that the hostile person is more likely to engage in poor health behaviors, and that these behaviors relate to CHD (Houston & Vavak, 1991; Leiker & Healy, 1988; Scherwitz & Rugulies, 1992). The health–behavior model is often opposed to other explanatory systems as a candidate for understanding hostility/CHD relationships (see Siegler, Peterson, Barefoot, & Williams, 1992; Smith & Christensen, 1992). This is a "truly false" organization as each health behavior could have multiple pathways to account for the association of the particular risk factor with CHD.

The limitation of hostility/risk factor associations to those of risk with CHD, is an important decision in this chapter. Scherwitz and Rugulies (1992) argued for the importance of risk factors determining a lifestyle. They define a risk factor as one which reduces the lifespan (or has an impact on all-cause mortality). The issue of risk behavior and lifestyle is related to the relationship between all-cause mortality and CHD. When the two are nearly identical (when men die in the 40s and 50s) then the distinction is less critical. Whereas some risk factors are related to both CHD and all-cause mortality (smoking, obesity), others are not (marital status, social support, sleep patterns, daily eating patterns and major life events). The major CHD risk factors with hostility data reviewed below are: smoking, lipid parameters, caffeine, diseases that increase the risk of CHD, family history, exercise, alcohol, and obesity.

FINDINGS ON THE RELATIONSHIPS BETWEEN MEASURES OF HOSTILITY AND DEMOGRAPHIC FACTORS

Demographic attributes of individuals are also CHD risk indicators. They are different from the other risk indicators in that they have a more permanent (except for social class) or less controllable aspect to them. They are not bad habits that have the potential for intervention. These demographic factors also interact with each other. However, without CHD outcome data to use as a criterion, the relative contributions of the risk factors discussed is difficult to assess. The references for findings on the relationship of various measures of hostility to demographic factors (age, period/cohort, gender, race, socio-economic status [SES]) are found in Table 10.1.

Age/Period/Cohort. Age has a curvilinear relationship to hostility. Hostility is high in late adolescence, falls through adulthood reaching a minimum at middle age and then starts rising again in later life. This relationship with age holds for cross-sections of persons measured in the 1960s and in the 1980s (see Fig. 10.1).

These cross-sectional age relationships suggest that age at baseline is a potentially important factor when comparing across study populations. No longitudinal data on age changes in hostility and associations with risk factors have been published.

TABLE 10.1

Citations on Demographics and Hostility

Age/Period Comparisons:
    Cook–Medley (Barefoot et al., 1991; Scherwitz et al., 1991; Swenson et al., 1973)
    MMPI Cynicism (Zonderman et al., 1993)
    PHN (Wrightsman, 1974)
    Framingham Anger-In (Haynes et al., 1978)

Gender Comparisons:
    Cook–Medley (Barefoot et al., 1991; Scherwitz et al., 1991)
    Framingham Anger-In (Haynes et al., 1978)

Race Comparisons:
    Cook–Medley (Barefoot et al., 1991; Scherwitz et al., 1991)
    Anger (Kumanyika & Adams-Campbell, 1991; Siegel, 1992)

Socioeconomic Status:
    Education:
        Cook–Medley (Barefoot et al., 1991; Scherwitz et al., 1991)
        Spielberger Trait Anger, Anger-In (Matthews et al., 1989)
    Occupation/Income:
        Cook–Medley (Barefoot et al., 1991)

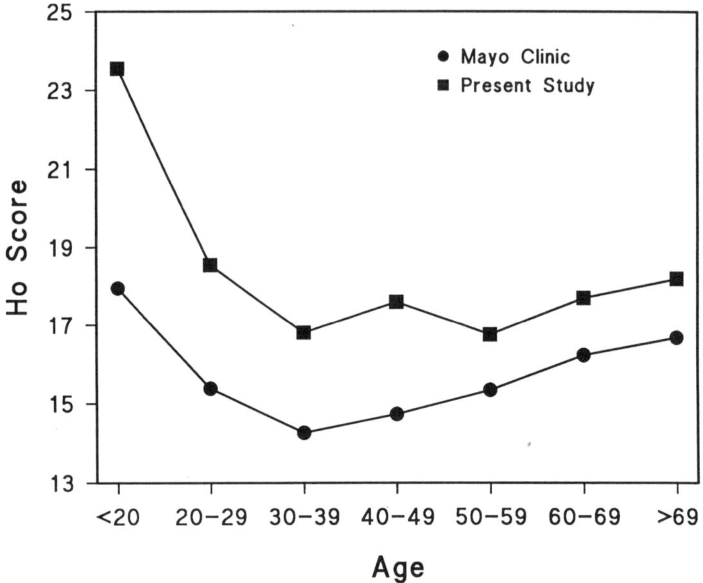

FIG. 10.1.   Mean Cook-Medley Hostility Score (adjusted for age) for data collected by Swensen, Pearson, and Osborne, 1973, Mayo Clinic, and data from the MMPI2 standardization sample, present study. From J. C. Barefoot, B. L. Peterson, W. G. Dahlstrom, I. C. Siegler, N. B. Anderson, and R. B. Williams, Jr. (1991). Adapted by permission.

Once we go beyond Cook–Medley and cynicism related measures to other types of measures of hostility the situation in terms of age gets more complex. Barefoot, Beckham, Haney, Siegler, and Lipkus (1993) gave a battery of standard paper-and-pencil measures of hostility to White, middle-aged, and older adults from a mixture of social classes. Hostility increased with age when the measures were from the cynicism domain (which included Cook–Medley and the hostile behavior index of the interview ratings from IHAT), decreased with age when they were primarily anger-based, and had no relationship to age when generally neuroticism-based.

We have very little data on cohorts tested with similar instruments. Wrightsman (1974) reported on successive cohorts of college students on the Trust subscale of the Philosophies of Human Nature and found that the mean level of trust declined from 1963 to 1974. Zonderman, Siegler, Barefoot, Williams, and Costa (1993) evaluated time of measurement, age, and gender effects for the MMPI content dimension of cynicism (Costa et al., 1985). There were no time of measurement effects comparing men of the same ages in 1960 versus 1980. There were significant gender contrasts with men higher on cynicism than women at each age studied, and age effects such that younger persons were higher on cynicism than older persons. As repeated measures of hostility are made on existing cohorts, we may be able to start to evaluate the cohort variation net of age and period variation. The available data suggest that cynicism has increased.

Gender. When gender differences are reported, men are usually higher on the measure of hostility than women. This also varies by the range of ages studied and by the type of hostility measured. Gender at various ages also may imply other factors that, if unmeasured, can be expected to influence the level of hostility and its association with coronary disease risk. For example, the use of oral contraceptives would be more prevalent in samples with premenopausal women (Davis & Matthews, 1990) and may also reflect cohort-specific birth control preferences. The exclusion of respondents who have CHD would result in the exclusion of men from the population at a younger age than the exclusion of women from that same population. Furthermore, there are gender differences in the patterns of most traditional risk behaviors (Baum & Gruenberg, 1991).

Race. Non-Whites tend to be higher on hostility than Whites. However, there are very few, if any studies of upper-class non-Whites. When multiple regression techniques are used to adjust for unequal social factors, race appears less important than social class indicators. James, Keenan, and Browning (1992) evaluated racial differences in health behaviors and health outcomes, but do not present any hostility data. Kumanyika and Adams-Campbell (1991) reviewed findings on anger and suppressed hostility and their association with hypertension in Blacks. Scherwitz, Perkins, Chesney, and Hughes (1991) and Barefoot et al. (1991) presented data on Cook–Medley hostility in Blacks and Whites.

Socioeconomic Status (SES). Hostility is inversely related to indices of higher SES: income, education, occupational achievement, and prestige. House and his colleagues (1992) detailed the centrality of SES in our society as a critical factor in the relationship of health status to age. Their data show an age by status interaction from ages 35–74 such that the level of poor health reached by a lower SES person in middle age (45–50) is not reached for a higher SES person until age 75! Even though these data do not focus on coronary disease outcomes, they provide a powerful model to use to study the impact of social class factors on hostility. Hostility data from Barefoot, Peterson, Dahlstrom, Siegler, Anderson, and Williams (1991) are shown by the House et al. (1992) categories of social class in Table 10.2.

The "hostility space" implied by the means in Table 10.2 puts lower SES Black men and women at the highest ranges of hostility; lower SES White men and women and higher SES Black men and women in the middle range and higher SES White men and women in the lowest range. The interactions

TABLE 10.2
Mean Cook–Medley Hostility Scores at Ages 18–24, 25–30, and 30+ for
Race/Gender Groups of Persons Defined by Income and Educational Level

Lower SES: < High School Graduate and < $20,000 Per Year

| | Age Group | | |
Race/Gender Group	18–24	25–30	30+
Black men	27.4(6.1)	27.9(7.7)	25.0(9.1)
	$n = 22$	$n = 7$	$n = 32$
Black women	25.7(9.9)	23.0(6.2)	25.8(8.9)
	$n = 19$	$n = 11$	$n = 46$
White men	24.5(3.1)	22.3(7.6)	22.1(8.6)
	$n = 8$	$n = 8$	$n = 41$
White women	22.2(8.6)	19.3(7.2)	18.5(7.9)
	$n = 17$	$n = 18$	$n = 93$

Higher SES: High School Graduate and > $20,000 Per Year

| | Age Group | | |
Race/Gender Group	18–24	25–30	30+
Black men	17.8(10.8)	22.9(7.6)	18.3(8.2)
	$n = 5$	$n = 11$	$n = 57$
Black women	24.1(9.2)	21.6(7.8)	16.3(5.6)
	$n = 13$	$n = 12$	$n = 56$
White men	18.7(7.5)	18.8(8.5)	15.79(7.62)
	$n = 28$	$n = 91$	$n = 445$
White women	14.4(6.8)	14.9(6.9)	14.5(6.8)
	$n = 44$	$n = 103$	$n = 458$

Adapted from Barefoot et al. (1991); Butcher et al. (1989).

of SES with race and sex may be important conceptually in understanding behavior patterns associated with disease risk.

Table 10.3 shows the regression results of these data in Barefoot et al. (1991), which allows a comparison of the relative strength of the demographic effects. Race and income interacted such that there was a strong hostility effect for non-Whites because of income levels; but no effect for Whites. This data from the national standardization sample for the MMPI2 (Butcher et al., 1989) has helped to close some gaps in our understanding of the impact of socio-demographic factors on hostility; however, it is also limited in representativeness.

We need to get measures of hostility and anger into ongoing national data collection efforts so that we have behavioral measures to use in monitoring the national health in the coming decades, with a full representation across the demographic groups in the population. Costa and McCrae (1986) discussed

TABLE 10.3
Main Effects Models

Source	df	F	p
Sex	1	31.69	.0001
Age	2	3.55	.0288
Income	1	9.14	.0025
Occupation	5	4.78	.0002
Education	1	71.05	.0001
Race	1	90.52	.0001

Note. From Barefoot et al. (1991, p. 20). Reprinted by permission.

the development of the short personality scales that were included as markers of neuroticism, extraversion, and openness in the NHANES data collection (Costa et al., 1986). Whereas it is our loss that the agreeableness/antagonism domain was not part of the data they collected, the Costa et al., 1986, work provides a model for future efforts.

FINDINGS ON THE RELATIONSHIP OF HOSTILITY TO ESTABLISHED CHD RISK FACTORS

The relationship of hostility to CHD risk factors remains confused in the literature. There is even a lack of agreement about what should be considered a traditional CHD risk factor (Hopkins & Williams, 1981). Part of the complexity is that each study operationalizes the same risk factor differently. Another part of the complexity comes from the analysis strategy that reports crude associations, associations controlled for demographic factors, or associations controlled for other CHD risk factors. Different statistical procedures are employed to evaluate the hostility risk association. Although there are design differences among studies including cross-sectional, case control, longitudinal, and prospective study designs that evaluate hostility and risk, the overall design of the study does not always indicate the nature of the contrast that measures the association between the measure of hostility and the measure of CHD risk. These differences make the kind of summary that looks at the preponderance of the evidence as number of positive versus negative studies impossible. Table 10.4 provides a shorthand review of the literature by describing the measures used in 14 study populations. Table 10.5 defines the study populations reported in Table 10.4, and gives citations to the papers reviewed.

Smoking. There is little controversy that smoking is a major CHD risk factor. The literature on hostility and smoking is less consistent. In both the UNCAHS and CARDIA, hostility is related to the prevalence of smoking.

TABLE 10.4

Major CHD Risk Factors and Hostility Associations

Smoking (Generally cigarettes only):
- prevalence (CARDIA+) (UNCAHS+) (UNCDRS−) (MINN53−) (MCGDRS−) (KANUG−)
- ever smoker (UNCAHS+) (UNCDRS−)
- stop smoking (UNCAHS+)
- # per day (CARDIA−) (WES+) (MRFIT+) (FHAM;M+W−)
- pack years (UNCDRS−)
- history (at least 10/day in past 5 years) (DLS2−)

Lipids (Net/controlled for demogs):
- total serum cholesterol (WES−) (DLS2−) (FHAM−)
- Ratio Total/HDL (UNCAHS+)
- self-report as hypercholesteremia (MCGDRS−)

Lipids (Controlled for BMI, Alcohol, Physical Activity):
- total serum cholesterol (CARDIA−) (KANLIP+)
- LDL (CARDIA−) (KANLIP+)M
- HDL (CARDIA−)

Caffeine:
- amount in diet per day (CARDIA−)BWi
- coffee and beverages only (UNCAHS+)

Hypertension:
- SBP (FHAM−) (CARDIA−)WWi (WES−)
- DBP (FHAM;M−W+) (MINN53−) (CARDIA−)BWi
- Hypertensive: (TORONTO+) (CARDIA−)BM+
- Self-report of diagnosis by MD (UNCAHS−)P; (UNCAHS+)C (UNCDRS+) (MCGDRS−)

Family history for CHD:
- (UNCDRS−) (MINN53−)

Exercise/Fitness:
- # hours (UNCHASi)P; (UNCAHS−)C (KANUG−)
- leisure time (CARDIA−)WWi
- aerobic exercise/walk/bike (MISS+)
- treadmill performance (CARDIA−)WW+
- Forced Expiratory Volume (CARDIA+)

Alcohol:
- consumption in past year (CARDIA−)
- average weekly intake in drinkers (CARDIA+) (UNCAHS+) (WES+)
- > 2 drinks/day (DLS2−)

Obesity:
- "Obesity" (MCGDRS−)
- BMI (weight/height2) (CARDIA−) (UNCAHS+) (HWS+)
  (UNCAHS−;@ baseline) (KANUG+?)
- Waist-to-Hip Ratio/Abdominal Fat (CARDIA+) (HWS+)

Note. The sign after the abbreviated study name is given as "+" when hostility is associated in the risky direction; "−" when the association is not statistically significant; and "i" when the association is inverse or protective.

TABLE 10.5

Abbreviations Used in Table 10.4 with References and Brief Descriptions

CARDIA	(Scherwitz et al., 1991, 1992) All four race/sex groups have the same relationship unless noted by initials. Cross-sectional analysis. Higgins et al. (1991) pulmonary data. Cook–Medley controlled for age, education analyzed within race/sex groupings.
DLS2	(Barefoot et al., 1987) Duke Second Longitudinal Study. Cattell 16PF- Factor L- suspiciousness; 502 men and women mean age 58; all White.
FHAM	(Haynes et al., 1978) Framingham Type-A Anger-in (suppressed hostility) as the measure of hostility.
HWS	(Wing et al., 1991) Healthy Women Study. Random sample middle-aged women aged 42–50 in Pittsburgh. Examined in laboratory. Speilberger Trait Anger and Anger-in as measures of hostility (Speilberger et al., 1983; 1985).
KANLIPS	(Dujovne & Houston, 1991) Lipid clinic patients. Cook–Medley and Buss–Durkee hostility.
KANUG	(Houston & Vavak, 1991) Kansas undergraduates. Cook–Medley. MANOVA on hostility and risk factors nonsignificant with ANOVA for BMI $p < .05$.
MCGDRS	(McCranie et al., 1986) Cook–Medley, 435 men and 12 women physicians from Medical College of Georgia tested 1953–61 as part of admission. Mean age at baseline 22, age at follow-up 47.
MINN53	(Hearn, Murray, & Luepker, 1989) 1399 White men. Aged 19–52, prospective. Time 1 = 1953. Baseline risk factors tested in case control study of 220 men.
MISS	(Leiker & Heily, 1988) Cook–Medley, undergraduates in Mississippi.
MRFIT	(Dembroski et al., 1989) Potential for hostility from Structured Interview in high-risk men (all smokers, all hypertensive, all high lipids and BMI @ 150% of normal).
TORONTO	(Irvine et al., 1991) Case control study hypertensives versus normotensives; potential for hostility from Structured Interview.
UNCAHS	(Barefoot et al., 1990; Siegler et al., 1990; Siegler et al., 1992; Siegler, Peterson, Barefoot, & Williams, 1992) 4710 men and women (99% White); Cook–Medley controlled for age and sex. Prospective (age 19–42)P and Concurrent (age 41/42)C analyses have same relationship unless noted. Hostility measured both at baseline and at follow-up. All risk factors measured at follow-up only except for BMI, which was calculated at baseline from other records (College).
UNCDRS	(Barefoot, Dahlstrom, & Williams, 1983; Barefoot, Smith, Dahlstrom, & Williams, 1989) 225 White men. Aged 25–52, prospective. Smoking, Family History, and Hypertension at follow-up as covariates for Cook–Medley/CHD relationship.
WES	(Shekelle, Gail, Ostfeld, & Paul, O., 1983) All White men. Same relationships of MMPI Content Dimension Cynicism (Almada et al., 1991).

Among smokers, the number smoked per day is related to hostility in the WES and MRFIT (but not CARDIA). Hostility was not related to smoking in a number of study populations (UNCDRS, FHAM, DLS2, MINN53, MCGDRS, KANUG). The association appears to vary as a function of the type of measure of smoking and the ages of the participants.

Lipids. This literature is particularly hard to review because many studies present the hostility/lipid associations only controlled for other risk factors (e.g., Dujovne & Houston, 1991; Scherwitz et al., 1992). Generally, relationships between total cholesterol and hostility are nonsignificant. Data from

UNCAHS prospectively and concurrently found a positive relationship of hostility to the ratio of Total to HDL cholesterol, whereas CARDIA found no relationships for Total, HDL, or LDL after controlling for physical activity, BMI, and alcohol use. The KANLIP study found mixed findings depending on the lipid, sex, and measure of hostility used.

Other risk factors are associated with lipid risk profiles—indexed by total cholesterol (TC)/HDL ratios. For example, in the UNCAHS, higher TC/HDL ratios are associated with male gender ($p < .0001$); higher body mass index ($p < .0001$); less time spent in exercise per week ($p = .017$); higher caffeine use ($p = .002$); *less* alcohol consumed per week ($p = .003$); and being a current smoker ($p < .0001$). These associations suggest that the associations between hostility and lipids may be the results of shared behaviors that are more directly related to hostility. Until we have CHD outcome data, it will be difficult to sort out the pathways.

Caffeine. CARDIA reported no relationship to hostility except an inverse relationship for Black women. UNCAHS found a positive relationship between the amount of caffeine and hostility both prospectively and concurrently for White men and women. As the risk of caffeine on CHD is generally thought to operate through lipids, this may provide a potential explanation for the findings.

Diseases. There is a large literature on anger-based measures and hypertension, particularly in minority communities, which generally finds consistent associations with measures of anger and increased rates of hypertension in Blacks (see Kumanyika & Adams-Campbell, 1991). The CARDIA data varied by race and sex of the respondent and in the UNCAHS hostility measured at middle age was associated with hypertension; but not prospectively. Part of the complexity in this area is illustrated with a finding reported by Siegel (1992). In a study of middle-aged male factory workers, there was no association between anger measures and diastolic blood pressure controlling for BMI, smoking, alcohol use, and family history. However, hostile outlook and Anger-in were associated with higher diastolic blood pressure in interaction with anxiety for persons higher in anxiety. There is no data on hostility and prevalence of diabetes.

Family History. There are no positive reports of data on family history and hostility (UNCDRS; MINN53). However, in both studies the respondents were young enough (ages 19–25), so that their parents may not have been old enough to have disease.

Exercise/Fitness. Associations between hostility and exercise behavior measured as "hours per week for fun or fitness" were inconsistent in UNCAHS. Prospectively, those who were more hostile exercised more, even controlling for age and sex, and concurrently, there was no relationship. In our more detailed analysis of personality and exercise (Siegler et al., 1991), we found that exercise was associated with measures of extraversion both prospectively and cross-sectionally; but not with cynicism. In CARDIA, hostility was negatively related to lung function, which can be considered an index of fitness. Relationships between hostility and lung function (FEV) were maintained controlling for other risk indices (Higgins et al., 1991). Hostility was also related to reports of aerobic exercise, walking, and biking (Leiker & Healy, 1988). Thus, leisure and modest levels of exercise may not be related to hostility, whereas more strenuous exercise or measures of fitness may be.

Alcohol.   Among drinkers, hostility is related to amount of alcohol consumed in CARDIA, UNCAHS, and WES. However, when the comparison is over a fixed amount (DLS2) or includes nondrinkers in the contrast (CARDIA), there is no association reported.

Weight.   Obesity, or larger Body Mass Indexes (BMIs) is generally not associated with hostility in younger populations (CARDIA, UNCAHS, when in college) but is associated when the samples are middle-aged (UNCAHS, HWS). Waist-to-hip ratio was positively associated with hostility/anger, in the two studies that employed it.

Clues for Reconciling Disparate Findings

There are no obvious factors that emerge from Table 10.4 that fully explain the discrepancies noted. There are, however, a number of clues suggested by the patterns of findings reviewed earlier.

Age at Time of Measurement of the Hostility Risk Factor Association.   When the risk factors are measured at baseline and the baseline measure is in young adulthood, the probability of significant associations is reduced. It may take time for the operation of hostility to insure the persistence of the risk factor. When the samples are middle-aged at baseline and elderly at follow-up, removal of persons who develop disease from the study may reduce the probability of finding an association.

Multiple Risk Factors and Hostility.   Lane, Barefoot, Williams, and Siegler (1991) looked at the relationship between caffeine (split at 3 servings per day) and cholesterol (split at 240 MG%) as a function of a median split in hostility. We found that in persons with low hostility, caffeine and cholesterol were associated with a relative risk = 1.93, whereas for those with high hostility caffeine and cholesterol were not significantly associated (relative risk = .93).

This finding suggests that there may be idiosyncratic effects when considering risk factors jointly. There is also a well-known inverse relationship between smoking and obesity (Kannel & Cupples, 1989). As both smoking and obesity are often associated with higher levels of hostility, understanding their joint operation will prove to be a challenge. There may be individual differences in the way that persons use the habits we consider to be risk factors to control stress. If this is true, then particular combinations of risky behaviors may have associated personality profiles. Furthermore, as the data of Siegel (1992) illustrated, hostility constructs may themselves interact with other individual difference factors such that associations between hostility and risk are modified by another psychological factor.

Secular Trends. An additional trend that requires explaining is that whereas rates of CHD appear to be going down, prevalence of hostility appears to be increasing. Sprafka, Burke, Folsom, Luepker, and Blackburn (1990) reported mixed findings on risk factor change in the Minnesota Heart Survey. From 1981 to 1986, smoking, blood pressure, and total cholesterol declined, whereas levels of HDL decreased (increasing risk), as did body mass index. We need to understand the changes in the prevalence of these risk factors and their time course.

Consensus on Measuring Hostility. The differences in the ways we measure hostility are not enough to account for the mess in the literature. However, it would be useful to have a consensus of items that would be short enough to be widely used and long enough to be reliable, as candidates for inclusion in future national population studies, and as markers to be used in conjunction with whatever measure of theoretical interest is being employed in a more limited study.

Obesity as a Model for Hostility. Kannel and Cupples (1989), in discussing obesity findings from the Framingham Study, "indicate that the prognostic importance of obesity varies by age, smoking status, duration of followup, and whether the mortality is from cardiovascular or noncardiovascular causes" (p. 115). Furthermore, there is controversy about the status of obesity as a risk factor for CHD, because obesity does not always emerge as an independent statistical predictor.

> However, it is important to recognize that a variable such as obesity can be an important intermediary in the pathogenesis of disease, even though it is not a significant predictor in multivariate analysis when other covariates are taken into account (Keys, 1980). Because obesity predisposes to hypertension, low-HDL cholesterol, and glucose intolerance, the public health significance of obesity is not refuted by its poor performance in a multivariate statistical model. It is

likely that obesity predisposes to cardiovascular disease precisely by promoting these atherogenic traits. (p. 124)

Thus, obesity might be a model for understanding the emergent data on hostility and heart disease. This finding is further supported by data suggesting that multiple ways of indexing obesity behave differently, and that obesity originating early in life may be more detrimental than that acquired later in life (Kannel & Cupples, 1989).

What is clear from this chapter is that there is no simple relationship between hostility and coronary risk. As the populations being followed prospectively develop disease, we will be able to observe the role that hostility plays in the prediction of coronary heart disease. If it is true that obesity is a good model for hostility, then we can expect a controversy about the status of hostility as an independent risk factor. Irrespective of the outcome of that controversy, searching for mechanisms to understand how hostility contributes to risky behavior will enhance the importance of behavioral medicine.

ACKNOWLEDGMENTS

This work was supported by the National Heart, Lung, and Blood Institute, Grant #HL36587; National Institute of Aging, Grant #AG09276; and the Duke University Behavioral Medicine Research Center.

REFERENCES

Almada, S. J., Zonderman, A. B., Shekelle, R. B., Dyer, A. R., Davligus, M. L., Costa, P. T. Jr., & Stamler, J. (1991). Neuroticism and cynicism and risk of death in middle-aged men: The Western Electric Study. *Psychosomatic Medicine, 53,* 165–175.

Barefoot, J. C. (1992). Developments in the measurement of hostility. In H. S. Friedman (Ed.), *Hostility coping and health* (pp. 13–32). Washington, DC: American Psychological Association.

Barefoot, J. C., Beckham, J. C., Haney, T. L., Siegler, I. C., & Lipkus, I. M. (1993). Age differences in hostility among middle-aged and older adults: A multimethod analysis. *Psychology and Aging, 8,* 3–9.

Barefoot, J. C., Dahlstrom, W. G., & Williams, R. B. (1983). Hostility, CHD incidence and total mortality: A 25-year follow-up study of 225 physicians. *Psychosomatic Medicine, 45,* 59–64.

Barefoot, J. C., Dodge, K., Peterson, B. L., Dahlstrom, W. G., & Williams, R. B. (1989). The Cook–Medley hostility scale: Item content and ability to predict survival. *Psychosomatic Medicine, 51,* 46–57.

Barefoot, J. C., Peterson, B. L., Dahlstrom, W. G., & Siegler, I. C. (1990, November). *Prospective prediction of smoking initiation and cessation.* Paper presented at the American Heart Association, Dallas, TX.

Barefoot, J. C., Peterson, B. L., Dahlstrom, W. G., Siegler, I. C., Anderson, N. B., & Williams, R. B., Jr. (1991). Hostility patterns and health implications: Correlates of Cook–Medley hostility scale scores in a national survey. *Health Psychology, 10,* 18–24.

Barefoot, J. C., Siegler, I. C., Nowlin, J. B., Peterson, B. L., Haney, T. L., & Williams, R. B., Jr. (1987). Suspiciousness, health and mortality: A follow-up study of 500 older adults. *Psychosomatic Medicine, 49*, 450–457.

Barefoot, J. C., Smith, R. H., Dahlstrom, W. G., & Williams, R. B., Jr. (1989). Personality predictors of smoking behavior in a sample of physicians. *Psychology and Health, 3*, 37–43.

Baum, A., & Gruenberg, N. E. (1991). Special Issue on Gender and Health. *Health Psychology, 10*, 79–153.

Brand, R. J. (1978). Coronary-prone behavior as an independent risk factor for coronary heart disease. In T. M. Dembroski, S. M. Weiss, J. L. Shields, S. G. Haynes, & M. Feinleib (Eds.), *Coronary-prone behavior* (pp. 11–24). New York: Springer-Verlag.

Buss, A. H., & Durkee, A. (1957). An inventory for assessing different kinds of hostility. *Journal of Consulting Psychology, 42*, 155–162.

Butcher, J. N., Dahlstrom, W. G., Graham, J. R., Tellegen, A., & Kaemmer, B. (1989). *MMPI-2 manual for administration and scoring.* Minneapolis: University of Minnesota Press.

Cattell, R. B., Eber, H. W., & Tatsuoka, M. M. (1970). *Handbook for the Sixteen Personality Factor Questionnaire (16PF).* Champaign, IL: Institute for Personality and Ability Testing.

Chesney, M. A., & Rosenman, R. H. (Eds). (1985). *Anger and hostility in behavioral medicine.* New York: Hemisphere.

Cook, W., & Medley, D. (1954). Proposed hostility and pharisaic-virtue scales for the MMPI. *Journal of Applied Psychology, 38*, 414–418.

Costa, P. T., Jr., & McCrae, R. R. (1985). *The NEO-personality inventory manual.* Odessa, FL: Psychological Assessment Resources.

Costa, P. T., Jr., & McCrae, R. R. (1986). 1. Development and validation of survey measures. *Psychology and Aging, 1*, 140–143.

Costa, P. T., Jr., McCrae, R. R., Zonderman, A. B., Barbano, H. E., Lebowitz, B., & Larson, D. M. (1986). Cross-sectional studies of personality in a national sample: 2. Stability in neuroticism, extraversion, and openness. *Psychology and Aging, 1*, 144–149.

Costa, P. T., Jr., Stone, S. V., McCrae, R. R., Dembroski, T. M., & Williams, R. B. (1987). Hostility agreeableness–antagonism and coronary heart disease. *Holistic Medicine, 2*, 161–167.

Costa, P. T., Jr., Zonderman, A. B., McCrae, R. R., & Williams, R. B. (1985). Content and comprehensiveness in the MMPI: An item factor analysis in a normal adult sample. *Journal of Personality and Social Psychology, 48*(14), 925–933.

Davis, M. C., & Matthews, K. A. (1990). Cigarette smoking and oral contraceptive use influence women's lipid, lipoprotein, and cardiovascular responses during stress. *Health Psychology, 9*, 717–736.

Dawber, T. R. (1980). *The Framingham Study.* Cambridge, MA: Harvard University Press.

Dembroski, T. M., MacDougall, J. M., Costa, P. T. Jr., & Granditis, G. A. (1989). Components of hostility as predictors of sudden death and myocardial infarction in the Multiple Risk Factor Intervention Trial. *Psychosomatic Medicine, 51*, 514–522.

Dujovne, V. F., & Houston, B. K. (1991). Hostility-related variables and plasma lipid levels. *Journal of Behavioral Medicine, 14*, 553–563.

Feinleib, M., Brand, R. J., Remington, R., & Zyanski, S. J. (1978). Section summary: Association of the coronary-prone behavior pattern and coronary heart disease. In T. M. Dembroski, S. M. Weiss, J. L. Shields, S. G. Haynes, & M. Feinleib (Eds.), *Coronary-prone behavior* (pp. 2–9). New York: Springer-Verlag.

Fletcher, R. S., Fletcher, S. W., & Wagner, E. H. (1982). *Clinical epidemiology the essentials.* Baltimore: Williams & Wilkins.

Friedman, H. S. (Ed.). (1992). *Hostility coping & health.* Washington, DC: American Psychological Association.

Friedman, M., & Rosenman, R. (1974). *Type A behavior and your heart*. New York: Knopf.

Hathaway, S. R., & McKinley, J. C. (1943). *Booklet for the Minnesota Multiphasic Personality Inventory*. Minneapolis: University of Minnesota Press.

Haynes, S. G., Levine, S., Scotch, N., Feinleib, M., & Kannel, W. B. (1978). The relationship of psychosocial factors to coronary heart disease in the Framingham Study. I. Methods and risk factors. *American Journal Epidemiology, 107*, 362–383.

Hearn, M. D., Murray, D. M., & Luepker, R. V. (1989). Hostility, coronary heart disease and total mortality: A 33-year follow-up study of university students. *Journal of Behavioral Medicine, 12*, 105–121.

Higgins, M., Keller, J. B., Wagenknecht, L. E., Townsend, M. C., Sparrow, D., Jackobs, D. R., Jr., & Hughes, G. (1991). Pulmonary function and cardiovascular risk factor relationships in Black and in White young men and women. *Chest, 99*, 315–322.

Hopkins, P. N., & Williams, R. R. (1981). A survey of 246 suggested coronary risk factors. *Atherosclerosis, 40*, 1–52.

House, J. S., Kessler, R. C., Herzog, A. R., Mero, R. P., Kinney, A. M., & Breslow, M. J. (1992). Social stratification, age and health. In K. W. Schaie, D. G. Blazer, & J. S. House (Eds.), *Aging, health behaviors, and health outcomes* (pp. 1–32). Hillsdale, NJ: Lawrence Erlbaum Associates.

Houston, B. K., & Snyder, C. R. (Eds.) (1988). *Type-A behavior pattern: Research, theory, and intervention*. New York: Wiley.

Houston, B. K., & Vavak, C. R. (1991). Cynical hostility: Developmental factors, psychosocial correlates, and health behaviors. *Health Psychology, 10*, 9–17.

Irvine, J., Garner, D. M., Craig, H. M., & Logan, A. G. (1991). Prevalence of Type-A behavior in untreated hypertensive individuals. *Hypertension, 18*, 72–78.

James, S. A., Keenan, N. L., & Browning, S. (1992). Socioeconomic status, health behaviors and health status among Blacks. In K. W. Schaie, D. G. Blazer, & J. S. House (Eds.), *Aging, health behaviors, and health outcomes* (pp. 39–58). Hillsdale, NJ: Lawrence Erlbaum Associates.

Kannel, W. B., & Cupples, L. A. (1989). Cardiovascular and noncardiovascular consequences of obesity. In A. J. Stunkard & A. Baum (Eds.), *Perspectives in behavioral medicine: Eating, sleeping and sex* (pp. 109–130). Hillsdale, NJ: Lawrence Erlbaum Associates.

Keys, A. (1980). Overweight, obesity, coronary heart disease and mortality. *Nutrition Reviews, 38*, 297–307.

Kumanyika, S., & Adams-Campbell, L. L. (1991). Obesity, diet and psychosocial factors contributing to cardiovascular disease in Blacks. *Cardiovascular Clinics, 21*, 47–73.

Lane, J. D., Barefoot, J. C., Williams, R. B., & Siegler, I. C. (1991, March). *Caffeine and cholesterol: Interactions with hostility*. Paper presented at the meetings of the Society of Behavioral Medicine, Washington, DC.

Leaverton, P. E., Sorlie, P. D., Kleinman, J. C., Dannenberg, A. L., Ingster-Moore, L., Kannel, W. B., & Cornoni-Huntley, J. C. (1987). Representativeness of the Framingham risk model for coronary heart disease mortality: A comparison with a national cohort study. *Journal of Chronic Disease, 40*, 775–784.

Leiker, M., & Healy, B. J. (1988). A link between hostility and disease: Poor health habits? *Behavioral Medicine, 14*, 129–133.

Matthews, K. A., Kelsey, S. F., Meilahn, E. N., Kuller, L. H., & Wing, R. R. (1989). Educational attainment and behavioral and biologic risk factors for coronary heart disease in middle-aged women. *American Journal Epidemiology, 129*, 1132–1144.

McCranie, E. W., Watkins, L. O., Brandsma, J. M., & Sisson, B. D. (1986). Hostility, coronary heart disease (CHD) incidence and total mortality: Lack of association in a 25-year follow-up study of 478 physicians. *Journal of Behavioral Medicine, 9*, 119–125.

MRFIT Research Group. (1982). Multiple risk factor intervention trial: Risk factor changes and mortality results. *Journal of the American Medical Association, 248*(12), 1465–1477.

Scherwitz, L., Perkins, L., Chesney, M., & Hughes, G. (1991). Cook–Medley hostility scale and subsets: Relationship to demographic and psychosocial characteristics in young adults in the CARDIA study. *Psychosomatic Medicine, 53,* 36–49.

Scherwitz, L., Perkins, L., Chesney, M., Hughes, G., Sidney, S., & Manolio, T. (1992). Hostility and health behaviors in young adults: The CARDIA study. *American Journal of Epidemiology, 136,* 136–145.

Scherwitz, L., & Rugulies, R. (1992). Lifestyle and hostility. In H. S. Friedman (Ed.), *Hostility coping and health* (pp. 77–98). Washington, DC: American Psychological Association.

Shekelle, R. B., Gale, M., Ostfield, A., & Paul, O. (1983). Hostility, risk of coronary heart disease and mortality. *Psychosomatic Medicine, 45,* 109–114.

Siegel, J. M. (1992). Anger and cardiovascular health. In H. S. Friedman (Ed.), *Hostility coping and health* (pp. 49–64). Washington, DC: American Psychological Association.

Siegler, I. C., Blumenthal, J. A., Costa, P. T., Jr., Dahlstrom, W. G., Peterson, B. L., Barefoot, J. C., & Williams, R. B. (1991, March). *Personality prediction of exercise in the UNC Alumni Heart Study.* Paper presented at the American Psychosomatic Society, Santa Fe, NM.

Siegler, I. C., Peterson, B. L., Barefoot, J. C., Harvin, S. H., Dahlstrom, W. G., Kaplan, B. H., Costa, P. T., Jr., & Williams, R. B. (1992). Using college alumni populations in epidemiologic research: The UNC Alumni Heart Study. *Journal of Clinical Epidemiology, 45*(11), 1243–1250.

Siegler, I. C., Peterson, B. L., Barefoot, J. C., & Williams, R. B. (1992). Hostility during late adolescence predicts coronary risk factors at mid-life. *American Journal of Epidemiology, 136,* 146–154.

Siegler, I. C., Zonderman, A. B., Barefoot, J. C., Williams, R. B., Jr., Costa, P. T., Jr., & McCrae, R. R. (1990). Predicting personality in adulthood from college MMPI scores: Implications for follow-up studies in psychosomatic medicine. *Psychosomatic Medicine, 52,* 644–652.

Smith, T. W., & Christensen, A. J. (1992). In H. S. Friedman (Ed.), *Hostility coping and health* (pp. 33–48). Washington, DC: American Psychological Association.

Spielberger, C. D., Jacobs, G., Russel, S., & Crane, R. (1983). Assessment of anger: The State–Trait Anger Scale. In J. N. Butcher & C. D. Spielberger (Eds.), *Advances in personality assessment* (Vol. 2, pp. 161–189). Hillsdale, NJ: Lawrence Erlbaum Associates.

Spielberger, C. D., Johnson, E. H., Russell, S. F., Crane, R. J., Jacobs, G. A., & Worden, R. J. (1985). The experience and expression of anger. In M. A. Chesney & R. H. Rosenman (Eds.), *Anger and hostility in behavioral medicine* (pp. 5–30). New York: Hemisphere.

Sprafka, J. M., Burke, G. L., Folsom, A. R., Luepker, R. V., & Blackburn, H. (1990). Continued decline in cardiovascular disease risk factors: Results of the Minnesota Heart Survey, 1980–82 and 1985–87. *American Journal of Epidemiology, 132,* 489–500.

Swenson, W. M., Pearson, J. S., & Osborne, D. (1973). *An MMPI Sourcebook: Basic item, scale and pattern data on 50,000 medical patients.* Minneapolis: University of Minnesota Press.

Williams, R. B. (1989). *The trusting heart.* New York: Times Books.

Wing, R. A., Matthews, K. A., Kuller, L. H., Meilahn, E. N., & Plantinga, P. (1991). Waist to hip ratio in middle-aged women. Associations with behavioral and psychosocial factors and with changes in cardiovascular risk factors. *Arteriosclerosis and Thrombosis, 11,* 1250–1257.

Wrightsman, L. S. (1974). *Assumptions about human nature: A social-psychological approach.* Monterey, CA: Brooks-Cole.

Zonderman, A. B., Siegler, I. C., Barefoot, J. C., Williams, R. B., & Costa, P. T., Jr. (1993). Age and gender differences in MMPI Content Scales. *Experimental Aging Research.*

11

ANGER AND HOSTILITY: POTENTIAL MEDIATORS OF THE GENDER DIFFERENCE IN CORONARY HEART DISEASE[1]

Catherine M. Stoney
Tilmer O. Engebretson
The Miriam Hospital, Brown University School of Medicine

The three main constructs that we address in this chapter are gender, anger and hostility variables, and coronary heart disease. The literature suggests that their interrelationships are complex, and might be conceptualized in a variety of ways. If we consider heart disease as the endpoint of interest, two ways of considering the interrelationship of all three constructs emerge. One, we can examine the mediating effect gender has on the hostility–disease relationship or, two, we can examine the mediating effect hostility has on the gender–disease relationship. We have elected to conceptually view the literature in the latter manner for two reasons. First, gender is a biological factor, which is more basic to our identities than the higher order psychological constructs of hostility. Second, the relationship of gender with heart disease is more clearly established than the relationship of hostility with heart disease. Research has clearly documented, for example, that males have about a two-fold greater risk of dying of coronary heart disease than do females, although the reasons for this are still largely unknown. The relationship of hostility with coronary heart disease, on the other hand, is still being examined.

The aims of this chapter are, therefore, several-fold. First, we review the epidemiologic data of gender differences in coronary heart disease, with the aim of presenting several postulated explanations for the differences. Second, we review the data on gender differences in anger and hostility. Here we propose guidelines by which the multidimensional aspects of anger and hostility might be framed and provide a theoretical model for examining relation-

---

[1]Supported in part by NIH Grant HL 48363.

ships between these aspects. Third, we briefly discuss the major hypotheses concerning the developmental basis for gender differences in anger and hostility. Fourth, we discuss the mechanisms by which anger and hostility might mediate the gender differences in coronary heart disease, including discussion of reactivity data. Fifth and finally, we conclude by providing some remarks regarding the implications of this literature for research.

EPIDEMIOLOGY OF GENDER DIFFERENCES IN CORONARY HEART DISEASE

In the United States, as well as in all other industrialized nations in the world, men experience twice the age-adjusted mortality and morbidity rates from coronary heart disease, relative to women. Cross-sectional studies that have analyzed coronary heart disease mortality rates of the major race–gender groups in the United States suggest that the gender ratio of age-adjusted mortality rates for Whites is about 2, whereas for Blacks, it is just under 2 (Sempos, Cooper, Kovar, & McMillen, 1988). Prevalence data such as these have been substantiated by at least four population-based prospective studies also conducted in the United States (Friedman, Dales, & Ury, 1979; Lerner & Kannel, 1986; Wingard, 1982; Wingard, Suarez, & Barrett-Connor, 1983). Although some discrepancies between the studies emerged, data from all four studies demonstrated that males die from coronary heart disease at a faster rate than do females, independent of gender differences in all known cardiovascular risk factors. In all studies, the age-adjusted gender ratio is about 2.0. The gender difference is largest among younger age groups and approaches 1 in older age groups. This is because of an increase in female mortality after 45 years of age, and a tapering of male coronary heart disease mortality after this age. In fact, data from the Framingham study suggests that there is approximately a 10-year difference in mortality rates between the sexes. Thus, the onset of coronary heart disease appears to be delayed in women, relative to men. It is important to understand that, despite the widely documented gender differences in rates of coronary heart disease, it is still the number one killer of both men and women in this country.

At least four major hypotheses have been proposed to explain the gender difference in heart disease mortality rates. It should be noted that no proposed explanation is mutually exclusive with any other. Further, none has been adequately tested, and it is unlikely that any one explanation will fully account for the large and consistent gender differences in coronary heart disease morbidity and mortality.

The first hypothesized explanation for the gender difference in coronary heart disease is that females may be more biologically fit than males (Madigan, 1957). This hypothesis initially emerged from demonstrations that males show both a generally larger fetal death rate and a greater mortality rate during the first year of life than do females, presumably because of some as-of-yet unidentified biological factors. However, it is not the case that women do not die of coronary heart disease; it is simply the case that the disease is delayed in women. Further, when adjusting for gender differences in biological variables that influence coronary heart disease (e.g., cholesterol, blood pressure, body weight), a gender ratio of about 2 remains (Wingard et al., 1983). Thus, the genetic explanation is probably not an adequate explanation for the gender difference in coronary heart disease.

The second hypothesis suggests that males may engage in more health-damaging behaviors and roles relative to women (Waldron, 1976; Wingard, 1984). To the extent that such behaviors impact on disease progression, the greater incidence of smoking behaviors, aggressive behaviors, and alcohol consumption by men relative to women, may help to explain the gender difference in coronary heart disease. In a similar vein, the gender difference in roles (marriage, parenthood, employment) may impact on disease rates. Two lines of evidence argue against this hypothesis. First, the age-adjusted gender ratio has been gradually increasing from below 1 at the turn of the 20th century, to nearly 2 currently. Most of the behaviors that have been implicated in contributing to heart disease (smoking, diet, sedentary lifestyle), however, have also increased among women during this time. Thus, the widening of the gender ratio in the latter portion of the 20th century probably cannot be attributable to widening of gender differences in health-damaging behaviors. Second, in the previously mentioned prospective studies examining gender differences in the incidence of coronary heart disease mortality, the gender difference remained after controlling for all known (and even some less traditional) risk factors. Thus, the gender difference in health-damaging behaviors cannot adequately explain the gender difference in coronary heart disease.

A third hypothesis suggests that reproductive hormones (particularly the estrogens) may confer a protective effect on women, relative to men (Bush & Barrett-Connor, 1985). Evidence for the effects of the estrogens on cardiovascular disease has come from both animal and human studies in which the presence of endogenous estrogens appears to be associated with a relatively lower incidence of coronary heart disease. In female animals and humans, the loss of those endogenous estrogens (during natural or surgical menopause) is associated with an increase in coronary heart disease. Although it was suggested that the protective effect of the estrogens is a function solely of their influence on lipid metabolism (Bush & Barrett-Connor, 1985), this explanation is not entirely adequate because the exogenous administration of estrogens to males (Coronary Drug Project Research Group, 1970) and some females (Mann et al., 1975) resulted in an increase, not a decrease in cardiovascular events and mortality.

A final hypothesis has been proposed to explain the gender difference in heart disease. Specifically, males may experience increased cardiovascular and physiological reactivity to stress, relative to females, and to the extent that such reactivity is relevant to the disease process, this may result in greater coronary heart disease in men. Related to this and the previous hypothesis, Wingard (1982) and Stoney, Davis, and Matthews (1987) postulated an interaction of biological and behavioral risk factors to explain the gender difference in coronary heart disease mortality. Specifically, reproductive hormones may interact with individual differences in psychological or personality variables to result in individuals at particularly high risk for the development and progression of coronary heart disease. Two psychological variables that have been strongly associated with heart disease are anger and hostility. There has, therefore, been increasing interest in examining both anger and hostility as mediating the gender difference in coronary heart disease.

GENDER DIFFERENCES IN ANGER AND HOSTILITY

A small series of studies published over the last 35 years strongly indicate that anger and hostility are clearly multidimensional constructs (Bendig, 1962; Buss & Durkey, 1957; Sarason, 1961; Zelin, Alder, & Myerson, 1972). This multidimensionality, however, is only recently receiving widespread recognition. The existence of three broad aspects of hostility and anger have been documented recently (Musante, MacDougall, Dembroski, & Costa, 1989). Experiential aspects of anger and hostility encompass the subjective and emotional components of anger processes, and they are episodic in nature. Attitudinal aspects of hostility encompass cognitions of resentment, suspiciousness, guilt, and mistrust, and have sometimes been grouped with experiential aspects of hostility. These aspects are more cognitive and enduring in nature than is experiential hostility. Finally, expressive aspects of hostility encompass the expressive and antagonistic outward behavioral manifestations of anger processes. Throughout this chapter, we make a somewhat artificial but important distinction between these three broad aspects of anger and hostility by referring to the emotional experience of anger and hostility as *experiential anger*; referring to the cognitive experience of anger and hostility as *attitudinal hostility*; and referring to the behavioral manifestations of anger and hostility as *expressive anger and hostility*. We further propose that within this latter category, two forms of expressive anger and hostility might be suggested. *Communicative expression* includes the nonthreatening expression of anger and hostility, whereas *aggressive expression* incorporates the expression of anger and hostility with the intent of inflicting harm (either physical or verbal). In this case, aggressive expression is most similar to the construct of hostile aggression, but not of instrumental aggression described by Bandura (1973) and Berkowitz (1978). Figure 11.1 provides a schematic illustration of how these broad aspects of anger and hostility might be experienced in response to an environmental stimulus. Note the manner in which each construct might interconnect. For example, attitudinal hostility might impact on both the experience and expression of anger and hostility, albeit to differing degrees. The distinction between attitudinal hostility, experiential anger, and expressive anger becomes particularly important when describing gender differences in anger and hostility, because it appears likely that the magnitude and possibly even the direction of gender differences in each of these parameters differs.

It is important to note that the particular mode of assessing anger and hostility can impact on the specific aspects of anger that are evaluated. Although a comprehensive evaluation of different assessment instruments is not possible in the scope of this chapter (for a more detailed discussion of these instruments, see Matthews, Jamison, & Cottington, 1985), we detail some of the more commonly used assessment instruments for each of the aforementioned aspects of anger and hostility.

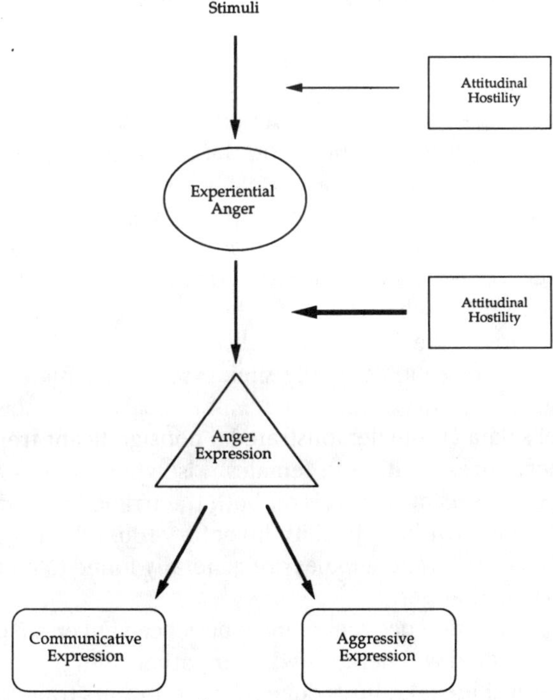

FIG. 11.1. Broad aspects of anger and hostility.

Experiential Anger.   It is not possible to directly determine an individual's level of experiential anger because it is subjective in nature. Therefore, researchers infer levels of experienced anger based on other indicators. The most commonly used indicator, and that which has the greatest face validity, is self-reports. Commonly used self-report trait measures, which appear to assess experiential anger, include Spielberger's Trait Anger scale (Spielberger, Jacobs, Russell, & Crane, 1983); Hostile Affect, a subscale derived from the Cook–Medley (Barefoot, Dodge, Peterson, Dahlstrom, & Williams, 1989); Irritability and Negativism subscales derived from the Buss–Durkee Hostility Inventory (Buss & Durkee, 1957); Neurotic Hostility, a factor score also derived from the Buss–Durkee Hostility Inventory (Siegman, Dembroski, & Kingel, 1987); and Anger Arousal, a factor score derived from the Multidimensional Anger Inventory (Siegel, 1986).

Although direct gender comparisons of all these scales are not yet available in the literature, there is a prevailing belief that women experience anger different from men; specifically, women are believed to be less able to recognize anger as such. However, studies that are available testing gender comparisons suggest that men and women generally experience similar levels of anger. For example, studies that employed Spielberger's Trait Anger scale generally reported that males and females experience similar amounts of trait anger (Engebretson & Matthews, 1992; Girdler, Turner, Sherwood, & Light, 1990; Matthews, Manuck, & Saab, 1986; Spielberger et al., 1983), although elsewhere males were reported to experience greater levels of trait anger, relative to females (Blumenthal, Barefoot, Burg, & Williams, 1987). Using the Hostile Affect subscale from the Cook–Medley scale, Barefoot and colleagues (1991) found, in a large national survey, that males and females endorsed similar amounts of trait anger across all ages from 18 to 90 years. However, slightly higher scores for males relative to females on the Hostile Affect subscale were reported by Scherwitz and colleagues (1991) in a sample of 18- to 30-year-olds. Use of the Anger Arousal subscale of the Multidimensional Anger Inventory resulted in generally similar scores for males and females (Siegel, 1986; Kneip, Delamater, Ismond, Milford, Salvia, & Schwartz, 1991), although Siegel's data (1986) demonstrated a nonsignificant trend for males to obtain higher scores relative to females. Elsewhere, males and females were found to endorse similar levels on both the Irritability and Negativism subscales of the Buss–Durkee Hostility Inventory (Buss & Durkee, 1957; Biaggio, 1980). Thus, males and females are generally found to endorse similar levels of experiential anger.

Another source of inference regarding experienced anger are other-ratings of observed behavior. Two methods whereby other-ratings are made of experienced anger include (a) ratings done by expert raters trained in an interview assessment method; and (b) ratings done by individuals familiar with the person in question, that is, spouses or teachers who have regular contact with the individuals. The expert-rater method reported here is the hostility rating derived from the Type A Structured Interview (SI). Although originally developed to assess the Type A Behavior Pattern, recent refinements have allowed for expert-ratings to be made of two anger aspects that fall in the domain of experiential anger: Hostile Content and Hostile Intensity (Dembroski & Costa, 1987). Only one study to date reports gender comparisons for these two constructs. This study (Engebretson & Matthews, 1992) found that during the SI, male and female adults reported similar amounts of experiential anger as determined by both Hostile Content and Hostile Intensity. It should be kept in mind, however, that these expert-ratings of experiential anger are largely derived from self-reports during the SI. We know of only one study in which ratings of an individual's experiential anger has been carried out by an individual familiar with that individual, and in which gender comparisons were presented (Kneip et al., 1991). In this study, hostility of the individuals in question was rated by their spouses through their completion of the Multidimensional Anger Inventory. These other-ratings indicated that males experience greater experiential anger than do females, based on gender differences on the Anger Arousal subscale.

In summary, based on a small collection of studies employing both self-report and other-rating methodologies, the literature generally indicates that males and females experience similar levels of experiential anger, a conclusion that is reinforced by the lack of reports indicating that females experience greater levels of experiential anger than do males. The few studies that do find gender differences suggest that the gender difference is in a consistent direction; that is, males encounter greater levels of experiential anger relative to females. Explanations for these somewhat discrepant findings will most likely come from examining differences in the characteristics of the subject sample. In particular, we propose that these variations in the literature may at least partly arise from the presence of gender differences in anger expression, rather than from gender differences in the experience of anger. This might come about because self-reports are a form of expression and, thus, self-reports of experiential anger are always dependent to some degree on anger expression. If there are gender differences in anger expression (discussed in a subsequent section), then there is the potential for those gender differences in anger expression to confound the self-reports of experiential anger. This should be kept in mind, therefore, when the amount of self-reported anger experience of males and females are compared.

Attitudinal Hostility. Attitudinal hostility is a cognitive experience, and, like experiential anger, must, therefore, be inferred from other indicators. As with experiential anger, the most commonly used indicator is self-reports. The most commonly used self-report measures of attitudinal hostility are five scales derived from the Cook–Medley Hostility Inventory, including Total

Hostility (Cook & Medley, 1954), the factor-derived scales of Cynical Mistrust and Paranoid Alienation (Costa, Zonderman, McCrae, & Williams, 1986), and the rationally derived subscales of Cynicism and Hostile Attribution (Barefoot et al., 1989). Other self-report measures that appear to assess attitudinal hostility include the Resentment and Suspicion scales of the Buss–Durkee Hostility Inventory (Buss & Durkee, 1957), and the Hostile Outlook subscale derived from the Multidimensional Anger Inventory (Siegel, 1986).

As with the experiential anger data, direct comparisons of males and females on levels of attitudinal hostility using these various measures are somewhat sparse. Gender comparisons that are available, however, suggest that males have greater levels of attitudinal hostility than females, although null findings are also reported. For example, when adult males and females are compared on total Cook–Medley Hostility Inventory scores, males receive higher scores than females (Barefoot et al., 1991; Blumenthal et al., 1987; Colligan & Offord, 1988; Engebretson & Matthews, 1992; Scherwitz et al., 1991; Weidner, Istvan, & McKnight, 1989). No published gender comparisons are yet available for the Cynical Mistrust and Paranoid Alienation factors derived by Costa and colleagues (1986). Two recent reports, however, provide gender comparisons for the rationally derived scales of Cynicism and Hostile Attribution (Barefoot et al., 1991; Scherwitz et al., 1991). One report suggested that males and females achieve similar levels on the Hostile Attribution subscale (Barefoot et al., 1991), whereas the other study indicated that relative to females, males produce higher scores on both Cynicism and Hostile Attribution (Scherwitz et al., 1991). Overall, the data suggested that males demonstrate greater attitudinal hostility than do females.

When gender comparisons on subscales from other self-report measures are examined, this conclusion is further supported. For example, among college undergraduates completing the Buss–Durkee Hostility Inventory, Resentment scores were found to be higher in males relative to females (Biaggio, 1980; Buss & Durkee, 1957). Suspicion scores, also from the Buss–Durkee Hostility Inventory, however, were found to be higher in males relative to females in one study (Buss & Durkee, 1957), but similar between males and females in another (Biaggio, 1980). Elsewhere, self-reports using the Hostile Outlook subscale from the Multidimensional Anger Inventory produced no gender differences in two different reports (Kneip et al., 1991; Siegel, 1986).

Finally, we know of only one report where attitudinal hostility was produced from an other-rating. In this study (Kneip et al., 191), spouses of patients completed the Multidimensional Anger Inventory, with regard to the patient. Results indicate that males were rated as having higher Hostile Outlook scores than females. This is particularly interesting in light of the finding reported in the previous paragraph that gender differences on this scale did not emerge when the same scale was completed as a self-report. Whether the absence or presence of gender differences as a function of self- versus other-report, respectively, is due to problems with self-reports, differences in the gender of the raters (all male patients were rated by their female spouses and all female patients were rated by their male spouses), or some unknown factor is currently not known.

In summary, the literature fairly strongly indicates that males have higher levels of attitudinal hostility relative to females. This is strongly supported by findings based on the Cook–Medley Hostility Inventory and generally supported by other measures that also appear to measure attitudinal hostility.

Expressive Anger and Hostility. Our current understanding of gender differences in the manner in which individuals express anger is largely based on self-reports to such measures as the Anger-In and Anger-Out subscales from the Anger Expression scale (Spielberger, Johnson, Russell, Crane, Jacobs, & Worden, 1985); Harburg's Anger Expression scales (Harburg, Erfurt, Hauenstein, Chape, Schull, & Schork, 1973); the subscales of Physical Assault, Indirect Hostility, Verbal Hostility (Buss & Durkee, 1957) and Expressive Hostility (Siegman et al., 1987), derived from the Buss–Durkee Hostility Inventory; the anger expression scale used in the Framingham study (Haynes, Levine, Scotch, Feinleib, & Kannel, 1978); the Anger-In and Anger-Out subscales from the Multidimensional Anger Inventory (Siegel, 1985); the Anger Expression Style score derived from Spielberger's Anger Expression scale (Engebretson, Matthews, & Scheier, 1989); and the Aggressive Responding subscale from the Cook–Medley Hostility scale (Barefoot et al., 1989).

It is usually tacitly assumed that women are more likely than men to suppress their anger, and this assumption has some empirical support. In the Framingham Heart Study, for example, middle-aged women who worked were more likely to inhibit anger expression than middle-aged men who worked (Haynes & Feinleib, 1980). Other studies, however, failed to find gender differences in anger expression. For example, in a community-based study of middle-aged men and women, there were no gender differences in Anger-In or Anger-Out (Engebretson & Matthews, 1992). Similarly, differences were not apparent in a study examining male and female responses to Spielberger's Anger Expression scale, although gender role identity impacted on anger expression (Kooper & Epperson, 1991). In this study, masculine gender role types were more likely than others to express their anger. Finally, a study of over 500 adults demonstrated no gender differences in self-reports of anger expression (Balswick & Avertt, 1977).

The bulk of the data suggest, however, that males are more likely than females to suppress emotions, including anger (cf. Ryckman, Stone, & Elam, 1971). For example, normative data on the Anger Expression scale suggested that whereas male and female adults report similar levels of Anger-Out responses, males report higher levels of Anger-In responses (Matthews et al., 1988; Spielberger et al., 1985). In a similar fashion, normative data for the

Multidimensional Anger Inventory showed that males and females endorse similar levels of Anger-Out characteristics, but that males endorse higher levels of Anger-In responses than do females (Siegel, 1985). When unidimensional scales of emotional expressiveness are used, females are more expressive of emotion in general than are males (Kennedy-Moore & Stone, 1990; King & Emmons, 1990).

The findings of greater emotional expression among females are further reinforced by results from the Emotional Survey, which Allen and Hoccoun (1976) administered to male and female undergraduates. These data showed that females were more expressive of every emotion, including anger, than were males. In a slight variation, a survey of 263 male and 260 female undergraduate students indicated that females were more expressive of feelings of happiness, love, and sadness, but that males and females were equally expressive of anger (Balswick & Avertt, 1977). In a survey of 412 university employees, Weidner and colleagues (Weidner, Istvan, & McKnight, 1989) found that females endorsed lower amounts of Anger-In behaviors and more Anger-Discuss behaviors than did males. Elsewhere, results of a survey administered to a combined community and undergraduate sample (Averill, 1982) indicated that females reported wanting to talk over an angering situation with the involved individual more so than males (i.e., Anger-Discuss). Finally, in a survey of 744 adults, females reported significantly more reflective responses (i.e., problem solving) to a hypothetical scenario with an angry boss than did males (Harburg, Blakelock, & Roeper, 1979).

In a study exploring how mode of anger expression is mediated by measures of assertion and social desirability, Delamater and McNamara (1987) found that unassertive women were more likely to have elevated Anger-In scores (based on the Spielberger scale) and depressed Anger-Out scores, and that both anger expression and assertion appeared to be susceptible to social desirability responding. Similarly, an early investigation examining the relationship between assertiveness and Buss–Durkee Hostility found that females scoring high on assertion were more likely to directly express their hostility (assertiveness was positively correlated with verbal hostility, negatively correlated with resentment and suspiciousness), whereas males scoring low on assertion were less likely to directly express anger. However, a similar study found no association between anger, hostility, and assertion (Wyrick, Gentry, & Shows, 1977). Elsewhere, in a study of college-aged men and women, males self-reported more physical aggression, verbal aggression, and assault (based on subscores of the Buss–Durkee) relative to females (Doyle & Biaggio, 1981), suggesting that self-reports of aggression may, in fact, be distinct from experiential anger.

When gender differences in anger expression were investigated under conditions of harassment or anger induction, a similar pattern of findings emerged. When criticized for their performance on a simple skill task, females expressed more irritation and embarrassment than did males (Ryckman et al., 1971). Females, relative to males, were found to be more verbally hostile when insulted, but less verbally hostile when complimented (Atkinson & Polivy, 1976; Simpkins, 1961). Under conditions of intense harassment, however (i.e., trying to work cooperatively with a condescending, verbally insulting, same-gender confederate), males and females expressed similar levels of experienced anger (Engebretson & Matthews, 1991). Thus, based on this literature, it appears that under most conditions males tend to inhibit the expression of anger relative to females, and females tend to express anger outwardly relative to males.

Most of the aforementioned examples represent studies of communicative expression, but a separate body of research examined gender differences in aggressive expression. Frodi, Macaulay, and Thome (1977) suggested that self-reports of aggressive responses to hypothetical situations often do produce gender differences, despite the fact that gender differences do not consistently emerge in actual aggressive behaviors. Their conclusions supported the data by Sarason (1961) and Biaggio (1980), who found that males score higher on subscales of the Buss–Durkee Hostility Inventory that indicate a tendency for aggressive expression (i.e., verbal hostility and assault), whereas females tend to score higher on subscales that indicate a tendency to inhibit anger expression (i.e., guilt). Barefoot and colleagues (Barefoot et al., 1991) found that, across all ages examined, males score higher on the Aggressive Responding subscale of the Cook–Medley, relative to females. We believe that, taken together, these findings indicate that males are more likely to express their anger as aggression, whereas females are more likely to express their anger in other ways.

A more recent review of the literature examining gender differences in aggression suggests, using a meta-analytic approach, that males are more likely than females to engage in aggressive expression behaviors, but the magnitude of the gender difference is associated with the specific characteristics of aggression studied (Eagly & Steffen, 1986). For example, the gender difference was most pronounced when examining aggression that produces physical harm and least pronounced for aggression causing psychological harm. Because Frodi and colleagues (Frodi et al., 1977) asserted that gender differences in self-report data may reflect gender stereotyping rather than actual gender differences in aggressive behaviors, these researchers based their conclusions on studies that did not employ self-report measures of aggression, and, thus, the data are less likely to be subject to self-report biases. Taken together, these data suggest that, in general, females appear to express their anger in a communicative fashion to a greater degree than males, but are less likely to express their anger in an aggressive fashion, relative to males.

In summary, these literatures suggest that there are gender differences in both anger expression and aggression, but that the direction of the gender differences are different for the two behavioral constructs; that is, the expression literature suggests that males inhibit and females express feelings of anger, whereas the aggression literature suggests that males are more physically, and, possibly, more verbally aggressive than are females. It is important to note that the magnitude and even direction of the gender difference may be influenced by the age of the cohorts studied, because the difference appears to be less robust in middle-aged or older populations, relative to young adult populations. These differential gender differences highlight, therefore, the potential value of distinguishing between communicative expressions of anger and aggressive expressions of anger.

BASIS FOR THE GENDER DIFFERENCE IN ANGER AND HOSTILITY

Several competing hypotheses have been proposed to explain the theoretical bases for the development of aggressive behaviors, but which are also clearly applicable to explaining the development of experiential anger and attitudinal hostility. The majority of the literature in this area has focused on examining the development of aggressive behaviors, rather than on the development of anger and hostility per se, because of the historical emphasis in the literature on studying observable behaviors as opposed to subjects or cognitive aspects. That this is changing may be seen in the work of researchers like Patterson (1985), where the study of subjective constructs is being integrated with that of aggressive behaviors. To the extent that aggressive behaviors are motivated by anger and hostility, the term *aggressive expression* is appropriate. Our aim in this chapter is not to provide an exhaustive review of each proposed explanation, but rather to briefly mention each of the major hypotheses, with special emphasis on theories that are particularly relevant to gender comparisons of experiential anger and attitudinal hostility.

It is clear that biological and genetic factors play an important role in shaping aggressive expression behaviors, and these factors might be immediately thought of as being most relevant to a discussion of gender differences in anger and hostility. However, it is also the case that situational and environmental influences impact on the development of patterns of anger and hostility, and may do so in gender-specific ways. The major hypotheses concerned with the development, maintenance, and control of anger and hostile behaviors include biological theories, social learning theory, social–cognitive theory, and drive theory. Theories most likely to be cited as relevant to the study of gender differences in anger and hostility are the biological theories, social learning theory, and social–cognitive theory.

The biologically based models of aggressive expression incorporate several physiological factors potentially related to the development of hostile and aggressive expression behaviors, including genetic markers or determinants of aggression, hormonal and other biochemical factors related to aggression, and central nervous system influences on aggression. Critical developmental periods can be identified that impact on some of these biological markers of aggressive expression. In addition, physical appearance, strength, or body muscle mass are other biological factors that may influence aggressive expression behaviors. The impact of biological influences such as these on the development of gender differences in anger and hostility are clear, because most of these biological determinants also differ according to gender.

The social learning theory of aggressive expression focused on environmental or external cues, cognitive factors, and self-regulatory influences (Bandura, 1973). Although the role of biological factors are acknowledged in social learning theory, humans are presumed to be less constrained by biologic factors than are nonhumans. Because environmental and external cues are frequently different among males and females, social learning theory might be particularly relevant with regard to gender differences in anger and hostility.

The social–cognitive model of aggressive expression developed as an aggregate of several models of social interaction, and it integrates concepts of self-regulatory processes, cognitive theories, theories of problem solving, and social learning theories (Dodge & Frame, 1982). This theory is, in many ways, ideal for examining gender differences in the development of anger and hostility, because it takes into account social expectations regarding gender roles, internal processes mediated by environmental and internal (biologic) cues, and learning theories.

Although not specifically relevant to discussions of gender differences in the development of anger and hostility, drive theory is another important model for the development of these constructs. Drive theory postulates that anger and aggressive expression are a function of internal drives stimulated by external cues. Most proponents of drive theory postulate that external stimuli that are frustrating in nature often lead to aggressive expression behaviors. More recently, a reformulation of this hypothesis has been somewhat modified by Berkowitz (1974), who suggested that the presence of aggressive cues, along with frustration, is necessary for aggressive expression to be manifest (but not necessarily experienced).

MECHANISMS

A relationship between measures of anger and hostility and the development of coronary heart disease has been suggested by several lines of evidence. For example, a number of investigations documented that anger and anger expression are associated with angiographically documented coronary heart disease (Dembroski, MacDougall, Williams, Haney, & Blumenthal, 1985;

Siegman et al., 1987) and hypertension (Esler et al., 1977; Kahn, Medalie, Neufeld, Riss, & Goldbourt, 1972), albeit somewhat inconsistently. A few important studies, although not directly comparing men and women, suggested that the relationship between anger and hostility and disease may be different for men and women. For example, in the Framingham Study (Haynes & Feinleib, 1980), suppression of anger was more commonly found in women with coronary heart disease than in healthy women. In contrast, suppression of anger in men was associated with both higher (Dembroski et al., 1985; MacDougall, Dembroski, Dimsdale, & Hackett, 1985) and lower (Siegman et al., 1987) incidence of coronary atherosclerosis. Thus, there may be gender differences in the role that anger plays in disease progression. Nonetheless, the specific mechanisms by which anger and hostility are linked to coronary heart disease are not yet firmly established.

One mechanism by which hostility and anger may impact on the progression and development of coronary heart disease has been suggested in the health psychology literature. Specifically, individuals scoring high on some measure of hostility may exhibit exaggerated cardiovascular and neuroendocrine reactivity in response to behavioral stressors, relative to individuals low in anger and hostility (Williams, Barefoot, & Shekelle, 1985). For example, Smith and Allred (1989) showed that during a current events debate task, men higher in attitudinal hostility (total Cook–Medley Hostility scores) displayed greater systolic and diastolic blood pressure responses, relative to men lower in attitudinal hostility. In a similar manner, Engebretson et al. (1989) demonstrated that anger expression, operationalized as a unipolar "style" score derived from the difference between scores on the Anger-Out and Anger-In subscales, was related to cardiovascular reactivity. Results show that Anger-Out style individuals displayed elevated systolic blood pressure and heart rate responses during harassment relative to Anger-In style individuals. In both studies, the situational condition was important. The reactivity hypothesis is among the most widely cited mechanisms underlying the association between anger and coronary heart disease (e.g., Houston, Smith, & Cates, 1989). To the extent that exaggerated physiological adjustments to stress are associated with the progression of heart disease, the further examination of gender differences in stress responses is warranted.

Males have generally been used almost exclusively in studies of the health consequences of anger and hostility. However, a small but growing body of literature documents the existence of gender differences in cardiovascular and neuroendocrine responses to laboratory-based stressors. A meta-analytic review was conducted recently to examine the early (prior to 1986) literature specifically examining gender differences in stress responses (Stoney et al., 1987). This meta-analysis included sufficient numbers of studies to test gender differences in heart rate, systolic and diastolic blood pressure, and urinary epinephrine and norepinephrine. After correction for baseline differences, results indicated that males, overall, displayed larger systolic blood pressure and urinary epinephrine responses to stress than did females, whereas females displayed a trend toward larger heart rate responses to stress, relative to males.

Several quite recent studies have further documented the complex nature of the gender differences in physiological stress responses. For example, we have reported significant gender differences in blood pressure (Matthews & Stoney, 1988; Stoney & Matthews, 1988; Stoney, Matthews, McDonald, & Johnson, 1988), plasma norepinephrine and LDL-cholesterol responses to stress (Stoney et al., 1988), with males demonstrating the largest elevations in each of these parameters, relative to females. Also important, we demonstrated in children that gender differences in cardiovascular reactivity are apparent after the age of puberty, but not before (Matthews & Stoney, 1988), suggesting that the gender differences may be, in part, a function of the influence of reproductive hormones.

More recently, Girdler and colleagues (1990) examined the nature of the gender difference in cardiovascular stress responses by examining gender differences in estimates of cardiac output, total peripheral resistance, and blood pressure using transthoracic cardiac impedance techniques. They reported that males showed elevations in total peripheral resistance responses to stress, relative to females, whereas females demonstrated elevations in cardiac output to stress. They concluded that males were primarily vascular reactors and females were primarily myocardial reactors. Despite the fact that this study did not report significant gender differences in blood pressure responses, these findings are relatively consistent with previous findings suggesting enhanced pressor responses in males and enhanced heart rate responses in females.

With few exceptions, the stressful tasks used in studies of gender differences are achievement-oriented. Although achievement tasks undoubtedly represent a significant portion of daily activities, individuals also spend significant amounts of time engaging in other types of challenges. A notable example most relevant for this particular discussion is interpersonal social interaction, especially that which may induce anger and hostility. Examination of the cardiovascular reactivity patterns of males and females during interpersonal social interactions also clearly warrants attention.

Only a small handful of studies exist that have examined gender differences in cardiovascular reactivity during and following interpersonal interactions. Most of this work was done by Hokanson and colleagues and was derived from their efforts to evaluate whether or not the expression of aggression per se results in decreases in physiological arousal (Hokanson & Edelman, 1966; Hokanson, Willers, & Koropsak, 1968). In the first of these studies, Hokanson and Edelman (1966) demonstrated that males who counteraggressed (i.e., delivered a shock) in a response choice interaction with a punitive confederate showed significantly faster systolic blood pressure recovery from harassment-induced levels than males who did not have an opportunity to respond, chose not to respond, or responded in a friendly manner (i.e., delivery of a reward point). Females, however, did not show differential systolic blood pressure recovery as a function of response choice. Responses of females were faster, however, than when females made no response at all (i.e., sat still). Also, males who responded with counteraggression had earlier recoveries than any mode of response carried out by the females.

In a subsequent study, males were again shown to produce faster physiological recovery, although this time in peripheral vasoconstriction, when responding to harassment with aggressive expression responses, relative to responding with friendly responses (Hokanson et al., 1968). In the same study, however, a reverse finding was reported for females such that females produced faster recoveries in peripheral vasoconstriction when responding to harassment with friendly responses, relative to responding with aggressive responses. In this study, Hokanson and colleagues further demonstrated that among both males and females, rapid vascular recoveries from harassment-induced levels could be conditioned to occur with a new behavioral response. This was done by having males' friendly responses and females' aggressive responses followed, 90% of the time over a total of 60 conditioning trials, by a friendly response from the confederate. This conditioning procedure resulted in males then showing faster vascular recoveries with friendly responses and females showing faster vascular recovery with aggressive expression responses. The importance of learning in these processes was, therefore, clearly documented.

The research by Hokanson and colleagues was the first to demonstrate gender differences in cardiovascular reactivity during interpersonal interactions, albeit highly structured ones. The nature of the interaction was one of conflict, and the manner in which the frustrated individual responded to that conflict emerged as an important moderator of the concomitant pattern of cardiovascular reactivity. This experimental situation is a close analogue of an angering interpersonal interaction and the individual's manner of dealing (i.e., aggressing, expressing anger, or no response) with their own experienced anger. These studies, however, failed to focus on patterns of physiological responses during the angering situation itself, and rather focused on cardiovascular responses following the interpersonal conflict.

More recently, gender differences in cardiovascular reactivity during social interaction were tested by Van Egeren (1979). Although not clearly conflictual in nature, the heart rate responses of males and females were compared during a mixed-motive game (cooperative vs. competitive) played with a confederate. During this social interaction, males and females exhibited different heart rate changes as a function of whether the interaction was competitive or cooperative. Females displayed greater heart rate change during the competitive interaction relative to the cooperative interaction, whereas males displayed greater heart rate change during the cooperative interaction relative to the competitive interaction. Unfortunately, the interpretation of these gender differences is confounded by the use of a male confederate in the interactions with both male and female participants.

In our own work, gender differences in cardiovascular reactivity were examined during an interaction with a condescending, verbally insulting, same-sex confederate. Under these conditions of high harassment, females exhibited greater heart rate and diastolic blood pressure responses but similar systolic blood pressure responses, relative to men. Additional data indicate that this type of harassing interaction is experienced more frequently by males than females. This suggests that the unexpected findings of a lack of gender difference in systolic blood pressure, in conjunction with the greater diastolic blood pressure reactivity among females, may be partly arising from a novelty effect (Engebretson & Matthews, 1991).

Taken as a whole, these data are provocative findings and suggest that gender differences do exist in cardiovascular responses to interpersonal and/ or angering situations. Clarification of these findings and further examination of the relationships between gender, different aspects of anger and hostility, and cardiovascular reactivity will help elucidate the mechanisms by which anger and hostility are associated with cardiovascular disease, and whether these behavioral parameters mediate the anger/aggression/disease relationship.

It is also possible that anger and hostility variables mediate stress-associated physiological responses differently in men and women. A direct test of this possibility was recently made in a large group of young adults (Weidner, Friend, Ficarrotto, & Mendell, 1989). Participants scoring high and low in hostility, based on scores from the Cook–Medley Ho scale, were asked to perform unsolvable anagrams that were described as being "easy to solve." Systolic blood pressure, diastolic blood pressure, and heart rate were measured every minute during the 3-minute task. A multiple regression analysis demonstrated that, although males had significantly higher stress-related systolic blood pressure than did females, and females had higher stress-associated heart rate than did males, gender did not influence the relationship between hostility scores and reactivity. Subjects with high Ho scores demonstrated higher systolic blood pressure and diastolic blood pressure during stress, relative to subjects with low Ho scores, although self-reports of anger during the task did not significantly correlate with reactivity. Using a different approach to this question, Lundberg, Hedman, Melin, & Frankenhaeuser (1989) found that potential for hostility (from the Structured Interview) was positively correlated with heart rate reactivity in men, but not women. Among extreme Type A and Type B individuals, high hostile men had greater changes in systolic blood pressure, heart rate, and cortisol during stress than did low hostile men, whereas hostility did not differentiate the women in their sample.

Anger and Blood Pressure at Rest. Anger and hostility may be associated with resting blood pressure levels, and this relationship may be different for men and women. A variety of studies have identified a relationship between blood pressure and anger and hostility. For example, elevations in blood pressure were noted among individuals who suppress the expression of anger (Harburg et al., 1973; Sullivan et al., 1981). Fewer studies have specifically tested whether or not such effects are the same in males and females. In contrast to the data for adults, blood pressure correlated positively with expressed hostility and negatively with experienced hostility in children (Treiber et al., 1989).

In a study designed to examine the relationship between expressed anger, using the Survey of Affective States and blood pressure, gender differences emerged (Goldstein, Edelberg, Meier, & Davis, 1988). Specifically, females scoring high on Suppressed Anger had larger systolic and diastolic blood pressure, whereas the association for males was only significant for diastolic blood pressure. However, other data was contradictory. In a large community study, a positive and significant relationship between systolic blood pressure and suppressed anger (measured by a modified version of the Harburg scale) was found only in men and not in women (Dimsdale, Pierce, Schoenfeld, Brown, Zusman, & Graham, 1986).

Other Mediating Factors. It is likely that other factors mediate the effects of anger and hostility on reactivity patterns and, ultimately, disease. Until recently, constitutional factors such as age and race and demographic factors such as socioeconomic status and education have not been examined systematically, although Cook–Medley hostility scores have been shown to vary with age (Colligan & Offord, 1988). Other related factors, such as lifestyle and behavioral variables, are also not well-explored, but may mediate the anger/hostility and disease relationship differently in men and women. Interesting and valuable results from the CARDIA study (Scherwitz et al., 1991) were reported recently. In this study, the relationships between participant age, gender, educational level, and a variety of psychosocial variables with Cook–Medley hostility scores were examined in healthy men and women. Age, race, gender, and education were all related to Cook–Medley scores in a pattern that followed the association of these variables with coronary heart disease. Thus, the biobehavioral mechanisms linking anger and hostility with the development and progression of coronary heart disease is only beginning to be understood.

CONCLUSIONS AND IMPLICATIONS FOR RESEARCH

The substantial gender difference in coronary heart disease, which remains largely unexplained, has prompted efforts to identify factors that may underlie the difference. We have discussed how the notion that gender differences in anger and hostility variables may contribute to this gender difference in disease via cardiovascular reactivity. Several broad points are suggested by the literature. First, there are very few studies in which direct gender comparisons are systematically made. Second, examination of gender differences in anger and hostility requires a recognition of the multidimensionality of anger and hostility, that is, experiential anger, attitudinal hostility, and anger expression (see Fig. 11.1). We believe that, within the latter category, distinguishing between communicative expression and aggressive expression may be critical when examining gender differences in anger expression. Future research may well suggest further refinements in these different aspects of anger and hostility.

Third, gender comparisons within each of these different aspects of anger and hostility produce different findings. Males and females appear to experience similar levels of anger. Males, however, appear to experience greater levels of attitudinal hostility relative to females. Regarding anger expression, it appears that females display more communicative expression, relative to males, but males display more aggressive expression relative to females. Finally, the basis for these gender differences rests on both biological and social learning factors.

These gender differences in hostility and anger expression are consistent with the gender difference in coronary heart disease if: (a) having high attitudinal hostility increases one's risk of coronary heart disease; (b) expressive anger in a communicative fashion reduces one's risk; or (c) if expressing anger in an aggressive fashion increases one's risk. The first and third points appear to be supported by the current literature, whereas the second point still requires adequate testing. If cardiovascular reactivity is the mechanism linking these behaviors with coronary heart disease, then these gender differences in hostility and anger expression should also be consistent with higher or lower reactivity in accord with their association with heart disease. To date, there are insufficient numbers of studies directly testing gender differences in these areas making conclusions premature. Overall, however, the literature suggests that gender differences in certain types of anger and hostility constructs are at least consistent with gender differences in coronary heart disease.

REFERENCES

Allen, J. G., & Hoccoun, D. M. (1976). Sex differences in emotionality: A multidimensional approach. *Human Relations, 29*, 711–722.

Atkinson, C., & Polivy, J. (1976). Effects of delay, attack, and retaliation on state depression and hostility. *Journal of Abnormal Psychology, 85*, 570–576.

Averill, J. R. (1982). *Anger and aggression: An essay on emotion.* New York: Springer-Verlag.

Balswick, J., & Avertt, C. P. (1977). Differences in expressiveness: Gender, interpersonal orientation, and perceived parental expressiveness as contributing factors. *Journal of Marriage and Family, 39*, 121–127.

Bandura, A. (1973). *Aggression: A social learning theory.* Englewood Cliffs, NJ: Prentice-Hall.

Barefoot, J. C., Dodge, K. A., Peterson, B. L., Dahlstrom, W. G., & Williams, R. B., Jr. (1989). The Cook–Medley Hostility scale: Item content and ability to predict survival. *Psychosomatic Medicine, 51,* 46–57.

Barefoot, J. C., Peterson, B. L., Dahlstrom, W. G., Siegler, I. C., Anderson, N. B., & Williams, R. B., Jr. (1991). Hostility patterns and health implications: Correlates of Cook–Medley Hostility scale scores in a national survey. *Health Psychology, 10,* 18–24.

Bendig, A. W. (1962). Factor analytic scales of covert and overt hostility. *Journal of Consulting Psychology, 26,* 200.

Berkowitz, L. (1974). Some determinants of impulsive aggression: The role of mediated associations with reinforcements for aggression. *Psychology Review, 81,* 165–176.

Berkowitz, L. (1978). Is criminal violence normative behavior? Hostile and instrumental aggression and violent incidents. *Journal of Research in Crime and Delinquency, 15,* 148–181.

Biaggio, M. K. (1980). Assessment of anger arousal. *Journal of Personality Assessment, 44,* 289–298.

Blumenthal, J. A., Barefoot, J., Burg, M. M., & Williams, R. B., Jr. (1987). Psychological correlates of hostility among patients undergoing coronary angiography. *British Journal of Medical Psychology, 60,* 349–355.

Bush, T. L., & Barrett-Connor, E. (1985). Noncontraceptive estrogen use and cardiovascular disease. *Epidemiologic Reviews, 7,* 80–104.

Buss, A. H., & Durkey, A. (1957). An inventory for assessing different kinds of hostility. *Journal of Consulting Psychology, 21,* 343–349.

Colligan, R. C., & Offord, K. P. (1988). The risky use of the MMPI Hostility scale in assessing risk for coronary heart disease. *Psychosomatics, 29,* 188–196.

Cook, W. W., & Medley, D. M. (1954). Proposed hostility and pharisaic-virtue scales for the MMPI. *Journal of Applied Psychology, 38,* 414–418.

Coronary Drug Project Research Group. (1970). The Coronary Drug Project: Initial findings leading to modifications of its research protocol. *Journal of the American Medical Association, 214,* 1303–1313.

Costa, P. T., Jr., Zonderman, A. B., McCrae, R. R., & Williams, R. B., Jr. (1986). Cynicism and paranoid alienation in the Cook and Medley Ho scale. *Psychosomatic Medicine, 48,* 283–285.

Delamater, R. J., & McNamara, J. R. (1987). Expression of anger: Its relationship to assertion and social desirability among college women. *Psychological Reports, 61,* 131–134.

Dembroski, T. M., & Costa, P. T., Jr. (1987). Coronary-prone behavior: Components of the Type A pattern and hostility. *Journal of Personality, 55,* 211–235.

Dembroski, T. M., MacDougall, J. M., Williams, R. B., Haney, T. L., & Blumenthal, J. A. (1985). Components of Type A behavior, hostility and anger-in: Relationship to angiographic findings. *Psychosomatic Medicine, 47,* 219–233.

Dimsdale, J. E., Pierce, C., Schoenfeld, D., Brown, A., Zusman, R., & Graham, R. (1986). Suppressed anger and blood pressure: The effects of race, sex, social class, obesity, and age. *Psychosomatic Medicine, 48,* 430–436.

Dodge, K. A., & Frame, C. L. (1982). Social cognitive biases and deficits in aggressive boys. *Child Development, 53,* 620–635.

Doyle, M. A., & Biaggio, M. K. (1981). Expression of anger as a function of assertiveness and sex. *Journal of Clinical Psychology, 37,* 154–157.

Eagly, A. H., & Steffen, V. J. (1986). Gender and aggressive behavior: A meta-analytic review of the social psychological literature. *Psychological Bulletin, 100,* 309–330.

Engebretson, T. O., Matthews, K. A., & Scheier, M. F. (1989). Relationships between anger expression and cardiovascular reactivity: Reconciling inconsistent findings through a matching hypothesis. *Journal of Personal and Social Psychology, 57,* 513–521.

Engebretson, T. O., & Matthews, K. A. (1991). *Sex differences in cardiovascular, affective, and behavioral responses to interpersonal harassment.* Paper presented at the 12th annual meeting of the Society of Behavioral Medicine, Washington, DC.

Engebretson, T. O., & Matthews, K. A. (1992). Dimensions of hostility in men, women, and boys: Relationships to personality and cardiovascular responses to stress. *Psychosomatic Medicine, 54*, 311–323.

Esler, M., Julius, S., Zweiffer, A., Randall, O., Harburg, E., Gardiner, H., & DeQuattro, V. (1977). Mild high-renin essential hypertension: Neurogenic human hypertension? *New England Journal of Medicine, 296*, 405–411.

Friedman, G. D., Dales, L. G., & Ury, H. K. (1979). Mortality in middle-aged smokers and non-smokers. *New England Journal of Medicine, 300*, 213–217.

Frodi, A., Macaulay, J., & Thome, P. R. (1977). Are women always less aggressive than men? A review of the experimental literature. *Psychological Bulletin, 84*(4), 634–660.

Girdler, S. S., Turner, J. R., Sherwood, A., & Light, K. C. (1990). Gender differences in blood pressure control during a variety of behavioral stressors. *Psychosomatic Medicine, 52*, 571–591.

Goldstein, H. S., Edelberg, R., Meier, C. F., & Davis, L. (1988). Relationship of resting blood pressure and heart rate to experienced anger and expressed anger. *Psychosomatic Medicine, 50*, 321–329.

Harburg, E., Blakelock, E. H., & Roeper, P. J. (1979). Resentful and reflective coping with arbitrary authority and blood pressure: Detroit. *Psychosomatic Medicine, 41*, 189–202.

Harburg, E., Erfurt, J. C., Hauenstein, L. S., Chape, C., Schull, W. J., & Schork, M. A. (1973). Socio-ecological stress, suppressed hostility, skin color, and Black–White male blood pressure: Detroit. *Psychosomatic Medicine, 35*, 276–296.

Haynes, S. G., & Feinleib, M. (1980). Women, work and coronary heart disease: Prospective findings from the Framingham Heart Study. *American Journal of Public Health, 70*, 133–141.

Haynes, S. G., Levine, S., Scotch, N., Feinleib, M., & Kannel, W. B. (1978). The relationship of psychosocial factors to coronary heart disease in the Framingham study. *American Journal of Epidemiology, 107*, 362–383.

Hokanson, J. E., & Edelman, R. (1966). Effects of three social responses on vascular processes. *Journal of Personality and Social Psychology, 3*, 442–447.

Hokanson, J. E., Willers, K. R., & Koropsak, E. (1968). The modification of autonomic responses during aggressive interchanges. *Journal of Personality, 36*, 386–404.

Houston, B. K., Smith, M. A., & Cates, D. S. (1989). Hostility patterns and cardiovascular reactivity to stress. *Psychophysiology, 26*, 337–342.

Kahn, H. A., Medalie, J. H., Neufeld, H. N., Riss, E., & Goldbourt, U. (1972). The incidence of hypertension and associated factors: The Israeli ischemic heart disease study. *American Heart Journal, 84*, 171–182.

Kennedy-Moore, E. & Stone, A. A. (1990). *Emotions, gender, and health.* Poster presented at the 11th annual meeting of the Society of Behavioral Medicine, Chicago, IL.

King, L. A., & Emmons, R. A. (1990). Conflict over emotional expression: Psychological and physical correlates. *Journal of Personality and Social Psychology, 58*, 864–877.

Kneip, R., Delamater, A. M., Ismond, T., Milford, C., Salvia, L., & Schwartz, D. (1991). *Self and spouse ratings of anger as predictors of CHD.* Society for Behavioral Medicine. Paper presented at the 12th annual meeting of the Society for Behavioral Medicine, Washington, DC.

Kooper, B. A., & Epperson, D. L. (1991). Women and anger: Sex and sex-role comparisons in the expression of anger. *Psychology of Women Quarterly, 15*, 7–14.

Lerner, D. J., & Kannel, W. B. (1986). Patterns of coronary heart disease morbidity and mortality in the sexes: A 26-year follow-up of the Framingham population. *American Heart Journal, 111*, 383–390.

Lundberg, U., Hedman, M., Melin, B., & Frankenhaeuser, M. (1989). Type-A behavior in healthy males and females as related to physiological reactivity and blood lipids. *Psychosomatic Medicine, 51*, 113–122.

MacDougall, J. M., Dembroski, T. M., Dimsdale, J. E., & Hackett, T. P. (1985). Components of Type A, hostility, and anger-in: Further relationships to angiographic findings. *Health Psychology, 4*, 137–152.

Madigan, F. C. (1957). Are sex differentials biologically caused? *Milbank Memorial Fund Quarterly, 35*, 202–223.

Mann, J. I., Vessey, M. P., Thorogood, M., & Doll, R. (1975). Myocardial infarction in young women with special reference to oral contraceptive practice. *British Medical Journal, 2*, 241–249.

Matthews, K. A., Jamison, W., & Cottington, E. M. (1985). Assessment of Type A, anger, and hostility: A review of measures through 1982. In A. M. Ostfeld & E. D. Eaker (Eds.), *Measuring psychosocial variables in epidemiological studies of cardiovascular disease.* (NIH publication No. 85-2270). Bethesda, MD: National Institutes of Health.

Matthews, K. A., Manuck, S. B., & Saab, P. G. (1986). Cardiovascular responses of adolescents during a naturally occurring stressor and their behavioral and psychophysiological predictors. *Psychophysiology, 23*, 198–209.

Matthews, K. A., Manuck, S. B., Stoney, C. M., Rakaczky, C. J., McCann, B. S., Saab, P. G., Woodall, K. L., Block, D. R., Visintainer, P., & Engebretson, T. O. (1988). Familial aggregation of behaviors associated with risk for coronary heart disease: I. Blood pressure and heart rate responses to physiological and exercise stress. *Psychosomatic Medicine, 50*, 341–352.

Matthews, K. A., & Stoney, C. M. (1988). Influences of sex and age on cardiovascular responses during stress. *Psychophysiology, 50*, 46–56.

Musante, L., MacDougall, J. M., Dembroski, T. M., & Costa, P. T., Jr. (1989). Potential for hostility and dimensions of anger. *Health Psychology, 8*, 343–354.

Patterson, G. R. (1985). A microsocial analysis of anger and irritable behavior. In M. A. Chesney & R. H. Rosenman (Eds.), *Anger and hostility in cardiovascular behavioral disorders* (pp. 83–100). New York: McGraw-Hill.

Ryckman, R. M., Stone, W. F., & Elam, R. R. (1971). Emotional arousal as a function of perceived locus of control and task requirements. *Journal of Social Psychology, 83*, 185–191.

Sarason, I. G. (1961). Intercorrelations among measures of hostility. *Journal of Clinical Psychology, 17*, 192–195.

Scherwitz, L., Perkins, L., Chesney, M., & Hughes, G. (1991). Cook–Medley Hostility scale and subsets: Relationships to demographic and psychosocial characteristics in young adults in the CARDIA study. *Psychosomatic Medicine, 53*, 36–49.

Sempos, C., Cooper, R., Kovar, M. G., & McMillen, M. (1988). Divergence of the recent trends in coronary mortality for the four major race–sex groups in the United States. *American Journal of Public Health, 78*, 1422–1427.

Siegel, J. M. (1985). The measurement of anger as a multidimensional construct. In M. A. Chesney & R. H. Rosenman (Eds.), *Anger and hostility in cardiovascular and behavioral disorders* (pp. 59–82). New York: McGraw-Hill.

Siegel, J. M. (1986). The multidimensional anger inventory. *Journal of Personality and Social Psychology, 51*, 191–200.

Siegman, A. W., Dembroski, T. M., & Ringel, N. (1987). Components of hostility and the severity of coronary artery disease. *Psychosomatic Medicine, 49*, 127–135.

Simkins, L. (1961). Effects of examiner attitudes and type of reinforcement on the conditioning of hostile verbs. *Journal of Personality, 29*, 380–395.

Smith, T. W., & Allred, K. D. (1989). Blood pressure responses during social interaction in high and low cynically hostile males. *Journal of Behavioral Medicine, 12*, 135–143.

Smith, T. W., & Frohm, K. D. (1985). What's so unhealthy about hostility? Construct validity and psychosocial correlates of the Cook and Medley Ho scale. *Health Psychology, 4*, 503–520.

Spielberger, C. D., Jacobs, G. A., Russell, S. F., & Crane, R. J. (1983). Assessment of anger: The State–Trait anger scale. In J. Butcher & C. D. Spielberger (Eds.), *Advances in personality assessment* (Vol. 2, pp. 161–189). Hillsdale, NJ: Lawrence Erlbaum Associates.

Spielberger, C. D., Johnson, E. H., Russell, S. F., Crane, R. J., Jacobs, G. A., & Worden, T. J. (1985). The experience and expression of anger: Construction and validation of an anger expression scale. In M. A. Chesney & R. H. Rosenman (Eds.), *Anger and hostility in cardiovascular and behavioral disorders* (pp. 5–30). New York: McGraw-Hill.

Stoney, C. M., Davis, M. C., & Matthews, K. A. (1987). Sex differences in physiological responses to stress and in coronary heart disease: A causal link? *Psychophysiology, 24*, 127–131.

Stoney, C. M., & Matthews, K. A. (1988). Parental history of hypertension and myocardial infarction predicts cardiovascular response to behavioral stressors in middle-aged men and women. *Psychophysiology, 25*, 269–277.

Stoney, C. M., Matthews, K. A., McDonald, R., & Johnson, C. A. (1988). Sex differences in lipid, lipoprotein, cardiovascular, and neuroendocrine responses to acute stress. *Psychophysiology, 25*, 645–656.

Sullivan, P., Schoentgen, S., DeQuattro, V., Procci, W., Levine D., & Bornheimer J. (1981). Anxiety and neurogenic tone—At rest and in stress, in primary hypertension. *Hypertension, 3*, 125–130.

Treiber, F. A., Musante, L., Riley, W., Mabe, P. A., Carr, T., Levy, M., & Strong, W. B. (1989). The relationship between hostility and blood pressure in children. *Behavioral Medicine, 15*, 173–178.

Van Egeren, L. F. (1979). Cardiovascular changes during social competition in a mixed-motive game. *Journal of Personality and Social Psychology, 37*, 858–864.

Waldron, I. (1976). Why do women live longer than men? *Social Science Medicine, 10*, 349–362.

Weidner, G., Friend, R., Ficarrotto, T. J., & Mendell, N. R. (1989). Hostility and cardiovascular reactivity to stress in women and men. *Psychosomatic Medicine, 51*, 36–45.

Weidner, G., Istvan, J., & McKnight, J. D. (1989). Clusters of behavioral coronary risk factors in employed women and men. *Journal of Applied Social Psychology, 19*, 468–480.

Williams, R. B., Barefoot, J. C., & Shekelle, R. B. (1985). The health consequences of hostility. In M. A. Chesney, R. H. Rosenman (Eds.), *Anger and hostility in cardiovascular and behavioral disorders* (pp. 173–185). New York: McGraw-Hill.

Wingard, D. L. (1982). The sex differential in mortality rates: Demographic and behavioral factors. *American Journal of Epidemiology, 115*, 205–216.

Wingard, D. L. (1984). The sex differential in morbidity, mortality, and lifestyle. *Annual Review of Public Health, 5*, 433–458.

Wingard, D. L., Suarez, L., & Barrett-Connor, E. (1983). The sex differential in mortality from all causes and ischemic heart disease. *American Journal of Epidemiology, 117*, 165–172.

Wyrick, C., Gentry, W. D., & Shows, W. D. (1977). Aggression, assertion, and openness to experience: A comparison of men and women. *Journal of Clinical Psychology, 33*, 439–443.

Zelin, M. L., Alder, G., & Myerson, P. G. (1972). Anger self-report: An objective questionnaire for the measurement of aggression. *Journal Consulting Clinical Psychology, 39*, 340.

12

ANGER REDUCTION: ISSUES, ASSESSMENT, AND INTERVENTION STRATEGIES

Jerry L. Deffenbacher
Colorado State University

OVERVIEW

As reviewed in other chapters, epidemiological and physiological studies suggest that anger, hostility, and related processes are implicated in the development of cardiovascular diseases such as coronary artery disease and hypertension and in overall mortality and morbidity. Given the importance of the anger risk factor, it is reasonable that anger would be targeted for intervention and that the impact of its reduction would be related to cardiovascular disease.

Although there have been many intervention studies for Type A behavior and hypertension, few address the anger factor cleanly. Many programs simultaneously target multiple risk factors such as different components of Type A behavior. For example, one program (Friedman et al., 1984) led to powerful reductions of Type A behavior, anger and hostility, and myocardial infarction rates. However, because intervention addressed elements other than anger, it did not elucidate the impact of anger-related interventions. A study with hypertensives (Bennett, Wallace, Carrol, & Smith, 1991) had the same difficulty. Stress and Type A reduction programs lowered blood pressure, and the Type A program, which included anger components, showed significantly greater reduction of Type A behavior and anger. Other studies (e.g., Nakano, 1990) revealed a different methodological problem. In this study, a self-control relaxation procedure for anger control and an operant self-management program for speed/impatience lowered Type A behavior.

However, because no measure of anger was included and the measure of Type A behavior did not have a separate anger–hostility index, it was not possible to evaluate differential effects of the anger-focused intervention. A study of hypertensives (Achmon, Granek, Golomb, & Hart, 1989) partially overcame these problems by including blood pressure and anger measures in comparisons of cognitive therapy focused on anger reduction and heart rate biofeedback for stress management. Compared to controls, both interventions reduced blood pressure, but reductions were significantly greater for the heart rate feedback condition, whereas anger reduction was significantly greater for cognitive therapy. In addition to the mixed findings and methodological issues such as clinic versus nonclinic blood pressure measurement, the fact that targets of intervention were crossed with cognitive therapy focused on anger and heart rate biofeedback on applications to stress makes it difficult to evaluate differential contributions. Thurman (1985a), however, assessed both anger and Type A behavior in a comparison of a cognitive intervention and a cognitive intervention combined with assertiveness and found that, compared to controls, the combined condition reduced anger and hostility in Type A behavior and that these effects were maintained a year later (Thurman, 1985b). In summary, anger is a significant contributor to cardiovascular disease, yet few intervention studies in the area of cardiovascular disease have clearly assessed effects of anger reduction.

This chapter approaches anger reduction from a different direction, namely, the literature where anger has been targeted directly. This literature is reviewed briefly, but the bulk of the chapter has a decidedly clinical bent, focusing on conceptual, assessment, and treatment issues. It is hoped that both health psychology researchers designing intervention programs and practicing therapists dealing with angry patients, who may or may not show cardiovascular involvement, will benefit from this exploration of applied issues.

ANGER REDUCTION STUDIES

In spite of the importance of anger in psycho–social–health functioning of people, treatment studies of anger reduction have lagged significantly behind those of other emotional problems such as anxiety and depression. It was not until Novaco's (1975) component analysis of stress inoculation that the field had its first well-controlled treatment study. When relaxation and cognitive interventions were compared to their combination (stress inoculation) and to an attentional control, stress inoculation was most effective followed closely by the cognitive condition. Relaxation effects were limited, which led Novaco to conclude that the cognitive component was the major contributor to stress inoculation, and relaxation was a poorer intervention for anger reduction.

Subsequent research has supported most of Novaco's conclusions. For example, the combination of cognitive and relaxation coping skills proved effective with highly stressed, anger-involved occupational groups such as police (Novaco, 1977) and probation (Novaco, 1980) officers. In a study with angry juvenile delinquents (Schlichter & Horan, 1981), the combination of cognitive and relaxation skills effectively reduced anger and was slightly more effective than a relaxation intervention. A series of studies with generally angry college students (Deffenbacher, McNamara, Stark, & Sabadell, 1990a; Deffenbacher & Stark, 1992; Deffenbacher, Story, Brandon, Hogg, & Hazaleus, 1988; Deffenbacher, Story, Stark, Hogg, & Brandon, 1987) showed that this combination lowers anger, and gains are maintained at 12–15 month follow-ups (Deffenbacher, 1988; Deffenbacher & Stark, 1992; Deffenbacher et al., 1988, 1990a). Additionally, this combination was as effective as cognitive (Deffenbacher et al., 1988), social skills (Deffenbacher et al., 1987), process group (Deffenbacher et al., 1990a) and relaxation (Deffenbacher & Stark, 1992) interventions. Thus, cognitive–relaxation coping skills interventions lead to robust and lasting results.

Cognitive interventions also have proven effective. For example, in the study reviewed previously, Achmon et al. (1989) demonstrated that cognitive therapy reduced anger and blood pressure in hypertensives. The cognitive component of stress inoculation also reduced anger in college students (Deffenbacher et al., 1988; Hazaleus & Deffenbacher, 1986; Moon & Eisler, 1983). Another type of cognitive intervention, problem-solving training, was also effective in this population (Moon & Eisler, 1983). Cognitive interventions were as effective as relaxation (Hazaleus & Deffenbacher, 1986), combined cognitive–relaxation (Deffenbacher et al., 1988) and social skills (Moon & Eisler, 1983) treatments, and long-term follow-ups (Deffenbacher et al., 1986; Hazaleus & Deffenbacher, 1986) revealed maintenance. Thus, cognitively oriented interventions too are effective, although some studies (Deffenbacher et al., 1988; Hazaleus & Deffenbacher, 1986) suggest that combining them with relaxation interventions is easier for therapist and client alike, even though this may not improve their overall effectiveness.

Effects for relaxation interventions, however, may be stronger than those originally suggested by Novaco. Deffenbacher and his colleagues (Deffenbacher, Demm, & Brandon, 1986; Deffenbacher & Stark, 1992; Hazaleus & Deffenbacher, 1986) suggested that poor intervention design may have compromised the original study. For example, rationale (active, self-control) may have been at odds with training procedure (passive counterconditioning); insufficient time and attention may have been devoted to progressive relaxation and specific relaxation coping skills; little home practice, either of relaxation or of in vivo application, was apparently employed; and the short time frame of intervention may have worked against the development of relaxation coping skills. Anxiety management training (Suinn, 1977, 1990; Suinn & Deffenbacher,

1988), a relaxation self-management program that addresses these deficiencies, was, therefore, adapted to anger management. In the initial study (Deffenbacher et al., 1986), this approach revealed anger reduction stronger than that reported by Novaco (1975). Subsequent studies replicated these effects and showed this intervention to be as effective as cognitive (Hazaleus & Deffenbacher, 1986) and combined cognitive-relaxation coping skills (Deffenbacher & Stark, 1992) programs. Additionally, anger reduction in three studies was maintained at 12–15 month follow-ups. Schlichter and Horan (1981) also found stronger effects for a relaxation intervention, even though these effects were not quite as strong as those of the combined cognitive–relaxation condition. Thus, self-managed relaxation coping skills also appear to be a viable intervention for anger reduction.

The interventions described to this point focus on emotional control, either through cognitive or relaxation strategies or their combination. However, another general approach, social and communication skills training, approaches anger reduction through development of skills (e.g., communication, negotiation, assertiveness) through which to handle inevitable interpersonal conflict. Two studies in this area (Deffenbacher et al., 1987; Moon & Eisler, 1983) showed social skills and social problem-solving strategies to be effective and to be as effective as cognitive and cognitive–relaxation coping skills. Long-term maintenance of anger reduction was found (Deffenbacher, 1988), and cognitive–relaxation and social skills programs were successfully combined (Deffenbacher, McNamara, Stark, & Sabadell, 1990b). Thus, social skills interventions also appear to be an appropriate intervention, at least for interpersonally prompted anger.

In summary, a number of anger reduction interventions were evaluated in well-controlled designs. The remainder of this chapter outlines treatments in more detail, along with a discussion of conceptualizing anger problems and their assessment.

ANGER AS AN EMOTIONAL DISORDER

Anger, whether problematic or not, can be conceptualized as an internal state consisting of cognitive, emotional, and physiological responses. Emotionally, anger varies along a continuum from mild irritation and annoyance, through frustrated and angry, to rage and fury. Physiologically, anger is marked by sympathetic activation, adrenal release, and increased facial and skeletal muscle tone. Cognitive processes include appraisal of triggering events, ongoing reappraisals of situational and experiential processes, memory and information processing, self-dialogue, attributions, imagery, urges, and the like. Cognitively, anger is often a "moral" emotion that results from a sense of violation or trespass on the person's domain (Beck, 1976) or on his/her rules for living (Beck, 1988; Dryden, 1990; Ellis, 1977). That is, anger rises when values are compromised, promises and expectations are broken, goal-directed behavior is blocked, rules of conduct are violated, and personally defined freedoms and rights are abridged. Anger escalates further if the source is seen as intentional, preventable, unjustified, and/or something to be blamed and punished (Hazaleus & Deffenbacher, 1985; Lohr, Hamberger, & Bonge, 1988; Zwemer & Deffenbacher, 1984). In summary, the individual has experienced something he/she "should" not have to experience, and cognitive, emotional, and physiological systems are mobilized. Although these three response systems are separable for conceptual and treatment planning purposes, they typically appear together and interact rapidly such that they are experienced as a relatively singular state of anger.

Anger, however, is separable from the behavior motivated by or related to it and should not be conceptually or clinically confused with aggressive or other behavioral expressions (Spielberger, 1988; Spielberger et al., 1983). Unfortunately, anger has too often been confused with aggression. When angry, some individuals verbally and/or physically assault themselves, others, or objects. However, these are but two types of behavior that may be displayed. Other individuals may deflect anger into indirect expressions. Others suppress anger, showing little outward manifestation, but experiencing considerable internal arousal. Because anger is a negatively sanctioned emotion, and, consequently, elicits anxiety, still others withdraw physically or distance themselves cognitively from anger through defense mechanisms such as denial, intellectualization, projection, reaction formation, suppression, and repression. Although additional anger-related behaviors could be listed, the point is that anger can and should be separated from related behaviors, and dysfunctional anger should be conceptualized, assessed, and treated in its own right.

The diagnosis of anger emotional disorders is not an easy task. The DSM-IIIR (American Psychiatric Association, 1987) disorders, excluding organic and psychotic disorders, list anger as a secondary or contributing feature of dysthymia, psychological factors affecting a physical condition, posttraumatic stress disorder (PTSD), explosive impulse control disorders, and passive–aggressive, antisocial, and borderline personality disorders. Anger, however, does not stand freely as an emotional disorder, although there are extensive lists of anxiety and depressive emotional disorders. For example, a patient may be diagnosed for chronic, moderate depression (dysthymia) or worry and anxiety (generalized anxiety disorder), but not for chronic, moderate anger. A patient can be diagnosed for various situational anxieties (phobias), but not for an intense, situational anger reaction (e.g., in response to being reprimanded or to discourteous drivers). An individual may have a diagnosable adjustment disorder with anxiety, depression, or mixed emotional features, but not with anger alone, unless it is accompanied by conduct problems.

(But what of the person who is highly angry during a relationship breakup, but does not act out?) Just because we can officially diagnose depressive and anxious emotional disorders, but not angry emotional disorders, does not mean that meaningful anger disorders do not exist.

What then might define dysfunctional anger reactions? As with most diagnostic issues, designating anger as debilitating or dysfunctional is a judgment call, that is, judging where the individual's experience falls along different dimensions. These judgments can be facilitated by looking at three response dimensions—intensity, frequency, and duration (Novaco, in press)—and their outcomes or consequences across cognitive, emotional, and physiological response systems.

More intense anger is more likely to be dysfunctional. For example, emotions of mild annoyance and frustration, although disquieting, are not likely to be problematic, whereas fury and "mad as hell" are much more likely to be dysfunctional, as they are more upsetting to the individual and, perhaps, to those around him/her and may prompt negative behaviors.

Frequency is important. Occasional anger, assuming it is not intense or associated with negative consequences, is less problematic than frequent anger. For example, Averill (1982) reported that the average U.S. citizen became angry every three days or so. Thus, the individual who is angry several times a day or nearly always angry in frequently occurring events is at much greater risk for anger-related problems.

Duration is also an important dimension. Averill's (1982) data revealed considerable variability in how long people experience anger: About 15% indicated durations of 5 minutes or less, whereas 25% stayed angry a day or more. In general, the latter individuals are more likely to be impacted negatively by their anger. Duration can be important in another way as well. Anger is more dysfunctional if it is reexperienced even if the person is far removed in time from provocation. For example, if a person is easily angered about a divorce or job loss several years earlier, life is more likely to be impaired by this anger.

The final dimension of the consequences of anger is more qualitative. Anger outcomes also vary considerably. For example, generally angry individuals experience more frequent physical damage to themselves, others, and property, more frequent disturbances in interpersonal relationships and school/work performance, lowered self-esteem, and greater alcohol involvement and alcohol-related consequences (e.g., Deffenbacher, 1992; Deffenbacher & Stark, 1992; Deffenbacher & Thwaites, 1991; Hazaleus & Deffenbacher, 1986; Liebsohn, Deffenbacher, & Oetting, 1991). Dysfunctionality is more likely when anger expressions and consequences are more frequent and/or more severe.

Clearly, these dimensions are not independent. For example, intense anger often disrupts judgment, problem solving, and interpersonal functioning more than does mild anger (i.e., intensity influenced consequences). Additionally, anger response systems are correlated, and changes in one may influence the others. These issues of interdependence not withstanding, anger is more likely to be judged problematic or dysfunctional when response systems show: (a) greater intensity; (b) higher frequencies; (c) prolonged durations; and/or (d) increased frequencies and severities of negative consequences. Furthermore, greater involvement across response systems, response parameters, consequences, and time suggest more dysfunctionality. In summary, it is argued that dysfunctional anger may be associated with, but not defined by, aggressive behavior, and dysfunctional anger constitutes a legitimate group of emotional disorders in their own right.

ASSESSMENT OF DYSFUNCTIONAL ANGER

Although anger problems share commonalities, differences must be assessed to develop a comprehensive treatment plan. For example, primary triggers for anger, nature of response patterning, mode of expression, and consequences of anger vary from person to person and within the individual over time and across situations. This section outlines general issues in the assessment of anger problems, specific targets to be assessed, and several assessment strategies.

General Assessment Considerations

Four general issues should be considered when assessing anger problems:

1. Many angry patients are guarded, resistant, and easily angered when they feel others are controlling them or telling them what to do. This anger is compounded if the patient feels he/she has been coerced into therapy. It is, therefore, suggested that assessment activities foster a sense of collaboration and facilitate the working alliance. The therapist may initially want to decrease his/her expertness and authority and develop assessment strategies as natural extensions of working together to understand the client's anger. For example, self-monitoring activities might be developed from a patient statement of "needing to figure out what pisses me off," rather than being assigned by the therapist. Even when the therapist introduces specific assessment strategies such as paper–pencil questionnaires about which the patient is likely to have little knowledge, effort should be made to link these naturally to the person's concerns. For example, an anger scale that is part of a larger inventory (e.g., MMPI-2) might be framed in terms of seeing how anger fits with other emotions, or an anger expression scale could be discussed as

a means of helping the client figure out how he/she habitually deals with anger. The small amount of time needed for such framing of assessment activities seems to consistently pay off in increased cooperation and compliance.

2. Assessment should enhance self-understanding, as many angry individuals do not have a well-developed sense of what triggers anger and how/why they respond as they do. Anger just seems to "happen" to them. Thus, assessment that fosters self-awareness is beneficial and may be therapeutic in itself. As patients become aware of internal and external patterns, they may be able to interrupt anger arousal and initiate alternative coping skills they already possess. Enhanced awareness also provides the cues to initiate interventions developed in therapy.

3. Assessment should lead to a jointly developed, detailed conceptualization of patient anger. This working model provides the client and therapist the base from which to develop and target interventions and fosters patient involvement and follow-through, as it is his/her anger and his/her plan for dealing with it.

4. Assessment is not something completed at the beginning of therapy and never revised. To the contrary, it is a dynamic process unfolding over time. New information, sometimes serendipitously discovered, and treatment successes and failures revise the understanding of patient anger and the internal and external contexts in which it occurs.

Targets of Assessment

Response systems should be explored carefully along quantitative and qualitative parameters noted previously. For example, how does the patient respond emotionally (e.g., high frustration? furious? slow burn?), physiologically (e.g., clenched jaw? burning stomach? intense frowning?), and cognitively (e.g., What kinds of images and self-talk occur? Does the person ruminate? If so, what is the content? Does he/she curse to self? If so, what expressions and phrases are used?)? Anger should also be defined in terms of its *latency* (i.e., how long after or even before a provocation does the individual become angry), *frequency* (i.e., how often does anger occur), *intensity* (i.e., how strong is the response), and *duration* (i.e., how long does it last and does it return with minimal external prompting). Additionally, anger expression styles (e.g., What exactly does the patient do when angry? How does this change over time and why?) and outcomes (e.g., What happens to the patient and others as a result of his/her anger expression? Is the patient under vocational, family, or legal pressure to change? Does the client experience elevated blood pressure that is suspicioned to be a result of suppressed anger? Does the patient feel guilty or depressed about anger?) should be outlined in detail.

So far, the focus has been on the response side of anger, but the stimulus side needs attention as well. Anger results from complex interactions of (a) eliciting stimuli; (b) the individual's preanger state, both momentary and enduring characteristics; and (c) appraisal processes, including initial appraisals of eliciting stimuli and coping resources and reappraisals and interpretations of the experience of anger, anger-related behavior, and feedback from the environment as the anger episode unfolds. That is, anger results from rapid interactions and recyclings of person and environment variables over time, all of which are important to assess.

Although neurological, temperament, endocrine, and other physiological processes may influence the threshold for anger, clinically, we find anger to be related to four different types of stimuli. These categories are neither exhaustive nor mutually exclusive because more than one type may be present in any anger experience. However, we find them helpful in conceptualizing anger difficulties, in planning treatment, and in understanding treatment impasses.

Some anger appears to be elicited by clear, specific precipitants. The nature of these stimuli varies widely and may involve behavior of others (e.g., children, spouse, supervisor), specific situations (e.g., cut off in traffic or criticism), specific objects (e.g., equipment not operating properly), impersonal events (e.g., politics or the weather), and the individual's own behavior or characteristics (e.g., being avoidably late for a meeting or a characteristic like height or weight). What ties these stimuli together is a relatively clear, often external, event that elicits anger. Furthermore, the individual can usually identify the source of provocation, often using a phrase such as "X makes me angry."

Other anger also appears elicited by external events, but less by direct provocation and more by the anger-related memories and images evoked by them. Dramatic examples are seen in PTSD victims, who experience anger and rage when exposed directly or indirectly to trauma-related cues. For example, a partner's sexual behavior may trigger anger-related memories from childhood sexual abuse, or an individual of another nationality may elicit anger and tension in a veteran. There are, however, many other less dramatic, but clinically relevant examples of such indirect cuing. For example, a supervisor's gesture or tone of voice may remind one of a disliked parent, or good-natured teasing may trigger anger stemming primarily from memories of being teased as a youngster.

Anger in such circumstances is often marked by confusion in the individual and, perhaps, in others as the individual is unaware or only partially aware of the memories and images triggered. This anger can create three different sources of confusion. First, anger often is out of proportion to or inappropriate for current circumstances. The patient may acknowledge the exaggerated or inappropriate quality, but still not know what makes him/her so angry. Second, it leads to mixed emotions, as when a person has positive feelings toward another but is angered by some historically rooted behavior. Third, because the individual does not have accurate connections between images and memories triggered by external stimuli, he/she may inaccurately attribute anger to external events and, therefore, feel and behave inappropriately. All of these circumstances can be quite confusing and can take considerable time to unravel.

Other anger appears more internally stimulated. One common example of this type of anger elicitation is anger in response to other emotions (e.g., feeling hurt, rejected, slighted, or anxious). Another internal source of anger is worrying, brooding, or ruminating. For example, with little external stimulation, an individual may become angry when worrying about potential rejection or when ruminating about a prior love affair. In either case, anger is secondary to and elicited by other internal emotional or cognitive processes.

The degree of insight into these internal sources of anger elicitation varies widely. Some individuals know relatively clearly that they are angry about certain feelings or thoughts. In these cases thoughts and feelings may be treated much like external events, that is, emotions and/or cognitions are identified as precipitants and are targeted for intervention. Others, however, show relatively little awareness and experience confusion, mixed emotions, and/or inappropriate attributions, emotions, and behavior as the individual fails to deal effectively with the source of anger or anger itself. Such cases may take more therapeutic time and exploration to clarify and link to intervention.

A fourth class of anger eliciting or influencing stimuli is negative components of the immediate preanger state. Prior anger is one such element. If an individual is already angry and frustrated, he/she is more likely to react with continued anger or with greater intensity than if he/she was not angered previously. This may be true even if the next provocation has little or nothing to do with the prior one. For example, many angry workers and nearly all parents report becoming more angry because they were already angry and upset with another worker or child. Zillmann (1971; Zillmann & Bryant, 1974) documented this effect experimentally showing that excitation from prior anger arousal can transfer to and enhance anger to subsequent events. Such transfer or anger enhancing effects, however, are not limited to prior anger. It appears that nearly any aversive mental–emotional–physiological state such as being tired, ill, hungry, or stressed may alter the probability and/or intensity of anger (Berkowitz, 1990). That is, there appears to be a kind of negative transfer that lowers anger thresholds and increases the presence and salience of aversive images and memories which increase the probability of other negative reactions such as anger. In the case of prior anger or other aversive states, individuals with aversive preanger states are more vulnerable to additional anger.

In these circumstances, the patient may appear angry without cause, overreact to minor frustrations, or react with anger to situations that would not otherwise elicit anger. This may be confusing to the patient and to those around him/her, as from their perspective, things look the same, but receive different emotional responses. Variations in response to seemingly similar situations often hold the key to this type of anger elicitation. For example, exploring why the person was angry in dealing with a situation on Tuesday, but not Thursday, may reveal that he/she was stressed, ill, or tired on Tuesday, but not Thursday.

As anger prompt and response characteristics are mapped generally, clinicians should seek variations in experience and concrete examples. Regarding variations, it is important to understand why the individual becomes angry one time and not another in the presence of seemingly similar circumstances. Exploration often reveals different attitudes and attributions, coping skills, or, as noted earlier, preanger states. Times when less anger was experienced may point to positive coping resources, which may be integrated into intervention design, whereas greater arousal and negative consequences may elucidate vulnerabilities to be targeted for intervention.

The therapist should also have patients describe specific examples of anger, as details may otherwise be omitted. It is not being suggested that angry patients consciously distort descriptions of anger, although some may, but that there are several reasons why they may not provide as rich descriptions as some other clients do. First, some patients simply do not have enough self-awareness to summarize information well. Second, because anger is a socially taboo emotion, patients may be uncomfortable with or embarrassed by their anger. Usually, little prompting and encouragement leads to candid, detailed descriptions. Third, some angry patients hold attitudes about or have grown up in environments that "normalize" anger and aggression. Such patients simply may not code and, therefore, describe anger and anger-related behavior as another person might. Finally, some angry patients are guarded until therapeutic trust is developed. Steady requests for and concrete explorations of anger incidents, however, often enhances the working conceptualization of anger and builds trust as the clinician explores anger although still accepting the client.

Common Assessment Strategies

Although many different assessment strategies can be applied to dysfunctional anger, four strategies—interviewing, self-monitoring, simulation and imagery sampling, and paper–pencil tests—consistently yield quality information.

Interviewing is most frequently used. For reasons and characteristics noted earlier, the interview should stay as open-ended as possible (e.g., "Tell me about that kind of anger"). This allows the patient to describe anger in his or her own words, which maximizes rapport while minimizing resistance because of the need for control or guardedness. Therapist summaries and reflections can be used to check understanding and integrate themes. These are followed with further open-ended inquiries and clarifications until general patterns, contrasts, and examples are explored. Interviews with relevant others such as parents, spouses, children, and coworkers also can provide important information and should be considered.

Self-monitoring, that is, patient observation and recording anger in vivo, is an excellent means of supplementing other sources of information. It provides current, contextually rich data and may enhance patient self-awareness. Although self-monitoring is an excellent assessment strategy, it is an unusual behavior for most patients, and several things can be done to maximize its effectiveness. First, compliance and quality increase when self-monitoring is developed collaboratively (Meichenbaum & Deffenbacher, 1988; Meichenbaum & Turk, 1987), rather than being suggested by the therapist with forms pulled from his/her files. The small amount of time taken assisting clients in suggesting and in investing in self-monitoring saves time and resources devoted to noncompliance and resistance to externally imposed tasks. Second, self-monitoring is best when it starts simple and adds complexity over time (Deffenbacher, 1981). For example, initially patients might only record anger and the situation in which it occurred. Over time, differentiating response components and coping efforts might be added to recording. Third, self-monitoring should be flexible and tailored to the patient. Written diaries and logs are excellent, but other recording methods (e.g., frequency tallies or dictation of one's thoughts when angry) may be more appropriate. Finally, the therapist must not to get caught up in other therapeutic activities and fail to review and discuss self-monitoring. To fail in this may miss valuable information, undermine the working alliance, and discredit the general value of between session assignments.

Anger cannot only be sampled by self-monitoring between sessions, but also via imagery recall and simulation procedures within sessions. These procedures attempt to generate or recreate "hot" emotions and cognitions, as there is evidence (e.g., Persons & Miranda, 1991) that these are state dependent and assessment is improved if the individual is in the state at the time of assessment. In imagery recall procedures, patients visualize an angering event and experience it as vividly as possible. After a period of visualization, which may encompass the whole event or a portion of it, imagery is terminated, and patients are interviewed about experiences during the visualization. In simulation approaches the patient role-plays or otherwise enacts real or potentially provocative events. Then he or she is interviewed regarding thoughts, feelings, urges, physical sensations, and the like. The therapist may also offer his or her observations and reactions. In group settings, other clients may be involved in the enactment sequence and/or offer observations and feedback. Simulation assessments can also be aided by audio or video recording. Subsequently, tapes can be stopped at different places and client reactions explored. In some cases (e.g., family discussions), it may even be possible for patients to audio- or videotape anger provoking events live and bring in the tape for review.

Sometimes the therapeutic interview itself becomes an in vivo sample of anger; for example, the client comes to a session angered by external events or becomes angry with the therapist for things such as not being understanding or being late. Although it is probably not wise to provoke anger purposefully, it is very appropriate to take advantage of it should it happen naturally. The immediate experience of anger can be explored, and, where appropriate, the therapist may introduce additional elements such as alternative explanations of events (e.g., being late was due to being unavoidably held up in traffic vs. being out to lunch with a friend).

Another assessment strategy is use of anger inventories and questionnaires. Increasingly, there are diverse, psychometrically sound instruments which the therapist can select to address specific questions or issues. Although there are too many scales to review comprehensively, a few are described along with possible clinical uses.

The Trait Anger scale (Spielberger, 1988; Spielberger et al., 1983) is a 10-item scale of general anger on which patients report how they generally react. It provides not only a normative definition of general anger, but also two related clusters of items, one assessing angry temperament (e.g., fiery temper) and the other anger in certain social circumstances (e.g., being criticized or slowed by others). Thus, an informal item analysis may also assist in identifying themes in the individual's anger prompts.

General scales can be supplemented by scales that assess anger more situationally. For example, the Anger Inventory (Novaco, 1975) is a 90-item questionnaire on which patients rate the degree of anger provoked by 90 different situations. It too may be employed in a normative fashion to assess general reactivity, but also to screen quickly for situations missed in other assessments and to identify potential patterns of situations that elicit greatest anger. The Anger Situation scale (Deffenbacher et al., 1986; Hazaleus & Deffenbacher, 1986) provides even greater idiographic, situational information by asking the individual to describe, in detail, his or her two worst, ongoing angering situations. Earlier versions asked the person to then rate anger intensity on a 0–100 scale. Subsequently, it has been revised to include frequency of occurrence per month, duration in minutes of anger per episode, and degree to which anger in these situations interferes with the respondent's life (0–100 scale). The Anger Situation scale thus gives considerable detail about two chronically aggravating situations. This data base can be expanded by asking patients how they typically express their anger in these situations.

Anger expression styles can also be assessed by the Anger Expression Inventory (Spielberger, 1988), which asks patients to indicate how they generally expresses anger. The 24-item questionnaire yields three, 8-item scales of general anger expression, measuring the tendencies to: (a) suppress or hold anger in (e.g., angrier than others know); (b) express it outwardly and negatively (e.g., cursing and throwing things); and (c) express it in more controlled, socially acceptable ways (e.g., being patient and calm). Anger suppression is minimally correlated with outward negative and controlled expressive styles, whereas the latter two are inversely correlated, and these expression styles are associated with different types of consequences and other variables (Deffenbacher, 1992; Spielberger, 1988). As with other scales, anger expression scores can be compared normatively; however, comparison of the patient's relative use of the three styles may provide hypothesis about potential strengths and about skill deficits needing remediation. Inquiry regarding what determines the deployment of a given style may also prove useful.

Anger-related physiological involvement may be sampled by the Anger Symptom measure (Deffenbacher et al., 1986; Hazaleus & Deffenbacher, 1986) on which the individual describes his or her two most salient, physical signs of anger. Originally physiological responses were rated on a 0–100 severity scale, but the measure now includes ratings of frequency, duration, and interference as well. Response may not only suggest dominant physiological involvement, but may also provide hypotheses about potential psychosomatic and disease involvement.

TREATMENT OF DYSFUNCTIONAL ANGER

As noted at the beginning of the chapter, several interventions are effective. The remainder of the chapter outlines general issues and specific strategies.

General Treatment Considerations

When treating anger problems, one is advised to pay additional attention to certain ethical and legal issues. For example, very early on, therapists should clarify guidelines for breaking confidence and for legal duty to report issues such as child abuse, dangerousness to self and others, and, in some cases, illegal activities and substance abuse. Additionally, when assessment or therapy involves a third party such as schools, courts, family or employers, and when the therapist will communicate with these outside systems, he or she should carefully think through issues of confidentiality, informed consent, and professional relationships in negotiating an ethically acceptable contract among parties. It is suggested that the nature, frequency, and type of expected communication among parties be negotiated clearly in advance of assessment and treatment and that these conditions be discussed among the parties, written down, and signed by all to maximize cooperation and protect confidentiality and informed consent.

Anger reduction can be done individually or in small, mixed gender groups led by a single therapist. Group format needs to fit the type of patient and treatment setting, but it is suggested that outpatient groups for adults last at least 75–90 minutes. This allows sufficient time to track individual issues, yet still provides time for introduction and rehearsal of specific interventions. In group interventions, it is also important to guard against overloading the group with content, that is, introducing more material than there is time to integrate and rehearse. Rehearsal within and between sessions appears critical to lasting anger reduction. Thus, if the material is truly important, then it should be given its time, and the number of sessions extended to ensure adequate rehearsal.

Another general consideration is therapist style or characteristics. Angry clients may be more abrasive, active, challenging, and intimidating and less compliant and accepting than some other clients. It is important that therapists not be frightened or put off by these characteristics, and that they be approaching and accepting, yet quite willing to be confrontive and challenging. That is, therapists seem to do better when they genuinely like and accept the angry person, but good naturedly and doggedly confront issues, and when they are durable and persistent when the client's emotions and behaviors test their limits.

Specific Intervention Strategies

Several clinically effective strategies follow, along with suggestions for implementation and integration with other interventions.

1. Enhanced Personal Awareness

Assessment and many interventions increase the patient's awareness of anger. However, because many angry patients reveal lessened self-awareness, it is suggested that this area be targeted specifically. Heightened awareness may lead to changes as the client employs extant coping skills or begins to engage in self-questioning such as "What am I responding to?" "Is this what I am really angry about?" or "Is this the way I want to handle this?" Increased anger sensitivity also provides perception of early anger arousal cues from which to apply other strategies developed in therapy.

Patients often become more self-aware through assessment activities, and these can be extended to maintain this focus. For example, self-report instruments can be discussed, and patients can then observe themselves to check these impressions. Self-monitoring can be continued and refined, and additional observational assignments may be developed. For example, patients might observe someone who handles anger well and note how their behavior differs from this other person's, or might track "what's written on my buttons" or "whose finger is on my anger trigger" for a period of time. In a group setting, patients might be asked to develop a list of nonverbal cues that tell them that someone is very angry and another list of nonverbal cues which tell them that a person is handling provocation well. Then they might be asked to track nonverbal cues they routinely give off. Reactions to visualizations and simulations can be explored for what is the patient learning about him- or herself as he or she goes through rehearsal activities. Video and audio recordings of simulated or live events too can increase self-awareness as they provide patients with direct feedback about how the patient looks, sounds, and comes across to others. Interviews about how anger was experienced and dealt with in the family of origin and how this is related to the present may increase self-understanding. Although these are but a few strategies that might be chosen, it is suggested that enhanced personal awareness of anger be developed early and maintained throughout therapy.

2. Response Disruption and Interference

These are a cluster of strategies which actively disrupt or interfere with anger arousal. Anger is reduced as eliciting cues are removed, as cognitive–emotional–physiological cycles are disrupted, and as the individual is provided with the opportunity to cool down and engage in alternative behavior. Response interference should be tailored to the individual's anger prompts and response patterns. Several general strategies for such tailoring follow.

Some strategies involve *physical removal from the provocative scene*. For example, the patient announces that he or she is leaving, "I'm getting pissed and am going to start saying stupid things. I'll be back in a few minutes, and we can talk about it then," or he or she simply leaves without explanation. A variant on this theme is "negotiated time-outs" in which people in a system (e.g., spouses, parents and children, business partners, or an angry youth and teachers) agree in advance that it is permissible to take a time-out to prevent angry or aggressive outbursts. The negotiated time-out may be unilateral, with one individual removing him- or herself from the environment, or bilateral, as when partners agree to separate on cue or when both parents and children go to their rooms. Generally, a 20–30 minute time-out is sufficient to regain emotional control.

Other strategies involve *seeking a delay in responding* to lower or to prevent anger arousal and allow time for constructive alternatives. For example, the person may verbally seek a delay, indicating the need for time to think before responding, for example, "Let me check into that and get back to you later this afternoon." The patient may also quietly do this without a signal, as was the case of a businessman who became angry in departmental meetings, but chose to respond by memos that summarized his thoughts. The person may also consciously seek a delay by engaging in behavior unrelated

3. Applied Relaxation Coping Skills

Relaxation coping skills are an intervention strategy that develop skills with which the patient can actively reduce emotional and physiological arousal and thereby regain a sense of calmness and control. In turn, this calmness and control may free the patient to gain a different perspective and to employ other coping skills.

Although several relaxation strategies can be applied, it is recommended that anxiety management training (Suinn, 1977, 1990; Suinn & Deffenbacher, 1988) be adapted to anger control. This strategy is recommended because (a) detailed manuals and descriptions are available; (b) it provides consistent self-management training within and between sessions; (c) it can be flexibly deployed in heterogeneous groups because it uses individualized anger scenes for anger arousal; and (d) because it is effective alone (Deffenbacher et al., 1986; Deffenbacher & Stark, 1992; Hazaleus & Deffenbacher, 1986) or in combination with other interventions (Deffenbacher et al., 1987, 1988, 1990a, 1990b; Deffenbacher & Stark, 1992; Nakano, 1990).

Relaxation coping skills can be developed in 6–10 sessions after emotional and physiological arousal has been identified as a target for intervention. The first three sessions are devoted to developing and linking a personalized self-control rationale to the patient's anger, to progressive relaxation training, and to developing and rehearsing specific relaxation coping skills. Coping skills typically include: (a) relaxation without tension, that is, focusing on muscle groups and relaxing them without tension exercises; (b) unobtrusive adaptations of tension-release exercises, that is, tensing and releasing key muscles in ways unnoticed by others such as tightening the stomach or thighs; (c) breathing-cued relaxation, that is, taking three to five deep breaths and relaxing more deeply on each exhalation; (d) cue-controlled relaxation, that is, slowly repeating a calm word or phrase such as "relax" or "calm control"; and (e) relaxation imagery, that is, visualizing an image that elicits relaxation. Relaxation coping skills are tailored to the individual as he or she develops proficiency with one or a combination of these skills. Homework in these early session involves: (a) practicing progressive relaxation; (b) rehearsing relaxation coping skills in nonstressful environments such as watching television or waiting for a meeting; (c) self-monitoring anger with particular attention to emotional and physiological components; and (d) beginning to develop anger arousing scenes.

Remaining sessions are devoted to coping skill application for anger control within sessions, to transferring skills to the external environment and to disquieting other emotional and physical states, and to integration of relaxation coping skills with other interventions. At the beginning of sessions, therapist and client go over homework assignments, and coping skill application during the past week is reviewed, with support for successes and troubleshooting for difficulties. The bulk of the session is devoted to trials of anger arousal and relaxation retrieval. Anger is induced either through anger imagery or simulation. Although imagery is typically used because of its ease, simulation should be considered when it can be arranged (e.g., role-plays of name-calling, of a teenager talking back to a parent, or of an overbearing supervisor). If anger imagery is used, it should involve clear, real life experiences and should include sufficient concrete, situational, cognitive, emotional, and physiological detail to elicit anger arousal. Anger arousal within sessions typically starts in the mild to moderate range, generally about 40–50 on a 100-point intensity scale, and increases over sessions as the client demonstrates greater self-control. In the early sessions, the therapist assists the patient in relaxation retrieval, but fades this assistance over time as the patient demonstrates self-control within sessions. When anger reduction is strong within sessions, the focus shifts to application in naturally occurring events and in events with a predictable angering capacity (e.g., discussing rule violations with a teenager or performing supervisory feedback with difficult employees). Homework during later sessions involves application for in vivo anger control with application to other emotions and problems encouraged.

Relaxation coping skills are most appropriate for emotional and physiological components of anger arousal. They are a commonsense intervention for many clients that helps them cool out and calm down; therefore, they can be introduced early in therapy with many clients. They are integrated easily with other interventions such as cognitive restructuring or behavioral change, as patients can initiate relaxation and then engage in other strategies when they are calmer and more focused. Furthermore, preceding cognitive interventions with relaxation coping skill training seems to make the cognitive interventions more acceptable and easier to implement (Deffenbacher et al., 1988; Hazaleus & Deffenbacher, 1986). Relaxation interventions also may alleviate or reduce some aversive preanger states (e.g., physical pain, tension, headaches) and emotions (e.g., hurt, anxiety, stress, rejection), which may totally or partially trigger anger reactions.

4. Cognitive Restructuring

Cognitive change interventions address biased, anger-engendering information processing, that is, cognitive content and process errors and underlying negative schema. These strategies are, therefore, most appropriate for dysfunctional appraisal and cognitive elements of anger and for appraising how these contribute to other response systems. That is, patients are aided in becoming aware of "hot" cognitions and replacing them with "cooler" thinking, which reduces their contributions to anger arousal and frees problem solving and other appropriate behavior.

Clinically, we find seven different, anger-engendering cognitive processes that occur frequently and need attention.

Misestimating Probabilities. Angry individuals often over- or underpredict anger-related events. For example, they may think that nearly every one has negative, manipulative intentions, and they will be treated poorly and unfairly. They may also underestimate their own resources and the positive influence of others. That is, the world or a specific situation is predicted to be a negative, even hostile place, a place for which anger and defensiveness make intuitive sense to the individual. Patients who make these errors need to find out realistically and currently the nature of their world and to explore how their predictions may inadvertently contribute to their negative realities (e.g., when they expect the worst out of others, they may get it).

Demanding and Coercive Thinking. As noted earlier, angry individuals often have extensive personal boundaries and rigid rules for living. Because of these, their sense of insult, affront, trespass, frustration, and injustice increase dramatically. Exploration of these processes, however, shows that they have elevated personal preferences and desires into demands and commands of themselves, others, and the world. Things "should," "ought," "must," "need," or "are expected" to be a certain way. When desires are so framed, they become coercive dictates, and anger and wrath follow when these rules are broken. Patients need to replace these demands with realistic, personal preferences and to see how they have appointed themselves to dictatorial and godlike positions.

In dealing with demanding/coercive thinking, therapists should be ready to address the issue of values. Some clients either insist that certain things are just "right" (implying no need to change or adjust to differences) or that the therapist is valueless (implying that he or she is readily dismissed). The therapist should underscore the importance of values and preferences, of caring deeply about them and working hard for them, and of experiencing the natural disappointments and frustrations when they are not being achieved. However, he or she should be equally ready to assist clients by helping them to see how they are creating unnecessary anger by raising preferences to demands and by commanding the world meet their demands.

Catastrophization. Catastrophe often follows on the heels of unmet demands, that is, it is "terrible" when something does or does not happen when it should. Other angry patients simply evaluate the consequences of events in dramatic, negative terms (e.g., terrible, can't stand it, all hell breaking loose). Such patients need to realistically appraise events and their outcomes, which are often still in negative, but much less extreme terms (e.g., disappointing, frustrating, sad, annoying, bothersome). When realistic negative interpretations replace catastrophic ones, patients have a reality with which they can cope, one which they may not like, but with which they can cope, nonetheless.

In dealing with catastrophization and misattributions (discussion follows), therapists should be ready to deal with two different types of resistance. In the first case, patients implicitly or explicitly hold that they should not experience negative realities, that is, a demand that life be positive or at least the portion about which they are angry. This demand should be replaced by a desire for positive experiences, but a realistic acceptance that bad things happen to good people and that it will rain on his or her parade occasionally. The second type of resistance is the insistence that things really are awful and bad, and, therefore, his or her anger is justified; hence, the anger does not need to be changed. The therapist should not avoid this issue. The situation should be assessed as the therapist may decide the circumstances are negative enough to shift to crisis intervention, to environmental change strategies such as assisting the individual to remove him- or herself from a toxic environment, and/or to training in behavioral limit setting. However, in less extreme circumstances, the catastrophe involves an implicit demand that negative events not be experienced. This demand should be addressed if cognitive distancing is lessened and difficulties are resolved.

Overgeneralization.   Angry individuals often make sweeping generalizations and employ broad negative labels. Once the invalid inference is made or the label applied, the person responds to the emotive meaning, rather than the frustrations of reality. Dysfunctional overgeneralizations often involve time (e.g., always, never) or negative labeling (e.g., dumb, crazy, out of control, worthless). Angry clients often need assistance in becoming situational thinkers in which they focus on the specifics of the situation, that is, what is happening in a specific situation at a given point of time. In doing this, they can base their emotions and behaviors on the specifics of the situation, rather than their overgeneralized reality.

Categorical and Inflammatory Thinking.   Although some of these cognitions might technically qualify as overgeneralizations, they are so frequent in angry patients as to stand alone. Angry patients tend to think in highly negative, sometimes abusive, and often obscene ways (e.g., creep, slob, asshole, bastard, bitch/son of a bitch). As with overgeneralizations, anger escalates when events are coded in this manner and the individual responds to the meaning of the construct, rather than the specifics of reality. Again, patients need assistance in appraising situations in realistic, situation-specific ways, rather than their colorful terms. Exploration of the inflammatory thoughts often reveals how nonsensical they are, which makes humorous interventions appropriate.

Dichotomous Thinking.   Angry individuals often construe events in either-or terms. Things exist either at one or the other end of a highly positive-negative, evaluative continuum. Within this cognitive processing, evidence that an event is not positive automatically implies that it is negative, leading him or her to respond to the negative categorization. For example, if an individual codes events in terms of constructs such as strong–weak, winner–loser, or like me–hate me, anger is likely to rise when the positive polarity is not confirmed. Rarely, however, does the world exist in such black–white, all–none ways, and angry clients need to detect and respond to the shades of gray. They may need to learn to use qualifying adjectives, adverbs, and phrases (e.g., a little, somewhat, a lot), which place things relatively along emotional continua, and to discriminate complexity (e.g., somebody liking some of their behaviors but not others).

Misattributions and Mind Reading. Many angry patients tend to jump to egocentric, malevolent conclusions without entertaining other possibilities. Even in ambiguous situations, they may favor negative interpretations over less negative but equally plausible options. Often these attributions involve knowing or intuiting another's intentions or motivations, that is, they "know" what other people are thinking and why they behave as they do. For example, they may know that another person did something purposefully to hurt, embarrass, or anger them. They then react with anger as if this is true, but they may not have the facts and be basing their reactions on current, accurate information. Patients need to challenge these automatic explanatory systems and to entertain more benign possibilities.

Cognitive restructuring of these biased information processes involves five overlapping steps or therapeutic tasks. Multiple strategies are employed at each stage (e.g., Beck & Emery, 1985; Meichenbaum, 1985).

The first two steps involve assisting clients to become more aware of their cognitions and to accept that cognitions influence feelings and behavior. Not all angry patients are aware of their cognitions or their influence. For them, anger is a natural reaction to external events or wells up automatically from within. Self-monitoring, interviewing, and tracking reactions to imagery and simulations assist clients in becoming more aware. The connection, however, may not be obvious. It is often helpful to have clients explain how they reacted differently to similar situations. This often leads them to indicate that they saw things differently or had a different perspective. This observation is then linked to the possibility of changing attitudes and cognitions as a means of influencing anger reactions. In a group, different members' reactions to the same event can also be employed to make the contrast. As the importance of cognitions is established, clients begin to track them more systematically and to look for patterns.

The third therapeutic task is a clarification of the errors and distortions involved in patient cognitions. Once again, strategies are tailored to the client. Many clients respond well to Socratic questions that explore the limits of their thoughts. For example, a series of "And what's another way of looking at that?" questions may increase cognitive flexibility and provide alternative attributions. Questions like, "Where's the evidence?" or requests like "Show me how that follows" help in the exploration of catastrophic and misattributional thinking. Questions like "And why shouldn't that happen to you?" facilitate exploration of demandingness, and a series of "And then what would happen?" can reduce catastrophic predictions and enhance a sense of efficacy, as patients often indicate that if negative realities happened, they would be able to cope. Such questions may be fairly gentle in style or quite confrontational as in "And who appointed you God?" Experiments in which patients behaviorally test their cognitions are also effective. For example, an angry, powerless teenager might be asked to see if he or she can get his or her parents to be more giving and positive; an angry businessman might be asked to be nice to others and admit mistakes for a week and see if others took advantage of him; or an angry college student might be asked to develop a point/counterpoint written debate outline regarding reasons to assume that others will hurt and reject him or her. Cognitive modeling in which the therapist models alternative perspectives and ways of thinking provides not only the opportunity for contrasts with patient cognitions, but also concrete cognitive counterresponses for the next phase. A kind of role reversal in which the patient helps the therapist who is playing the role of a friend who is angry can also help patients access appropriate cognitions that can be adapted to the client's world.

The fourth therapeutic task is an extension of the prior step, namely, converting new insights and understanding into specific, cognitive counterresponses with which to counteract dysfunctional cognitive processes. These images, attitudes, and self-dialogue are honed and refined through discussion, homework, and rehearsal (next step) until the person has a new set of believable, realistic, value-centered cognitive responses with which to deal with anger.

The final step involves increasing response strength of these responses and transferring them to the external environment for reliable self-management of anger. Rehearsal strategies described previously for relaxation can be adapted. For example, new cognitions can be rehearsed to reduce anger induced by imagery. As with relaxation skills, it is suggested that rehearsal begins with low levels of anger provocation and high levels of therapeutic assistance and moves to lower therapist involvement and greater anger arousal as the client demonstrates anger control within sessions. Then, role-plays, in vivo experiments, and applications in natural events can be employed to transfer cognitive coping skills. The importance of this rehearsal phase cannot be overemphasized. Anger-engendering cognitive processes tend to be highly overlearned, automatic processes. It takes repetition and rehearsal, sometimes seemingly again and again over the same ground, for new cognitive processes to become strong and easily accessed in the face of provocation and anger arousal.

5. Humor

Humor is effective with many angry patients. It is not only appropriate for inflammatory labeling, but also for a number of other cognitive distortions. Humor lowers anger by inducing an anger-incompatible affect, by helping patients gain cognitive distance and a perspective shift, and by providing alternative, more benign interpretations of provocative situations.

Although humor is a variant of cognitive change, it has enough special relevance to anger management to warrant separate discussion. In general, humor follows the steps of cognitive restructuring, that is, first becoming aware of and exploring the impact of humor and then developing humorous self-dialogue and images as new responses that are rehearsed and transferred. Humorous images and self-dialogues are easily integrated with cognitive restructuring and other interventions. However, because some patients react to humor with anger, thinking they are being made fun of or laughed at, humor generally is introduced later in therapy when the therapeutic alliance is strong.

At the outset, two things should be noted about the use of humor. First, humor should be of the silly variety. If the humor is hostile or sarcastic, the client is learning an indirect, often dysfunctional means of expressing anger that prolongs and perhaps increases anger as others counterattack in response. Second, patients are not simply encouraged to laugh off or deny anger. On the contrary, patients are encouraged to develop humor as a way of gaining an emotional release and achieving control over anger so they can put the situation into perspective and cope with it. A few examples follow.

One of the simplest forms of humor is concretizing inflammatory labels and phrases. When working with individuals, the therapist listens for pet words or phrases, and with a group of adults a range of colorful phrases can be generated by asking group members what they call discourteous drivers. For example, it is not uncommon for angry patients to label others as "asses" or "assholes." In concretizing a term like *ass*, the patient is asked to define the term concretely or literally, which usually generates references to buttocks and donkeys. Then, the patient is asked to picture the term visually and to indicate how this definition accounted for the situation. Asshole, or the space between the buttocks, creates an even more ludicrous image. To further concretize the construct, the patient may be asked to draw a picture of it. For example, this procedure has led to pictures of a donkey driving a truck and two buttocks teaching a university class. Such conversations and images often give patients an immediate chuckle and an alternative perspective. With repetition and pushing patients to be specific in their use of language, many indicate that they simply cannot look at the situation in the old way without laughing and taking it less seriously.

Patients may also adapt humorous drawing to other content such as picturing themselves as gods, kings/queens, or dictators in relationship to demandingness. Provocative events can also be seen through the eyes of the patient's favorite cartoon character (e.g., Garfield dealing with the patient's boss), perhaps drawing out sketches of these characters as they deal with the situation.

Hyperbole and exaggeration may be useful in shifting perspective and misattributions. For example, a worker's interpretation that people intentionally make work difficult might be exaggerated into a conspiracy. First, the worker might be asked if work is well-organized, efficient, and planful, which usually draws a resounding "no." This can be followed by a hyperbolous account of the highly planned, well-organized, efficient way in which management ran things to make them difficult for the patient. As another example, someone who is angered by putdowns and rejection might be exposed to exaggerated putdowns (e.g., "Look, you creep, if you were the last person on the face of the earth, I would want to be at least one continent away!"). Usually, these putdowns draw a laugh. The contrast between the individual's reaction to lesser slights and the laugh at the exaggeration is explored.

Other humor involves reattribution. For example, the frustrating behavior of a child might be attributed to "doing his or her job," namely, to frustrate parents, rather than being a malevolent being. An individual's grouchiness and constant complaining might be attributed to being "totally constipated" complete with visceral image, rather than to a personal attack. Another's absent-mindedness might be attributed to "brain damage," rather than to purposeful inconsiderateness.

6. Task-Oriented Self-Instruction

Interventions described so far lower anger by reducing or disrupting cognitive, emotional, and physiological components of anger and their impact on associated behavior. Some angry patients, however, are deficit in initiating and maintaining appropriate task-oriented cognitions and behaviors, that is, they do not address provocations as problems and initiate effective problem solving. Such patients may benefit from task-oriented, problem-solving self-instruction (Meichenbaum, 1985; Moon & Eisler, 1983).

Self-instructional training assists patients in defining affronts and frustrations as problems to be solved and in initiating constructive problem solving. It follows the same general stages of cognitive restructuring and can be easily combined with other interventions (e.g., initiate relaxation, cognitive restructuring, and/or thought stopping followed by self-instruction to address the issue via problem solving). Type of self-instructions needed should emerge and be shaped collaboratively and should be based on the specific cognitive deficits observed. With this caveat in mind, possible types of such self-instruction (Meichenbaum & Deffenbacher, 1988) follow.

Cool, Calming Thoughts.   These prompt relaxation skills, focus attention in calm ways, and provide emotional palliatives, for example, "That's it, just kick in that relaxation image and ride this out." "Stay cool and focused. This won't last forever."

Orienting to Anger as a Problem to be Solved.   These inculcate an attitude that anger is just a hassle or a problem to be solved (e.g., "It's not 'the shits,' just a problem to solve. So, let's get on with it.") and assist the patient in beginning a problem-solving sequence, for example, "Develop a plan. That's better than getting all mad. Think straight and get organized. Screaming hasn't done any good before." On occasion, the clinician will need to recycle cognitive restructuring for clients who do not want to see problems as theirs and magically think that they should not have to deal with them or experience discomfort.

Breaking Anger Down.   Anger may result from a collage of different stressors, and some patients benefit from self-instruction to break things into smaller units (e.g., "Break it down. I can handle little ones. Get a piece of paper and list what's going on. Then, I'll know where the anger is coming from").

Planning and Problem Solving.   These self-instructions trigger planning (e.g., "What's may plan of attack? Let's develop a plan. So, the first step is") and follow-through ("Ok, so you think it's a good idea to call him, rather than confront him personally. Now make the notes on what you want to say and do it.") with the goal of developing, initiating, and evaluating quality solutions.

Terminating Problem Solving When No good Solutions Are Apparent.   Not all sources of anger have a good solution or, potentially, any solution at all. Nonetheless, some clients continue to press on angrily and may be helped by instructing themselves to abort problem solving efforts (e.g., "Looks like there is no good way out of this. The best thing I can do is not get all crazy about it. I'm stuck. Back away and try again another time. No use getting all bent out of shape about it."). A variant of these self-instructions focuses on ultimate control and escape routes for the patient who feels anger is escalating out of control. They need to see they have more control than they think and to initiate ultimate control self-instructions (e.g., "If I really start to lose it, I will walk away from it. I'm really mad and starting to go out of control. Feet take me out of here before I do something really dumb!"). Sometimes cognitive restructuring of the need to be in control and for catastrophes connected to not being in control also may be indicated.

Self-Reward/Self-Efficacy for Coping and Problem Solving. This set of self-instructions should support positive coping, reward attempts to reduce anger, provide self-attributions for such management, and set realistic, positive expectations for the future, for example, "Terrific! I kept my cool and didn't blow up. I'm getting better at this anger management stuff. If I keep practicing, I bet I can get even better."

7. Behavioral Skill Training

Just as some individuals do not possess cognitive problem-solving skills, others lack overt behavior with which to handle inevitable provocation. Anger escalates as they do not know how to resolve frustration and conflict. For example, generally angry clients tend to be more verbally abrasive and intimidating and to employ fewer listening, communication, and negotiations skills (Deffenbacher, 1992; Deffenbacher et al., 1986; Deffenbacher & Sabadell, 1992) and may benefit from social skill training programs (e.g., Deffenbacher et al., 1987, 1990b; Moon & Eisler, 1983). Many other skill deficits may be related to anger. For example, angry parents may benefit from parenting classes, angry spouses and partners from assertion and communication skills, or angry supervisors from training in supervision and team leadership. Clearly, the nature of contributing skill deficits vary widely, but their contribution should be assessed and a skill enhancement program either developed or located for referral.

Concluding Comments about Treatment

No two clients need exactly the same intervention. As indicated early in the chapter, therapist and client should develop a working model of anger, and intervention should be tailored to the components of this working model. However, with these general comments in mind, intervention strategies outlined previously can be sequenced into four, overlapping phases. First are interventions that enhance personal awareness of anger. These flow relatively easily out of assessment and lead to a continually revised understanding of anger and to the basis of application of skills already in the patient's repertoire or those developed in therapy. The second stage involves response disruption and relaxation. Response disruption is recommended because usually it can be developed rapidly and enhance a sense of self-efficacy and rudimentary control. Response interference may also break up cycles of systemic anger and aggression. Relaxation is recommended early because it is effective, because it fits many patients' presenting concerns, because it is nonconfrontive and generally experienced positively, and because it seems to lower resistance to and is integrated easily with other interventions. The third phase includes cognitive restructuring and humor. By this point, the patient is probably experiencing some anger reduction, and the relationship is strong enough to support the confrontation and dissonance elicited by cognitive restructuring and humor. The last phase involves cognitive (task-oriented problem solving) and behavioral skill enhancement. These are the natural action sides of lowered anger arousal. That is, as the individual is able to lower arousal, he or she is in a better place to learn and implement problem-solving and constructive behavior. Additionally, placing these last allows the therapist and patient alike to see if coping skills naturally emerge as interfering anger is reduced.

The goal of intervention should be *anger management*, not anger elimination. It is idealistic to believe that anger will or can ever be eliminated. Frustration, pain, injustice, and disagreement will continue. People become ill, jobs are lost, relationships end, others are inconsiderate and obnoxious. Even when anger regarding these events is well managed, a realistic residue of mild anger (e.g., frustration, disappointment, annoyance, irritation) remains, and difficult choices remain to be made and implemented. Acceptance and tolerance of these events are among the developmental and existential tasks of life. However, employing anger management strategies such as those described in this chapter can help patients lower their anger and move more freely and more healthfully through life, a life that still may be realistically painful and frustrating at times.

ACKNOWLEDGMENT

Preparation of this chapter was funded, in part, by the Tri-ethnic Center for Prevention of Drug Abuse, National Institute of Drug Abuse Grant #P50DA07074.

REFERENCES

Achmon, J., Granek, M., Golomb, M., & Hart, J. (1989). Behavioral treatment of essential hypertension: A comparison between cognitive therapy and biofeedback of heart rate. *Psychosomatic Medicine, 51,* 152–164.

American Psychiatric Association (1987). *Diagnostic and statistical manual (DSMIII-R)* (3rd ed., revised). Washington, DC: American Psychiatric Association.

Averill, J. R. (1982). *Anger and aggression: An essay on emotion.* New York: Springer-Verlag.

Beck, A. T. (1976). *Cognitive therapy and the emotional disorders.* New York: International Universities Press.

Beck, A. T. (1988). *Love is never enough.* New York: Harper & Row.

Beck, A. T., & Emery, G. (1985). *Anxiety disorders and phobias.* New York: Basic Books.

Bennett, P., Wallace, L., Carroll, D., & Smith, N. (1990). Treating Type-A behaviours and mild hypertension in middle-aged men. *Journal of Psychosomatic Research, 35,* 209–223.

Berkowitz, L. (1990). On information and regulation of anger and aggresssion: A cognitive-neoassociationistic analysis. *American Psychologist, 45,* 494–503.

Deffenbacher, J. L. (1981). Anxiety. In J. L. Shelton & R. L. Levy (Eds.), *Behavioral assignments and treatment compliance: A handbook of clinical strategies* (pp. 93–109). Champaign, IL: Research Press.

Deffenbacher, J. L. (1988). Cognitive-relaxation and social skills treatments of anger: A year later. *Journal of Counseling Psychology, 35*, 234–236.

Deffenbacher, J. L. (1992). Trait anger: Theory, findings, and implications. In J. N. Butcher & C. D. Spielberger (Eds.), *Advances in personality assessment* (Vol. 9, pp. 177–201). Hillsdale, NJ: Lawrence Erlbaum Associates.

Deffenbacher, J. L., Demm, P. M., & Brandon, A. D. (1986). High general anger. *Behaviour Research and Therapy, 24*, 481–489.

Deffenbacher, J. L., McNamara, K., Stark, R. S., & Sabadell, P. M. (1990a). A combination of cognitive, relaxation, and behavioral coping skills in the reduction of general anger. *Journal of College Student Personnel, 31*, 351–358.

Deffenbacher, J. L., McNamara, K., Stark, R. S., & Sabadell, P. M. (1990b). A comparison of cognitive-behavior and process oriented group counseling for general anger reduction. *Journal of Counseling and Development, 69*, 167–172.

Deffenbacher, J. L., & Sabadell, P. M. (1992). Leicht argerliche (high trait anger) personen und nur schwer zu argernde (low anger) personen: Ein vergleich. In M. Muller (Ed.), *Psychophysiologische risikofaktoren bei herz-kreislauferkrakungen: Grundlagen und therapie* (pp. 153–169). Gottingen, Germany: Hogrefe Verlag.

Deffenbacher, J. L., & Stark, R. S. (1992). Relaxation and cognitive-relaxation treatments of general anger. *Journal of Counseling Psychology, 39*, 158–167.

Deffenbacher, J. L., Story, D. A., Brandon, A. D., Hogg, J. A., & Hazaleus, S. L. (1988). Cognitive and cognitive-relaxation treatments of anger. *Cognitive Therapy and Research, 12*, 167–184.

Deffenbacher, J. L., Story, D. A., Stark, R. S., Hogg, J. A., & Brandon, A. D. (1987). Cognitive-relaxation and social skills interventions in the treatment of general anger. *Journal of Counseling Psychology, 34*, 171–176.

Deffenbacher, J. L., & Thwaites, G. A. (1991, April). *Consequences of trait anger.* Paper presented at Rocky Mountain Psychological Association, Denver, Colorado.

Dryden, W. (1990). *Dealing with anger problems: Rational–emotive therapeutic interventions.* Sarasota, FL: Practitioner's Resource Exchange.

Ellis, A. (1977). *Anger: How to live with and without it.* New York: Reader's Digest Press.

Friedman, M., Thoresen, C. E., Gill, J. J., Powell, L. H., Ulmer, D., Thompson, L., Price, V. A., Rakin, D. D., Breall, W. S., Dixon, T., Levy, R., & Bourg, E. (1984). Alteration of Type A behavior and reduction in cardiac recurrences in postmyocardial infarction patients. *American Heart Journal, 108*, 237–248.

Hazaleus, S. L., & Deffenbacher, J. L. (1985). Irrational beliefs and anger arousal. *Journal of College Student Personnel, 26*, 47–52.

Hazaleus, S. L., & Deffenbacher, J. L. (1986). Relaxation and cognitive treatments of anger. *Journal of Consulting and Clinical Psychology, 54*, 222–226.

Liebsohn, M. A., Deffenbacher, J. L., & Oetting, E. R. (1991). *Anger, alcohol and alcohol consequences.* Unpublished manuscript, Department of Psychology, Colorado State University, Fort Collins, CO.

Lohr, J. M., Hamberger, L. K., & Bonge, D. (1988). The relationship of factorially validated measures of anger proneness and irrational beliefs. *Motivation and Emotion, 12*, 171–183.

Meichenbaum, D. H. (1985). *Stress inoculation training.* New York: Pergamon.

Meichenbaum, D. H., & Deffenbacher, J. L. (1988). Stress inoculation training. *The Counseling Psychologist, 16*, 69–90.

Meichenbaum, D. H., & Turk, D. C. (1987). *Facilitating treatment adherence.* New York: Plenum Press.

Moon, J. R., & Eisler, R. M. (1983). Anger control: An experimental comparison of three behavioral treatments. *Behavior Therapy, 14*, 493–505.

Nakano, K. (1990). Effects of two self-control procedures on modifying Type A behavior. *Journal of Clinical Psychology, 46,* 652–657.

Novaco, R. W. (in press). A contextual perspective on anger with relevance to blood pressure. In E. Johnson & S. Julius (Eds.), *Personality, elevated blood pressure, and essential hypertension.* New York: Hemisphere.

Novaco, R. W. (1975). *Anger control: The development and evaluation of an experimental treatment.* Lexington, MA: Heath.

Novaco, R. W. (1977). A stress inoculation approach to anger management in training of law enforcement officers. *American Journal of Community Psychology, 5,* 327–346.

Novaco, R. W. (1980). Training of probation counselors for anger problems. *Journal of Counseling Psychology, 27,* 385–390.

Persons, J. B., & Miranda, J. (1991). Treating dysfunctional beliefs: Implications of the mood-state hypothesis. *Journal of Cognitive Psychotherapy, 5,* 15–25.

Schlichter, K. J., & Horan, J. J. (1981). Effects of stress inoculation on the aggression management skills of institutionalized juvenile delinquents. *Cognitive Therapy and Research, 5,* 359–365.

Spielberger, C. D. (1988). *State–Trait Anger Expression Inventory.* Orlando, FL: Psychological Assessment Resources.

Spielberger, C. D., Jacobs, G. A., Russell, S. L., & Crane, R. J. (1983). Assessment of anger: The State–Trait Anger Scale. In J. N. Butcher & C. D. Spielberger (Eds.), *Advances in personality assessment* (Vol. 3, pp. 112–134). Hillsdale, NJ: Lawrence Erlbaum Associates.

Spielberger, C. D., Johnson, E. H., Russell, S. F., Crane, R. J., Jacobs, G. A., & Worden, T. J. (1985). The experience and expression of anger: Construction and validation of an anger expression scale. In M. A. Chesney & R. H. Rosenman (Eds.), *Anger and hostility in cardiovascular and behavioral disorders* (pp. 5–30). New York: Hemisphere.

Suinn, R. M. (1977). *Manual—anxiety management training (AMT).* Fort Collins, CO: Rocky Mountain Behavioral Sciences Institute.

Suinn, R. M. (1990). *Anxiety management training.* New York: Plenum Press.

Suinn, R. M., & Deffenbacher, J. L. (1988). Anxiety management training. *The Counseling Psychologist, 16,* 31–49.

Thurman, C. W. (1985a). Effectiveness of cognitive-behavioral treatments in reducing Type A behavior among university faculty. *Journal of Counseling Psychology, 32,* 358–362.

Thurman, C. W. (1985b). Effectiveness of cognitive-behavioral treatments in reducing Type A behavior in university faculty—One year later. *Journal of Counseling Psychology, 32,* 445–458.

Zillman, D. (1971). Excitation transfer in communication-mediated aggressive behavior. *Journal of Experimental Social Psychology, 7,* 419–434.

Zillmann, D., & Bryant, J. (1974). Effect of residual excitation on the emotional response and delayed aggressive behavior. *Journal of Personality and Social Psychology, 30,* 782–791.

Zwemer, W. A., & Deffenbacher, J. L. (1984). Irrational beliefs, anger and anxiety. *Journal of Counseling Psychology, 31,* 391–393.

AUTHOR INDEX

SUBJECT INDEX

A

Age
   and anger-hostility and coronary disease
      association, 90, 183, 209
   and anger-hostility levels, 80, 201–206
Aggression. *See also* Anger-hostility
   in animal models, 127–145
   definition of, 25–26
Alcohol, 122, 206–207, 209
Anger. *See also* Anger-hostility
   definition of, 25–27, 242–243
   sources of, 246–249
Anger emotional disorders, 242–267
   assessment, 242–252
   treatment, 252–267
Anger-hostility and coronary disease associ-
      ation, studies of, 5–17, 67–92,
      182–187, 223–224. *See also* Psy-
      chophysiological reactivity
   cross-sectional, 71–78
   longitudinal, 79–85
   methodological issues in, 29–31, 69–70
Anger-hostility, components of, 10–16,
      25–27, 97–100, 199–200. *See also*
      Expression of anger-hostility
Angina, 69, 88

B

Behavioral medicine, history of, 1–17
Beta-adrenergic reception, 118–119,
      135–137, 145, 160
Biological mechanisms of anger-hostility
      and coronary disease association,
      31–33, 37, 118–124, 140–145, 157
Blood pressure reactivity. *See* psychophysio-
      logical reactivity
Blood pressure (resting), 232
Buss-Durkee Hostility Inventory (BDHI),
      48–49, 180

Angiography (right column)

Angiography studies, 30, 55, 69, 73–77, 184
Animal models, 118, 121, 127–145
Anxiety. *See* Neuroticism
Asymptomatic coronary disease, 55–56
Atherogenesis, 117–120, 135–145
Atherosclerosis, 69, 73–77, 127–145
Autonomic reactivity. *See* Psychophysiologi-
      cal reactivity

C

Caffeine, 17, 206–209
Cardiac death, 70